Pocket Companion for

Black and Matassarin-Jacobs

MEDICAL-SURGICAL NURSING

Clinical Management for Continuity of Care

Fifth Edition

Pocket Companion for

Black and Matassarin-Jacobs

MEDICAL-SURGICAL NURSING

Clinical Management for Continuity of Care

Fifth Edition

CATHERINE ROLLMAN SORRENTINO, RN, BSN

Assistant Patient Care Manager
University of Nebraska Hospital
University of Nebraska Medical Center
Omaha, Nebraska

CATHERINE CIHUNKA, MSN, ARNP

Neurology Department
University of Nebraska Hospital
University of Nebraska Medical Center
Omaha, Nebraska

W. B. SAUNDERS COMPANY

A Division of Harcourt Brace & Company

Philadelphia London Toronto Montreal Sydney Tokyo

W. B. SAUNDERS COMPANY
A Division of Harcourt Brace & Company
The Curtis Center
Independence Square West
Philadelphia, PA 19106

Pocket Companion for Black and Matassarin-Jacobs
MEDICAL-SURGICAL NURSING:
Clinical Management for Continuity of Care
ISBN 0-7216-7287-6

Last digit is the print
number: 9 8 7 6 5 4 3 2 1

PREFACE

The *Pocket Companion for Medical-Surgical Nursing: Clinical Management for Continuity of Care* was developed as a quick reference guide for nurses and nursing students in the clinical setting based on content from *Medical-Surgical Nursing: Clinical Management for Continuity of Care*, 5th Edition, edited by Black and Matassarin-Jacobs. Information on more than 325 adult medical-surgical disorders is included and organized in a format closely following the main textbook. Each condition concludes with a reference to the relevant page number(s) in the textbook.

The *Pocket Companion* provides concise, relevant information at your fingertips.

Special features to help you quickly locate information include:

- consistently styled format with easily identified subject headers for each condition
- inclusion of only pertinent information for each condition with exclusion of routine nursing care
- separate listing of medical and surgical nursing care
- alphabetical listing of conditions
- convenient pocket size
- comprehensive cross-referenced index grouping of nursing interventions according to whether the patient is receiving medical or surgical treatment

Disorders follow a format designed to assist the nurse to quickly locate information:

Overview—pertinent information such as a definition/brief description of the disorder, pathophysiology, incidence, and risk factors.

Clinical Manifestations—signs and symptoms commonly seen in clients with the disorder.

ACUTE AND SUBACUTE CARE

— **Medical Management**—medical interventions including pharmacological and dietary management.

— **Surgical Management**—operative procedures performed for palliative or curative treatment.
— **Nursing Management**—independent and collaborative nursing interventions specific for the condition. Interventions are grouped according to medical or surgical management where appropriate.

Community and Self-Care—discharge instructions for the client/family specific for the condition.

Several therapies frequently encountered in the clinical setting are also included:

- Mechanical Ventilation
- Endotracheal Tubes
- Tracheostomy
- Blood Component Transfusion
- Chemotherapy
- Pain Assessment and Intervention
- Radiation Therapy
- Enteral Feedings
- Closed Chest Drainage

Appendices are found at the end of the book as additional sources of information.

- Reference Values for Hematology
- Reference Values for Urinalysis
- Reference Values for Blood Plasma and Serum
- Analysis of Arterial Blood Gas Results
- Blood Components
- Comparison of Five Types of Viral Hepatitis
- Risk Predictors for Skin Breakdown
- Acid-Base Imbalances
- Functions and Types of Cranial Nerves
- Glasgow Coma Scale

We hope the *Pocket Companion* will serve as a beneficial source of information in your delivery of patient care.

Catherine Sorrentino

Catherine Cihunka

ACKNOWLEDGMENTS

We would like to thank Thomas Eoyang, Vice President and Editor-in-Chief, Nursing Books, Lee Henderson, Senior Developmental Editor, and Elizabeth Byrd, Associate Developmental Editor, of the W.B. Saunders Company for their guidance and support; and Alison Zaintz, The Production House, Inc., for her assistance.

CONTENTS

APPENDICES

A

Abdominal Aortic Aneurysm

OVERVIEW

- An aneurysm is a permanent localized dilation of an artery. A 50 per cent increase in the size of a vessel is the usual criterion. An aneurysm tends to enlarge gradually, and, if untreated, may rupture.
- The aorta is under greater stress than the rest of the arterial system because of its large diameter and exposure to high pressure during each systolic contraction. Abdominal aortic aneurysms (AAAs) occur about four times more often than thoracic aortic aneurysms.
- When an AAA reaches about 5 cm in diameter, it can usually be palpated. An AAA measuring 6 cm or greater in diameter has a 20 per cent chance of rupturing in 1 year.

CLINICAL MANIFESTATIONS

- most are asymptomatic; discovered on physical or x-ray examination
- awareness of a pulsating mass in the abdomen
- abdominal or back pain
- groin or flank pain

Ruptured AAA

- abdominal pain
- intense pain, typically in one or both flanks, with radiation to the lower abdomen, groin, or genitalia
- signs/symptoms of shock
- lightheadedness
- pulsating abdominal mass
- ecchymosis in the flank and perianal area
- decreased red blood cell count and elevated white blood cell count
- nausea

ACUTE AND SUBACUTE CARE

Medical Management

Surgery is usually not performed on clients with an asymptomatic AAA smaller than 4 to 5 cm.

- ultrasonographic examination every 6 months to determine any change in size
- antihypertensive therapy

Surgical Management

May be performed as an emergency (for ruptured AAA) or elective procedure.

- Excision is done through a midline incision that extends from the xiphoid process to the symphysis pubis. The aneurysm is exposed, clamps are applied above and below the area, the aneurysm is excised, and the segment is replaced with a Dacron graft.

Nursing Management

Surgical

In addition to routine preoperative care:

- Assess baseline peripheral pulses for comparison postoperatively.
- Administer fluids and vasoactive therapy (if ruptured AAA) and monitor for signs/symptoms of shock.

In addition to routine postoperative care:

- Monitor for signs/symptoms of hemorrhage.
- Assess pulses distal to graft at least hourly as ordered.
- Monitor for signs/symptoms of occlusion—change in pulses, severe pain, cool to cold extremity below graft, pallor or cyanosis.
- Monitor intake and output.
- Maintain patency of NG tube.
- Monitor for signs/symptoms of complications, including:
    - — myocardial infarction—clients often have underlying coronary artery disease
    - — renal failure—secondary to ischemia, sustained from decreased aortic blood flow
    - — emboli in arteries of lower extremities or mesentery

— bowel necrosis is exhibited as fever, leukocytosis, ileus, diarrhea, and abdominal pain
— spinal cord ischemia resulting in paraplegia, rectal and urinary incontinence, loss of pain and temperature sensation

- Monitor oxygen saturations and initiate pulmonary hygiene measures (location of incision).

COMMUNITY AND SELF-CARE

Instruct client regarding:

Medical

- antihypertensive therapy
- signs/symptoms of enlarging aneurysm and need to notify physician of:
  — pulsating abdominal mass
  — abdominal or back pain
  — flank pain
- importance of follow-up ultrasound examinations

Surgical

- wound care
- activity restrictions
- signs/symptoms of ruptured bypass graft and need to notify physician of:
  — abdominal pain with intense back, flank, and scrotal pain
  — pulsating abdominal mass
  — ecchymosis in the flank or perianal area
  — lightheadedness
  — nausea

(For more information, see pp. 1425–1428 of Black and Matassarin-Jacobs: *Medical-Surgical Nursing: Clinical Management for Continuity of Care,* 5th ed.)

Achalasia

OVERVIEW

- Achalasia is an idiopathic condition characterized by progressive increased dysphagia. It is due to impaired motility of the lower two-thirds of the esophagus.
- The lower esophageal sphincter (LES) fails to relax as it normally would with swallowing, causing food and fluid to accumulate in the lower esophagus. When hydrostatic pressure exceeds the force of resistance of the LES, the contents pass into the stomach.

CLINICAL MANIFESTATIONS

Signs/symptoms increase in severity as achalasia progresses.

- dysphagia
- substernal pain, inability to belch (in early stages)
- regurgitation of undigested food

ACUTE AND SUBACUTE CARE

Medical Management

Treatment is aimed at relieving the symptoms

- anticholinergic drugs, gastrointestinal hormones, and calcium channel blockers to relax the LES or lower esophageal pressures
- analgesics for pain
- dietary changes (see Nursing Management)

Surgical Management

- esophageal dilation (also called bougienage)—dilation of the lower esophagus and sphincter
- esophagomyotomy (Heller's procedure)—enlargement of the lower esophageal sphincter by incising the circular muscle fibers down to the mucosa. The incision is made via a thoracic approach, necessitating the use of chest tubes. Complications include reflux esophagitis and re-stenosis.
- gastrostomy tube placement—if the client will be unable to swallow for long periods

Nursing Management

Medical

- Discuss dietary changes:
  - — small frequent feedings
  - — use of semisoft, warm foods rather than cold, hard foods
  - — avoidance of hot, spicy, or iced foods
  - — avoidance of alcohol or tobacco
  - — chewing all foods thoroughly
  - — use of different positions to reduce pressure while eating
- Instruct client to sleep with head of bed elevated.
- Daily weights.
- Administer prescribed analgesics, antacids.

Surgical

Esophageal Dilation

- *Preoperative care*
  Instruct client regarding:
  - — procedure is done while awake with a local anesthetic and an analgesic or tranquilizer
  - — taking slow, deep breaths during passage of the tube
  - — possible brief discomfort when bag is inflated
- *Postoperative care*—Monitor for signs of perforation (chest or shoulder pain, elevated temperature, and subcutaneous emphysema). Report to physician immediately.

Esophagomyotomy

- *Preoperative care*
  In addition to routine preoperative care:
  - — Discuss purpose and care of chest and NG tubes.
- *Postoperative care*
  In addition to routine postoperative care:
  - — Monitor thoracotomy incision for excessive bleeding. Maintain clean and dry dressings.
  - — Maintain chest tube drainage system.
  - — Monitor for respiratory distress.
  - — Maintain nasogastric or gastric drainage system.

— Administer prescribed analgesics.

COMMUNITY AND SELF-CARE

Instruct client regarding:

- diet
- symptoms of respiratory complications related to esophageal reflux and aspiration
- signs/symptoms of perforation
- signs/symptoms of infection
- care of gastrostomy tube
- wound care
- sleeping with the head of bed elevated
- signs/symptoms of respiratory complications post chest tube placement
- when to call physician

(For more information, see pp. 1733–1737 of Black and Matassarin-Jacobs: *Medical-Surgical Nursing: Clinical Management for Continuity of Care,* 5th ed.)

Acidosis, Metabolic

OVERVIEW

- Metabolic acidosis may be caused by two different mechanisms: accumulation of fixed acid or loss of base.
- When acidosis is the result of addition of acid (as in lactic acidosis), bicarbonate is consumed in buffering. When acidosis is due to loss of bicarbonate, chloride levels increase to maintain electroneutrality.
- Causes of metabolic acidosis include:
  — acid excess:
    - renal failure—acid end products of protein metabolism cannot be excreted
    - diabetic ketoacidosis—ketoacids accumulate from accelerated lipid metabolism in the absence of insulin
    - lactic acidosis—lactic acid builds up as a consequence of anaerobic metabolism

  — ingested toxins (i.e., aspirin, antifreeze)

— base deficit:
  - renal tubular acidosis— kidneys are unable to reabsorb bicarbonate
  - enteric drainage tubes—lose gastric secretions high in bicarbonate
  - certain medications—Diamox interferes with bicarbonate reclamation during urinary buffering

CLINICAL MANIFESTATIONS

- hyperventilation (Kussmaul's respirations)
- stress response followed by lethargy
- abdominal pain and distention
- nausea/vomiting
- hypotension
- bradycardia or other dysrhythmias
- pH below 7.35
- bicarbonate (HCO_3) less than 22 mm Hg
- hyperkalemia

ACUTE AND SUBACUTE CARE

Medical Management

- determination/treatment of underlying cause
- sodium bicarbonate therapy
- ventilatory support

Nursing Management

- Monitor respiratory status.
- Administer bicarbonate therapy as ordered (observe IV site, as bicarbonate is a tissue irritant).
- Position for optimal ventilation.
- Monitor lab results—arterial blood gases, electrolytes, oxygen saturations.
- Monitor cardiac status.
- Monitor for signs of hyperkalemia:
  — irregular, slow heart rate
  — ECG changes—tall T waves, widened QRS complexes, prolonged PR interval
  — paresthesias
  — muscle twitching, cramps
  — weakness
- Assess ability to perform activities of daily living.
- Plan scheduled rest periods.

COMMUNITY AND SELF-CARE

Discharge care is based on the etiologic factor(s) causing metabolic acidosis.

(For more information, see pp. 336–339 of Black and Matassarin-Jacobs: *Medical-Surgical Nursing: Clinical Management for Continuity of Care,* 5th ed.)

Acidosis, Respiratory

OVERVIEW

- Respiratory acidosis is nearly always due to hypoventilation.
- The rate of carbon dioxide excretion by the lungs depends upon the rate of alveolar ventilation. As ventilation increases (i.e., as tidal volume or respiratory rate increases), carbon dioxide excretion increases and pH rises. Conversely, when ventilation is decreased, less acid is excreted and pH falls.
- Etiologic factors of respiratory acidosis include:
  - — COPD
  - — neuromuscular disease:
    - Guillain-Barré Syndrome
    - myasthenia gravis
  - — respiratory center depression:
    - drugs
      - barbiturates
      - sedatives
      - narcotics
      - anesthetics
  - — central nervous system lesions:
    - tumor
    - stroke
  - — iatrogenic disorders:
    - inadequate mechanical ventilation
    - carbon dioxide narcosis (excessive oxygen administration to clients with COPD)
  - — excess carbon dioxide production:
    - increased metabolic rate
      - sepsis
      - burns

- excessive carbohydrate intake:
  - total parenteral nutrition (TPN)
  - enteral feeding

CLINICAL MANIFESTATIONS

- hypoventilation
- dyspnea
- disorientation or coma
- headache
- hypertension
- dysrhythmias
- pH below 7.35
- $PaCO_2$ above 45 mm Hg
- hyperkalemia—acidosis at the tissue level causes extracellular hydrogen ions to shift into the cell while potassium moves into the blood
- hypoxemia

ACUTE AND SUBACUTE CARE

Medical Management

- determination/treatment of underlying cause
- ventilatory support
- intravenous sodium bicarbonate

Nursing Management

- Monitor respiratory status.
- Position for optimal ventilation; reposition frequently.
- Encourage coughing and deep breathing. Suction PRN.
- Administer sodium bicarbonate therapy as ordered (observe IV site as bicarbonate is a tissue irritant).
- Monitor oxygen therapy.
- Monitor laboratory results—arterial blood gases, electrolytes, oxygen saturations.
- Assess cardiac status.
- Assess ECG for rhythm changes.
- Assess neurologic status and institute appropriate safety measures.
- Monitor for signs/symptoms of hyperkalemia:
  - irregular, slow heart rate

— ECG changes — tall T waves, widened QRS complexes, prolonged PR intervals
— paresthesias
— muscle twitches, cramps
— weakness

- Assess ability to complete activities of daily living.
- Schedule activities to allow for rest periods.

COMMUNITY AND SELF-CARE

Discharge care is based on the etiologic factor(s) causing respiratory acidosis.

(For more information, see pp. 333–335 of Black and Matassarin-Jacobs: *Medical-Surgical Nursing: Clinical Management for Continuity of Care,* 5th ed.)

Acromegaly

- Acromegaly is a disturbance of growth that arises from an oversecretion of growth hormone (GH).
- Acromegaly results from growth hormone secreting adenomas of the anterior pituitary glands.
- Clinical manifestations include: coarsening of the facial features, enlargement of the hands and feet, headache, visual disturbances, lethargy, weight gain, paresthesias, glucose intolerance, irregular or absent menses.
- Medical management includes: radiation therapy and bromocriptine (Parlodel) to reduce the levels of growth hormone and decrease tumor size.
- Surgical management involves transphenoidal microsurgery.

(For more information, see p. 2063 of Black and Matassarin-Jacobs: *Medical-Surgical Nursing: Clinical Management for Continuity of Care,* 5th ed.)

Actinic Keratosis

OVERVIEW

- Actinic keratosis is the most common epithelial precancerous skin lesion in whites, caused by exposure to the sun.
- It occurs in areas of the body with chronic sun exposure like the face, ears, back of the neck, forearms, and the back of the hands.
- It affects nearly 100 per cent of the elderly white population.

CLINICAL MANIFESTATIONS

These lesions are irregularly shaped, flat, slightly erythematous macules or papules with indistinct borders and an overlying hard keratotic scale or horn.

ACUTE AND SUBACUTE CARE

Medical Management

- topical application of 5-fluorouracil (5-FU, Efudex)

Surgical Management

- Cryotherapy—using liquid nitrogen to freeze the lesion
- Electrodesiccation and Curettage—using bursts of electrical current to destroy the lesions
- Shave or excisional biopsy—used for large or suspicious lesions

Nursing Management

Surgery

- Cryosurgery:
  - — instruct client of possible slight discomfort while freezing lesion—apply warm damp cloth to area after procedure
  - — blister care after freezing
- Electrodesiccation and Curettage:
  - — done under local anesthesia
  - — keep wound moist with topical antibiotic ointment

- instruct client regarding side effects of 5FU—erythema, vesiculation, erosion, ulceration, necrosis, and epithelialization
- apply 5FU twice daily with gloved hand, avoiding contact with the eyes, nose, mouth, and scrotum
- place porous gauze dressing over the lesion

COMMUNITY AND SELF-CARE

Instruct client regarding:
- proper use of medications
- use of 5FU until the erosion, necrosis, and ulceration stage (usually 2-4 weeks)
- possible discomfort with 5FU use and the need for pain medications
- complete healing may take 1-2 months after therapy
- wound care, if applicable
- the signs and characteristics of new lesions and when to seek medical advice

(For more information, see p. 2225 of Black and Matassarin-Jacobs: *Medical-Surgical Nursing: Clinical Management for Continuity of Care,* 5th ed.)

Acute Myocardial Infarction

OVERVIEW

- Acute myocardial infarction (MI), also known as a heart attack, coronary occlusion, or "a coronary," is a life-threatening condition characterized by the formation of localized necrotic areas within the myocardium. MI usually follows the sudden occlusion of a coronary artery and the abrupt cessation of blood and oxygen flow to the heart muscle.
- The most common cause of MI is complete or nearly complete occlusion of a coronary artery due to ongoing atherosclerosis. The vessel lumen slowly occludes and is often blocked with a thrombus. When blood flow ceases abruptly, the myocardial tissue supplied by the artery dies and

becomes necrotic. Other causes of acute occlusion are coronary artery spasm or hemorrhage into a plaque.

- MI can be considered the endpoint of coronary artery disease (CAD). Unlike the temporary ischemia that occurs with angina, prolonged unrelieved ischemia causes irreversible damage to the myocardium. Cardiac cells can withstand ischemia about 20 minutes before cellular death occurs. Because the myocardium is very metabolically active, signs of ischemia can be seen within 8 to 10 seconds of decreased blood flow. When the heart is not sustained with blood and oxygen, it converts to anaerobic metabolism with lactic acid as a byproduct. Myocardial cells are very sensitive to changes in pH and become less functional, leading to conduction system disorders, dysrhythmias, and decreased contractility.
- Every year approximately 1,500,000 Americans fall victim to heart attacks. MI is the leading cause of death in America, resulting in an estimated 500,000 deaths each year.
- Approximately 45 per cent of all heart attack clients are under the age of 65 years and 5 per cent are under age 40 years.
- The risk factors that predispose a client to heart attack are the same as for all forms of coronary artery disease (see "Coronary Artery Disease," p.196).
- The infarcted site is called the zone of infarction and necrosis. Around it is the zone of hypoxic injury. This zone is able to return to normal but may necrose if blood flow is not restored. The outermost zone is called the zone of ischemia; damage to this area is reversible.
- The most common sites of infarction are: (1) the anterior wall of the left ventricle near the apex, (2) the posterior wall of the left ventricle near the base, and (3) the inferior surface of the heart.

CLINICAL MANIFESTATIONS

- chest pain (major symptom)
  - similar to angina but more severe in character and duration and unrelieved by nitroglycerin

— may radiate to neck, jaw, shoulder, back, or left arm

- hypotension
- gray facial color
- cold diaphoresis
- weak pulse
- peripheral cyanosis
- tachycardia or bradycardia
- weakness
- indigestion
- increased temperature within 24 hours lasting 3-7 days
- great fear of death, apprehension
- nausea and vomiting
- dyspnea, orthopnea
- palpitations
- ECG changes—pathologic Q wave and serial ST-segment and T-wave changes

ACUTE AND SUBACUTE CARE

Medical Management

The first 24 hours after an MI are the time of highest risk for sudden cardiac death. The crucial time frame for salvage of the myocardium is the first 6 hours. Pain control is a priority. Continued pain is a sign of myocardial ischemia. Pain also stimulates the autonomic nervous system and increases preload, increasing myocardial demands.

- Acute attack:
  - — analgesics and nitrates to alleviate pain
  - — supplemental oxygen
  - — fluids and vasopressors to reverse ensuing shock
  - — invasive hemodynamic monitoring
  - — bedrest and sedation to ease restlessness and fear
  - — anticoagulation therapy (reduce risk of embolism)
  - — continuous ECG monitoring
  - — antiarrhythmic therapy
  - — thrombolytic therapy (to lyse or dissolve the clot)—streptokinase, urokinase, tissue plasminogen activator (t-PA) and anisoylated plasminogen streptokinase activator complex

(APSAC)—must be administered within 3–6 hours after the onset of chest pain, followed by 5–7 days of heparin therapy

- Prevention of complications:

(1) Dysrhythmias (major cause of death after an MI): ventricular premature beats, ventricular tachycardia and fibrillation, supraventricular tachycardia and heart block secondary to ectopic foci near the area of ischemia, conduction system interference or reperfusion of a previously ischemic area.
— continuous cardiac monitoring
— oxygen therapy
— prompt intervention for dysrhythmias (procainamide, lidocaine, elective cardioversion, temporary pacemaker, etc.)

(2) Cardiogenic shock — secondary to decreased myocardial contraction, dysrhythmias, or sepsis.
— rapid pain relief
— intravenous fluid administration
— hemodynamic monitoring
— vasopressors (levarterenol, dopamine, dobutamine, etc.)

(3) Heart failure and pulmonary edema—secondary to decreased myocardial contraction
— low-sodium diet
— fluid restriction
— digitalis therapy and diuretics

(4) Pulmonary embolism—secondary to phlebitis of the legs or pelvic veins or from atrial flutter or fibrillation.
— anticoagulant therapy
— range of motion exercises during bedrest
— elastic stockings
— adequate hydration

(5) Recurrent myocardial infarction—secondary to overexertion, embolization, or further thrombotic occlusion of the coronary artery.
— strict, progressive activity program
— anticoagulation therapy

(6) Pericarditis—the inflamed area of infarction rubs against the pericardial surface, causing it to lose its lubricating fluid

— frequent assessment for early detection and intervention
- Cardiac rehabilitation program

Nursing Management

- Assess characteristics of chest pain and associated symptoms.
- Assess respirations and blood pressure.
- Obtain a 12-lead ECG.
- Administer analgesics and nitrates and monitor response to drug therapy.
- Administer thrombolytic therapy. See "Peripheral Vascular Disease: Chronic Arterial," p. 556.
- Provide restful, quiet environment.
- Maintain continuous cardiac monitoring.
- Administer antidysrhythmics as ordered.
- Monitor serial serum enzyme levels.
- Assess apical pulse for murmurs, rub, S_3 and S_4.
- Monitor serum potassium levels.
- Monitor hemodynamic parameters—cardiac output, pulmonary artery pressures, etc.
- Assess for signs of decreased cardiac output (decreased urinary output, change in mental status, hypotension, etc.).
- Assess for signs of congestive heart failure (rales, rhonchi, S_3 and S_4, dependent edema, etc.).
- Administer supplemental oxygen.
- Monitor oxygen saturations and arterial blood gas results.
- Maintain progressive activity schedule per cardiac rehabilitation program.
- Monitor cardiopulmonary response to activity.
- Monitor intake and output.
- Daily weights.
- Monitor effectiveness of stool softeners and laxatives to prevent straining.
- Facilitate Dietary consult.
- Assist client in identifying own risk factors.

COMMUNITY AND SELF-CARE

Instruct the client regarding:
- disease process and treatment
- importance of risk factor modification
  — dietary restrictions—decreased cholesterol, decreased saturated fat, low-calorie

— smoking cessation
— blood pressure reduction
— stress management
- importance of cardiac rehabilitation program
- antiplatelet aggregation therapy—one aspirin daily
- how to take pulse to monitor response to activity
- management of anginal episodes
  — lie or sit down
  — take nitroglycerin tablets sublingually, 5 minutes apart
  — if pain not relieved by three nitroglycerin, client is to be taken to emergency department
- activity limitations
- driving limitations
- importance of follow-up visits

(For more information, see pp. 1258–1276 of Black and Matassarin-Jacobs: *Medical-Surgical Nursing: Clinical Management for Continuity of Care,* 5th ed.)

Addison's Disease

OVERVIEW

- Chronic primary adrenal insufficiency, or Addison's disease, is the result of idiopathic atrophy or destruction of the adrenal glands by an autoimmune process or other disease.
- Addison's disease, a rare disorder, affects all age groups and both sexes.
- Seventy-five per cent of the cases are caused by an autoimmune process. Adrenal insufficiency is commonly seen in persons with AIDS. Tuberculosis is the cause of about 20 per cent of Addison's disease.
- Secondary adrenal insufficiency is hypofunction of the pituitary-hypothalamic unit. The most common cause is chronic treatment with glucocorticoids for nonendocrine uses.
- Adrenal hypofunction causes decreased levels of mineralocorticoids (aldosterone), glucocorticoids (cortisol), and androgens.

— Aldosterone normally promotes retention of sodium (and frequently water) and excretion of potassium. A deficiency of aldosterone causes increased sodium excretion as well as: (1) increased water excretion, (2) depleted extracellular volume (dehydration), (3) development of hypotension, (4) decreased cardiac output, and (5) increased potassium levels.

— Glucocorticoid deficiency causes decreased gluconeogenesis with resultant hypoglycemia and liver glycogen deficiency. Cortisol deficiency also results in failure to inhibit the anterior pituitary secretion of adrenocorticotropic hormone (ACTH), which increases levels of melanocyte-stimulating hormone (MSH), causing increased skin pigmentation.

— Androgen deficiency fails to produce symptoms in men because the testes supply adequate amounts of sex hormones. Women depend upon the adrenal cortex for an adequate secretion of androgens.

CLINICAL MANIFESTATIONS

The onset is usually insidious, and symptoms intensify as the disease progresses. The development of clinical manifestations requires the loss of over 90 per cent of both adrenal cortices.

- fatigue
- weight loss, nausea, vomiting
- postural hypotension
- bronzed skin discoloration
- emotional disturbances range from mild neurotic symptoms to severe depression
- decreased resistance to emotional or physical stress.

Addisonian Crisis (Acute Adrenal Insufficiency)

Manifestations are related to the degree of hormone deficiency and electrolyte imbalance.

- sudden, penetrating pain in the back, abdomen, or legs
- depressed or changed mentation
- volume depletion
- loss of consciousness
- shock

ACUTE AND SUBACUTE CARE

Medical Management

- Corticosteroid replacement
- For Addisonian crisis, medical management goals are to: (1) reverse shock, (2) restore blood circulation, and (3) replenish body with essential steroids.

Nursing Management

- Administer steroids as ordered.
- Monitor for signs of decreasing cardiac output.
- Monitor electrolyte levels and blood glucose results.
- Monitor intake and output.
- Assess for signs of infection as additional stress may necessitate an increase in steroid replacement dose.
- Monitor for signs and symptoms of Addisonian crisis (see above).
- Implement progressive activity schedule and monitor client's response.

COMMUNITY AND SELF-CARE

Instruct client regarding:

- actions of prescribed hormones
- importance of taking medications daily without fail
- signs of under- and over-dosage of medication
- importance of hydrocortisone self-injection when unable to tolerate oral medication
- need for intramuscular self-injection kit to be available at all times
- intramuscular injection technique
- need for a Medic Alert bracelet and card
- need to call physician to have dosage increased when experiencing stressful situations, e.g., emotional upheavals, dental extractions, upper respiratory infections, etc.

(For more information, see pp. 2041–2047 of Black and Matassarin-Jacobs: *Medical-Surgical Nursing: Clinical Management for Continuity of Care,* 5th ed.)

Adult Respiratory Distress Syndrome (ARDS)

OVERVIEW

- Adult respiratory distress syndrome (ARDS) is a sudden, progressive pulmonary disorder characterized by severe dyspnea, hypoxemia, and diffuse bilateral infiltrates.
- ARDS develops as a result of an insult, condition, or noxious event that traumatizes the lung tissue. The insult may be directly to the lung or indirectly through other body systems.
- After the initial insult occurs, normal lung function is maintained for approximately 1–96 hours. Then hypoxemia rapidly develops and progresses with decreasing lung compliance and the development of diffuse lung infiltrates, atelectasis and pulmonary edema.
- Mortality rates range from 40–60 per cent.
- Conditions at high risk of leading to ARDS are:
  - — direct pulmonary trauma
    - pneumonia
    - lung contusion
    - fat embolus
    - aspiration
    - massive smoke inhalation
    - prolonged exposure to high concentrations of oxygen
  - — indirect pulmonary trauma
    - sepsis
    - shock
    - multisystem trauma
    - disseminated intravascular coagulation
    - pancreatitis
    - drug overdose
    - massive blood transfusions
    - pregnancy-induced hypertension
    - increased intracranial pressure

CLINICAL MANIFESTATIONS

- increased respiratory rate, labored breathing

- air hunger, retractions, cyanosis
- adventitious breath sounds may or may not be present (crackles)

ACUTE AND SUBACUTE CARE

Medical Management

- endotracheal intubation with mechanical ventilation and use of positive end-expiratory pressure
- sedation to reduce anxiety and restlessness
- pharmacologic paralysis with pancuronium bromide or curare if the client is "bucking the ventilator" and sedation is ineffective
- inotropic agents to improve cardiac output and increase systemic blood pressure
- antibiotics if infection is present
- large doses of corticosteroids (controversial)

Nursing Management

- Follow principles of nursing management for clients with pneumonia, pulmonary edema, and other pulmonary disorders affecting gas exchange (see specific disorders).
- Provide continuous mechanical ventilation (see "Mechanical Ventilation," p. 467).
- Provide emotional support and frequent updates to client and significant other.

COMMUNITY AND SELF-CARE

Discharge instructions will vary depending upon client condition and post discharge needs.

(For more information, see pp. 1170–1173 of Black and Matassarin-Jacobs: *Medical-Surgical Nursing: Clinical Management for Continuity of Care,* 5th ed.)

Agranulocytosis

OVERVIEW

- Agranulocytosis is an acute, potentially fatal blood dyscrasia characterized by profound neutropenia resulting in greater susceptibility to bacterial invasion.
- Agranulocytosis results either from the failure of granulocyte production to keep pace with destruction of cells or increased granulocyte destruction.
- Causes of agranulocytosis include:
  - agents that produce neutropenia when given in large doses over time (chemotherapy, radiation, benzene)
  - agents that produce neutropenia only in clients sensitive to the drug (chlorpromazine, propylthiouracil, phenytoin, chloramphenicol, phenylbutazone)
  - aplastic anemia
  - megaloblastic anemia
  - certain diseases—tuberculosis, malaria, uremia

CLINICAL MANIFESTATIONS

- severe fatigue, weakness
- sore throat, ulcerations of the pharyngeal and buccal mucosa
- dysphagia
- fever, severe chills
- weak, rapid pulse
- WBC count 500 to 3000/mm^3 with an extreme reduction in polymorphonuclear cells
- bone marrow examination—absence of granulocytes, a maturational arrest of young cells, or an increased number of myeloid precursors (signifying peripheral granulocyte destruction)
- positive cultures (usually gram-negative cocci)

ACUTE AND SUBACUTE CARE

Medical Management

- identification/possible elimination of toxic agent or disease

- agranulocytosis caused by toxic substances usually reverses within 2–3 weeks after withdrawal of the causative agent
- surveillance cultures (collected at predetermined intervals [i.e., weekly] for detection of infectious organisms)
- antibiotic therapy
- colony-stimulating factors

Nursing Management

- Administer antibiotic and marrow-stimulating therapy.
- Maintain protective isolation.
- Monitor temperature and assess for signs/symptoms of infection.
- Monitor laboratory findings—CBC, WBC, culture reports, absolute granulocyte count.
- Encourage balanced diet with no raw fruits or vegetables.
- Provide adequate rest.
- Provide meticulous oral and physical care.
- Avoid rectal suppositories and rectal temperatures.
- Obtain cultures as ordered.

COMMUNITY AND SELF-CARE

Instruct client regarding:

- disease process and treatment regime
- measures to prevent infection:
  - good personal hygiene
  - avoid crowds and people with known infectious disease
  - wear a mask in public
  - no raw fruits, vegetables, or raw meats
  - change air conditioner and furnace filters weekly
  - remove additional sources of bacteria found in standing water—fish tanks, flower vases, humidifier
  - well-balanced diet
  - adequate rest
- signs/symptoms to report to physician
- importance of follow-up laboratory and clinic visits

(For more information, see pp. 1497–1498 of Black and Matassarin-Jacobs: *Medical-Surgical Nursing: Clinical Management for Continuity of Care,* 5th ed.)

Airway Obstruction, Foreign Body

- Foreign bodies usually enter the right main bronchus because its orifice is slightly wider than that of the left main bronchus. It also lies in a more direct line with the trachea.
- Clinical manifestations of an aspirated foreign body include: severe dyspnea; hemoptysis; fever; atelectasis; pulmonary infection; excessive mucous production; harsh, brassy cough; wheezing; and inspiratory stridor. If the obstruction is complete or nearly complete and at the laryngeal level, clinical manifestations include: obvious respiratory distress, inability to speak, ineffective ventilation efforts, and the international sign for distress (hands at the throat). Asphyxia follows rapidly.
- Complete airway obstruction is a life-threatening emergency requiring immediate intervention.
- The Heimlich maneuver and thrust techniques are used when clients are unable to speak, unable to elicit effective cough, or are unconscious.
- For incomplete obstruction, the client may be placed in Trendelenburg's position so that the foreign body will not move any lower into the airway.
- Some foreign bodies lodged in the laryngeal area may be removed with grasping forceps inserted through a laryngoscope under local or general anesthesia.
- A bronchoscope and special grasping forceps are used for objects that are deeper into the airway.

Alkalosis, Metabolic

OVERVIEW

- Metabolic alkalosis may be caused by either abnormal loss of fixed acid or excess accumulation of bicarbonate.
- Etiologic factors causing metabolic alkalosis include:
  — fixed acid loss:
    - hypokalemia secondary to diuretic or steroid therapy—when potassium is deficient, the kidneys excrete hydrogen in exchange for sodium and this in turn stimulates bicarbonate reabsorption
    - gastric fluid loss (vomiting, nasogastric suctioning); hydrochloric acid is lost

  — excessive bicarbonate intake:
    - overcorrection of acidosis with sodium bicarbonate
    - massive transfusion of whole blood; citrate anticoagulant used for storage is metabolized to bicarbonate

  — excessive bicarbonate reabsorption:
    - hyperaldosteronism—increased renal absorption of sodium and subsequent loss of hydrogen ions

CLINICAL MANIFESTATIONS

- hypoventilation (compensatory)
- increased bicarbonate level
- dysrhythmias
- hypocalcemia
- pH above 7.45
- confusion, decreasing level of consciousness
- hypokalemia
- hypotension
- seizures
- muscle tremors, cramping, or tetany
- numbness and tingling of extremities

ACUTE AND SUBACUTE CARE

Medical Management

- determination/treatment of underlying cause
- potassium replacement therapy
- ventilatory support
- electrolyte replacement therapy
- acidifying salts administration (in extreme cases)—ammonium chloride
- cardiac monitoring

Nursing Management

- Monitor respiratory status.
- Monitor cardiac status.
- Evaluate ECG for rhythm changes.
- Administer electrolyte replacement therapy.
- Monitor laboratory results—arterial blood gases, electrolytes.
- Monitor oxygen saturations.
- Monitor for signs/symptoms of hypokalemia:
  - — thready, weak pulse
  - — postural hypotension
  - — ECG changes:
    - ST depression
    - flattened or inverted T wave
    - prominent U wave
    - heart block
  - — anxiety, lethargy, confusion
  - — nausea, vomiting
- Monitor for signs/symptoms of hypocalcemia:
  - — anxiety, irritability
  - — paresthesias
  - — muscle twitching and cramps
  - — ECG changes:
    - prolonged ST interval
    - prolonged QT interval
  - — hypotension
  - — abdominal cramping
- Assess neurologic status and implement appropriate safety measures.
- Assess ability to perform activities of daily living.
- Plan scheduled rest periods.

COMMUNITY AND SELF-CARE

Discharge care is based upon etiologic factor(s) causing metabolic alkalosis.

(For more information, see pp. 336–339 of Black and Matassarin-Jacobs: *Medical-Surgical Nursing: Clinical Management for Continuity of Care,* 5th ed.)

Alkalosis, Respiratory

OVERVIEW

- Respiratory alkalosis is caused by alveolar hyperventilation, in which excess carbon dioxide (CO_2) is eliminated. The most common cause of respiratory alkalosis is hypoxemia.
- Low levels of oxygen partial pressure (PaO_2) in the blood are sensed by the peripheral chemoreceptors in the carotid bodies and aortic arch. These receptors then increase their rate of firing to the respiratory center in the medulla, and rate and depth of ventilation increase.
- Etiologic factors that cause respiratory alkalosis include:
  - hypoxemia
    - emphysema
    - pneumonia
    - adult respiratory distress syndrome (ARDS)
  - impaired lung expansion:
    - pulmonary fibrosis
    - ascites
    - scoliosis
    - pregnancy
  - thickened alveolar-capillary membrane:
    - congestive heart failure
    - adult respiratory distress syndrome (ARDS)
    - pneumonia
    - pulmonary embolism
  - chemical stimulation of the respiratory center:
    - sepsis
    - high level of ammonia (hepatic failure)
    - high level of salicylates (aspirin overdose)

- traumatic stimulation of the respiratory center:
  - central nervous system trauma
  - central nervous system tumor
  - increased intracranial pressure
  - stress
  - pain

CLINICAL MANIFESTATIONS

- tachypnea
- lightheadedness
- confusion
- giddiness, dizziness, syncope, convulsions, or coma
- weakness, paresthesias of the extremities and around the mouth
- pH above 7.45
- $PaCO_2$ below 35 mm Hg
- tachycardia
- hypokalemia—in alkalosis, potassium shifts into the cell
- hypocalcemia

ACUTE AND SUBACUTE CARE

Medical Management

- determination/treatment of underlying cause
- measures to increase carbon dioxide retention:
  - mechanical hypoventilation
  - carbon dioxide rebreathing
  - sedation
- ventilatory support
- electrolyte replacement therapy

Nursing Management

- Monitor respiratory status.
- Implement CO_2 retention measures as ordered.
- Assess for signs/symptoms of hypokalemia:
  - thready, weak pulse
  - postural hypotension
  - ECG changes:
    - ST depression
    - flattened or inverted T wave
    - prominent U wave
    - heart block

— anxiety, lethargy, confusion
— nausea, vomiting

- Assess for signs/symptoms of hypocalcemia:
  — anxiety, irritability
  — paresthesias
  — muscle twitches and cramps
  — ECG changes:
    - prolonged ST interval
    - prolonged QT interval
  — hypotension
  — abdominal cramping
- Monitor laboratory findings—arterial blood gases, electrolytes.
- Assess cardiac status.
- Assess ECG for rhythm changes.
- Assess neurologic status and implement appropriate safety measures.
- Assess ability to perform activities of daily living.
- Schedule activities to allow for rest periods.
- Implement measures to prevent or eliminate pain, fever, or anxiety, if present (these increase respiratory rate).

COMMUNITY AND SELF-CARE

Discharge care is based on the etiologic factor(s) causing respiratory alkalosis.

(For more information, see pp. 333–335 of Black and Matassarin-Jacobs: *Medical-Surgical Nursing: Clinical Management for Continuity of Care,* 5th ed.)

Alzheimer's Disease

OVERVIEW

- Dementia involves progressive change in personality and two or more areas of cognition, usually memory and one or more of the following: language, calculation, visual (spatial perception), judgment, abstraction. Dementia of the Alzheimer's type (DAT) comprises at least one-half of all the dementias.

- The actual cause of DAT has not been found. However, accumulation of abnormal proteins and neurotransmitter changes have been found.
- DAT occurs in 10 to 15 per cent of people over age 65, 19 per cent of people over age 75, and 47 per cent of people over 85.
- Risk factors identified include: (1) increasing age, (2) familial tendency, and (3) environmental and metabolic factors.

CLINICAL MANIFESTATIONS

First Stage

- memory loss
- poor judgment and problem-solving skills
- personality changes—irritability, suspiciousness, or indifference

Second Stage

- language disturbances — impaired word finding, circumlocution (talking around a subject), empty spontaneous speech, paraphasia (words used in wrong context), echolalia (repetition of words)
- motor disturbances — apraxia (difficulty using everyday objects like a toothbrush)
- increased memory loss
- forgetfulness
- hyperorality (desire to take everything into the mouth to suck, chew, or taste)
- increased irritability and depression
- delusions, hallucinations
- psychotic behavior
- wandering
- occasional incontinence

Third Stage

- virtual loss of all mental abilities
- minimal voluntary movement; limbs become rigid with flexor posturing
- frequent urinary and fecal incontinence
- lost ability for self-care

ACUTE AND SUBACUTE CARE

Medical Management

- low-dose antipsychotic agents — haloperidol
- antidepressants — nortriptyline, desipramine
- tacrine (Cognex) has been recently approved for delaying cognitive decline (increases nerve impulse transmission)

Nursing Management

- Adapt communication to the level of the client.
- Speak slowly and simply, with firm volume and low pitch.
- Assess nonverbal behavior.
- Intervene if client displays angry, hostile behavior by:
  - — decreasing environmental stimuli
  - — approaching in a calm, reassuring manner
  - — taking care not to place any more demands on the client
  - — distracting the client
  - — making sure all verbal and non-verbal cues are concordant
  - — using multiple sensory modalities (visual, auditory, and tactile) to communicate.
- Implement measures to enhance memory:
  - — reorient as necessary
  - — place a clock and calendar in client's room
  - — allow client to reminisce
  - — repeat instructions frequently.
- Institute appropriate safety measures:
  - — ensure that client cannot leave the premises without being noticed
  - — ensure that identification bracelet is worn at all times
  - — remove harmful objects.
- Encourage the client to do own activities of daily living as much as possible.
- Allow plenty of time to complete tasks.
- Anticipate elimination needs and schedule voiding and defecation times.
- Limit fluid intake after the dinner meal to decrease nocturnal incontinence.

- Provide emotional support to family members, particularly the caregivers.

COMMUNITY AND SELF-CARE

- Instruct the family regarding:
  — disease process and prognosis
  — providing a safe home environment
  — communication techniques
  — measures to enhance the client's memory and orientation
- Refer to available community resources—Alzheimer's Disease and Related Disorders Chapter, respite care, adult day care, Visiting Nurse Association.

(For more information, see pp. 863–872 of Black and Matassarin-Jacobs: *Medical-Surgical Nursing: Clinical Management for Continuity of Care,* 5th ed.)

Amputation

OVERVIEW

- Extremity amputation is the surgical removal of all or part of an extremity. Clients with peripheral vascular disease are the most frequent candidates for amputation of the lower extremities.
- Primary amputations are undertaken as definitive treatment for lower extremity ischemia. Secondary amputations follow a previous reconstructive vascular procedure. Amputations may also be required for acute limb-threatening conditions, mainly trauma, and for malignant tumors and congenital deformities.

ACUTE AND SUBACUTE CARE

Surgical Management

- Prior to amputation the surgeon and rehabilitative team considers the following:
  (1) client's physical condition
  (2) type of amputation to be performed

- closed or "flap"—stump is covered with a flap of skin sutured over the end of it
  - performed when there is no evidence of infection
- opened or "guillotine"— stump is not covered with a skin flap but left open to allow wound to drain
  - used when infection is present
  - requires a second surgery for stump closure once infection is eradicated

(3) level of amputation—should be as distal as possible

(4) peripheral vascular function test results to determine vascular patency

(5) client's attitude toward amputation

(6) client's rehabilitation potential

(7) type of postoperative prosthetic-fitting and rehabilitation program

NURSING MANAGEMENT

In addition to routine preoperative care:

- Assist the client in dealing with anticipated loss and body image change.
- Facilitate referral to Social Work or psychologist.
- Prepare the client for phantom limb sensation (peculiar sensation that missing limb is still present).
- Mark the sites where peripheral pulses can be palpated or assessed using the Doppler to assist with postoperative assessment.

In addition to routine postoperative care:

- Assess for signs of bleeding or oozing.
- Elevate stump for the first 24 hours if ordered to control edema, then place flat on bed to prevent hip contracture.
- Assess incision for signs of healing.
- Assist in adjusting to phantom sensations or pain.
- Encourage range of motion and muscle strengthening exercises.
- Follow weight-bearing guidelines prescribed by physician.
- Consult Physical Therapy for adaptive devices for ambulation, transfer techniques, and exercise instructions.

- Assist the client in coping with the loss and integrating the prosthetic device into the total body image.

COMMUNITY AND SELF-CARE

Instruct client regarding:

- stump care:
  - — inspect daily for redness, blistering, or abrasions
    - use a mirror to examine all sides
  - — perform daily stump hygiene
    - wash with mild soap, rinse, and dry
    - do not use oils, creams, or alcohol on the stump
    - wear woolen socks over the stump
    - put prosthesis on immediately when arising and keep on all day (once wound has healed completely) to reduce swelling
    - continue prescribed exercises to prevent weakness
- prosthesis care:
  - — remove sweat and dirt daily from inside of socket with warm water and soap
  - — never attempt to adjust prosthesis; consult a prosthetist
- available support groups and community resources

(For more information, see pp. 1415–1424 of Black and Matassarin-Jacobs: *Medical-Surgical Nursing: Clinical Management for Continuity of Care,* 5th ed.)

Amyloidosis

- Amyloid is a proteinaceous substance that can infiltrate the liver and other organs. Accumulation of amyloid deposits causes tissues to cease functioning.
- The liver generally receives the greatest damage. Hepatomegaly is the most noticeable effect of this pathologic process. Liver function remains relatively unaffected. Clinical jaundice rarely appears.
- Treatment consists of removing the primary cause

and administering antimicrobial therapy to relieve chronic infection. Chemotherapy may also be ordered.

(For more information, see pp. 1902–1903 of Black and Matassarin-Jacobs: *Medical-Surgical Nursing: Clinical Management for Continuity of Care,* 5th ed.)

Amyotrophic Lateral Sclerosis

OVERVIEW

- Amyotrophic lateral sclerosis (ALS) is the most common of the motor neuron diseases.
- ALS involves degeneration of both anterior horn cells and the corticospinal tracts. Consequently, both upper and lower motor neuron signs and symptoms are seen. The sensory system is not involved.
- The onset of ALS usually occurs in middle age. Men are affected more often than women.
- Weakness typically begins in the upper extremities and progressively involves the upper arms and shoulders and then the muscles of the neck and throat. The trunk and lower extremities are usually not affected until late in the disease.
- Cognition, as well as bowel and bladder sphincters, remain intact, even when the client is totally debilitated.
- The course of the disease is relentlessly progressive. Death usually results from pneumonia due to respiratory compromise within 2 to 5 years.

CLINICAL MANIFESTATIONS

- weakness, fatigue
- muscle atrophy
- muscle twitching
- spasticity and hyperreflexia
- dysphagia (difficulty swallowing)
- dysarthria (slurred speech)
- shallow respirations

- ineffective cough

ACUTE AND SUBACUTE CARE

Medical Management

- Supportive therapy is the only intervention for ALS.

Nursing Management

- Assess client's ability to perform self-care.
- Conserve client energy by spacing activities and allowing rest periods.
- Encourage fluid intake.
- Initiate aspiration precautions.
- Collaborate with Physical and Occupational Therapy for exercises and adaptive devices for ambulation and self care.
- Allow plenty of time to complete activities.
- Assure that suction equipment is maintained at the bedside.
- Monitor respiratory status and laboratory arterial blood gas results.

COMMUNITY AND SELF-CARE

- Instruct the client/family regarding:
  - — disease process and prognosis
  - — need for respiratory support equipment in the home (oxygen, suction set-up) and training of household members in its use
  - — methods to conserve energy
  - — avoidance of muscle stress, strenuous activity, and extremes of hot and cold
  - — importance of avoiding exposure to anyone with respiratory infections
  - — the need to use good posture and swallowing techniques while eating and drinking to avoid aspiration
  - — use of abdominal muscles to enhance respiration when the intercostal muscles and diaphragm become weak
  - — use of adaptive devices
  - — the importance of follow-up pulmonary function tests and clinic visits

- Refer to available community resources (Visiting Nurse Association, ALS support groups).

(For more information, see pp. 886–888 of Black and Matassarin-Jacobs: *Medical-Surgical Nursing: Clinical Management for Continuity of Care,* 5th ed.)

Anemia, Acute Hemorrhagic

OVERVIEW

- Acute posthemorrhagic anemia is a normocytic, normochromic anemia that develops after the rapid loss of red blood cells from hemorrhage.
- The adverse effects of acute hemorrhage result from a rapid decrease in blood volume and red blood cells, reducing the oxygen-carrying capacity of the blood and perfusion to vital organs. The severity of symptoms and the prognosis for acute hemorrhage depend upon (1) the rate of bleeding, (2) the site of the hemorrhage, and (3) the volume of blood lost.

CLINICAL MANIFESTATIONS

- restlessness
- dizziness, syncope
- thirst
- pallor
- diaphoresis
- rapid, thready pulse
- dramatic drop in blood pressure
- rapid, deep respirations, which later become shallow
- disorientation, coma

ACUTE AND SUBACUTE CARE

Medical Management

- determination of and intervention to control hemorrhage
- fluid replacement therapy
- blood component replacement therapy
- oxygen therapy

Nursing Management

- Administer fluid and blood component therapies. See "Blood Component Transfusion," p.88.
- Assess for signs/symptoms of decreased cardiac output.
- Monitor vital signs.
- Monitor laboratory findings—CBC.

COMMUNITY AND SELF-CARE

Acute anemia will be resolved prior to discharge.

(For more information, see p. 1481 of Black and Matassarin-Jacobs: *Medical-Surgical Nursing: Clinical Management for Continuity of Care,* 5th ed.)

Anemia, Aplastic

Overview

- Aplastic anemia describes bone marrow that is severely hypoplastic ("empty"), that is, devoid of erythroid, myeloid, and megakaryocytic cell lines. Hypoplastic bone marrow results in anemia, leukopenia, and thrombocytopenia. When all three cellular elements are suppressed, the condition is known as pancytopenia.
- The etiologic agents that cause aplastic anemia inhibit mitosis (cell division) or block the synthesis of purines or nucleic acids and thus impede blood cell production. Usually, the mechanism of marrow failure from these agents is unknown.
- In about one-half the cases of aplastic anemia, the cause is unknown. Factors identified as causing aplastic anemia are an autoimmune reaction or direct injury by myelotoxins. Myelotoxins include:
  - — agents that always cause marrow damage when received in large amounts (x-rays, radium, radioactive isotopes, benzene, alkylating agents, and antimetabolites used in cancer therapy)
  - — agents that occasionally cause marrow failure, such as chloramphenicol (the drug most com-

monly linked with aplastic anemia), sulfonamides, phenylbutazone, diphenylhydantoin
  - agents that have been linked to aplastic anemia in a few cases, such as streptomycin, tripelennamine, DDT
- The onset of aplastic anemia may be insidious or rapid.

CLINICAL MANIFESTATIONS

Manifestations of pancytopenia are particularly severe. Not only does the red blood cell count fall, but so do the leukocyte and platelet counts. The client consequently develops the following three conditions.

Normocytic Anemia

- progressive fatigue, lassitude, dyspnea

Granulocytopenia

- increased susceptibility to infection

Thrombocytopenia

- bleeding into the skin and mucous membranes
- hemorrhage

ACUTE AND SUBACUTE CARE

Medical Management

- identification and withdrawal of the offending agent or drug
- blood product replacement therapy
- bone marrow transplantation if autoimmune phenomenon is suspected or bone marrow fails to regenerate with withdrawal of myelotoxic agents (See "Bone Marrow Transplantation," p. 92)
- steroid and androgen therapy to stimulate bone marrow activity
- oxygen therapy

Nursing Management

- Administer blood products as ordered. See "Blood Component Transfusion," p. 88.

— Because the marrow of the aplastic client is so severely depressed, transfusions of blood components may be irradiated in order to inactivate lymphocytes and prevent transfusion associated graft-versus-host disease (GVHD).

- Monitor laboratory findings—CBC and platelet count.
- Monitor response to activity and provide rest periods.
- Maintain protective isolation.
- Monitor temperature and assess for other signs/symptoms of infection.
- Assess for signs/symptoms of bleeding—hematest positive stools, petechiae, epistaxis, change in level of consciousness, abdominal pain, etc.
- Maintain bleeding precautions—electric razor, soft toothbrush, assisted ambulation, etc.
- See "Bone Marrow Transplantation," p. 92.

COMMUNITY AND SELF-CARE

Instruct client regarding:

- the importance of follow-up clinic appointments
- need to avoid exposure to others with infections
- signs/symptoms to report to physician
- importance of adequate rest
- precautions to prevent bleeding:
  - — no contact sports
  - — soft toothbrush
  - — electric razor
  - — care when doing yardwork
  - — safety precautions
- see "Bone Marrow Transplantation," p. 92.

(For more information, see pp. 1477–1478 of Black and Matassarin-Jacobs: *Medical-Surgical Nursing: Clinical Management for Continuity of Care,* 5th ed.)

Anemia, Chronic Hemorrhagic

OVERVIEW

- Anemia due to chronic blood loss is a chronic, microcytic, hypochromic anemia.

- The results of chronic bleeding are (1) continuous loss of small numbers of erythrocytes, usually replaced by the bone marrow, and (2) continuous loss of iron.
- The major causes of chronic blood loss include bleeding peptic ulcers, prolonged or excessive menses, bleeding hemorrhoids and cancerous lesions within the gastrointestinal tract.

CLINICAL MANIFESTATIONS

- asymptomatic—mild cases
- dizziness, headaches
- sensitivity to cold
- pallor
- palpitations
- weakness, fatigue

ACUTE AND SUBACUTE CARE

Medical Management

- determination/treatment of cause
- fluid replacement therapy
- blood component replacement therapy
- oxygen therapy
- iron replacement therapy—ferrous sulfate
- dietary modification—high in iron and protein

Nursing Management

- Administer fluid/blood component replacement therapy. See "Blood Component Transfusion," p. 88.
- Administer iron replacement therapy.
  - Oral iron supplements should be administered with meals (to decrease gastric upset).
  - Liquid iron preparations should be taken through a straw (to prevent staining the teeth).
  - Intramuscular replacements should be given by Z-track technique (to prevent discoloration of the skin).
- Monitor laboratory findings—CBC.
- Monitor response to activity and schedule adequate rest periods.

COMMUNITY AND SELF-CARE

Instruct client regarding:

- importance of medication regime
- measures to prevent constipation if taking iron replacement (high fiber diet, stool softener, increased fluid intake)
- need for adequate rest

(For more information, see p. 1481 of Black and Matassarin-Jacobs: *Medical-Surgical Nursing: Clinical Management for Continuity of Care,* 5th ed.)

Anemia, Folic Acid Deficiency

OVERVIEW

- Folic acid deficiency causes a megaloblastic anemia.
- Folic acid deficiency impedes the formation of DNA precursors, which causes abnormal maturation of red blood cells (megaloblasts), leukocytes, and platelets.
- Factors causing folic acid deficiency include:
  - — diet lacking in foods such as green leafy vegetables, liver, citrus fruits, and yeast
  - — alcoholism (due to [1] inadequate dietary intake of folic acid and [2] high levels of alcohol in the blood, which partially block the response of the bone marrow to folic acid)
  - — malabsorption syndromes (sprue, celiac disease, steatorrhea)
  - — certain medications that impede folic acid absorption and utilization (phenobarbital, antimetabolites used in cancer therapy, certain contraceptives)
  - — times of increased demand for folate (pregnancy, adolescence, infancy)
- Anemia due to folic acid deficiency has a slow, insidious onset.

CLINICAL MANIFESTATIONS

- thin and emaciated appearance

- fatigue, weakness
- slight jaundice
- dyspepsia; smooth, beefy tongue

ACUTE AND SUBACUTE CARE

Medical Management

- determination/treatment of underlying cause
- folic acid replacement
- vitamin C therapy (increases role of folic acid in promoting erythropoiesis)
- dietary modification

Nursing Management

- Administer replacement therapy as ordered.
- Monitor laboratory findings—CBC, folate level.
- Monitor response to activity and provide rest periods.
- Monitor patient for signs/symptoms of delirium tremors (if history of alcohol abuse).

COMMUNITY AND SELF-CARE

Instruct client regarding:

- importance of medication regime
- dietary modifications
- importance of follow-up clinic appointments
- available community alcohol cessation programs (if history of alcohol abuse)

(For more information, see pp. 1476–1477 of Black and Matassarin-Jacobs: *Medical-Surgical Nursing: Clinical Management for Continuity of Care,* 5th ed.)

Anemia, Glucose-6-Phosphate Dehydrogenase (G6PD) Deficiency

OVERVIEW

- Glucose-6-phosphate dehydrogenase (G6PD) is an important red blood cell enzyme. G6PD anemia is

a genetic disorder that leaves red blood cells more susceptible to hemolysis after ingestion of medication and food classified as chemical oxidants (i.e., quinine, aspirin, sulfonamides, primaquine, phenacetin, Vitamin K derivatives, chloramphenicol, thiazide diuretics, fava bean). After exposure to any of these agents, the client with G6PD deficiency develops acute intravascular hemolysis lasting 7–12 days.
- Among Americans, G6PD deficiency affects about 20 per cent of the black population and 1–2 per cent of the white population. It is common among Sephardic Jews, Greeks, Italians, and Arabs.

CLINICAL MANIFESTATIONS

Clients with G6PD deficiency may remain completely asymptomatic throughout their lives. Typically, symptoms develop only after viral or bacterial infection or ingestion of certain medications or toxins.
- anemia
- jaundice (bilirubin accumulation)

ACUTE AND SUBACUTE CARE

Medical Management

- identification and elimination of the food or medication precipitating the hemolytic reaction
- fluid replacement therapy

Nursing Management

- Administer fluid replacement therapy.
- Encourage adequate rest.
- Monitor laboratory findings—CBC, bilirubin levels.
- Encourage nutritious diet.

COMMUNITY AND SELF-CARE

Instruct client regarding:
- foods or medications that may precipitate an attack
- importance of adequate rest
- importance of screening family members

(For more information, see p. 1483 of Black and Matassarin-Jacobs: *Medical-Surgical Nursing: Clinical Management for Continuity of Care,* 5th ed.)

Anemia, Hemolytic

Overview

- Major hallmarks of hemolytic anemia are:
  - — a shortening of the red blood cell life span
  - — an abnormal increase in the number of red blood cells destroyed by macrophages
  - — failure of the bone marrow to replace destroyed red blood cells
- Premature hemolysis of red blood cells results from:
  (1) trauma—when red blood cells are exposed to excessive turbulence in the circulation, they may fragment and are quickly destroyed by phagocytes.
    - — external trauma or burns
    - — prosthetic heart valve replacement (causes turbulence in blood flow)

  (2) chemical agents and medications—hemolytic reaction is due to the oxidant effects of the medication or chemical, or an immune reaction caused by the medication.
    - — benzene, nitrates, potassium chlorate, lead, quinine, quinidine, methyldopa, penicillin

  (3) infectious agents—infectious organisms cause hemolysis by releasing toxins, by entering the red cell and destroying it, or by promoting an antigen-antibody reaction.
    - — bacterial endocarditis, malaria, miliary tuberculosis, infectious hepatitis, infectious mononucleosis

  (4) systemic diseases—hemolytic anemia sometimes complicates the following systemic conditions.
    - — Hodgkin's disease, leukemias, lymphomas, systemic lupus erythematosus (SLE)

  (5) splenic overactivity

(6) isoimmune hemolytic reaction—an antigen-antibody reaction that destroys red blood cells when antibodies develop in response to antigens from another individual.
    — transfusion reaction

- Hemolytic anemia may be acute or chronic.

CLINICAL MANIFESTATIONS

- dyspnea
- palpitations, tachycardia
- chronic fatigue
- pallor
- sore mouth and tongue
- angina
- anorexia
- headache, dizziness
- jaundice—accumulation of bilirubin
- splenomegaly, hepatomegaly—macrophages in the spleen and liver become hyperactive due to increased demands to phagocytize defective erythrocytes
- cholelithiasis (gallstones)—due to excessive bilirubin
- signs/symptoms of renal failure—due to excretion of increased load of blood cell degradation products

ACUTE AND SUBACUTE CARE

Medical Management

- identification/elimination of causative factor
- fluid and electrolyte management
- oxygen therapy
- blood product replacement therapy
- corticosteroid therapy

Nursing Management

- Administer steroid therapy as ordered.
- Administer blood products as ordered. See "Blood Component Transfusion," p. 88.
- Monitor laboratory findings—CBC, renal panel, bilirubin levels.
- Monitor intake and output.

- Assess response to activity and provide rest periods.

COMMUNITY AND SELF-CARE

Instruct client regarding:

- importance of medication regime
- importance of rest
- need for follow-up clinic appointments

(For more information, see pp. 1478–1480 of Black and Matassarin-Jacobs: *Medical-Surgical Nursing: Clinical Management for Continuity of Care,* 5th ed.)

Anemia, Iron Deficiency

OVERVIEW

- Iron deficiency anemia is associated with either inadequate absorption or excessive loss of iron; it is a chronic, microcytic, hypochromic anemia.
- An inadequate supply of iron, which is needed to synthesize hemoglobin, decreases the oxygen-carrying capacity of heme. When this disorder becomes severe, the marrow produces red cells that are deficient in hemoglobin concentration and are hypochromic and microcytic.
- The poor of all nations suffer far more frequently from iron deficiency than do the middle and upper classes. Menstruating women and young children also are vulnerable to iron deficiency. These groups of clients must have a higher daily intake of iron to prevent this deficiency. Iron deficiency anemia also occurs with chronic blood loss (peptic ulcers, ulcerative colitis). Alteration in the mucosa of the duodenum and proximal jejunum (chronic diarrhea, celiac disease, gastrectomy) affects iron absorption, predisposing clients to iron deficiency states.
- The major risk factors for iron deficiency anemia are inadequate nutrition and blood loss.

CLINICAL MANIFESTATIONS

Mild cases may be asymptomatic:
- palpitations, tachycardia
- dizziness, headaches
- sensitivity to the cold
- brittle hair and nails
- weakness, fatigue
- sore mouth and tongue

ACUTE AND SUBACUTE CARE

Medical Management

- determination/treatment of the underlying cause
- supplemental iron preparations—ferrous sulfate (Feosol), ferrous gluconate (Fergon), iron-dextran (Imferon)
- dietary modification—increased iron

Nursing Management

- Administer ordered iron replacement therapy.
  - Oral iron salt replacement should be given with meals (to decrease gastric upset).
  - Liquid iron preparations should be taken through a straw (to prevent staining the teeth).
  - Intramuscular replacements should be given by Z-track technique (to prevent discoloration of the skin).
- Monitor response to activity and provide adequate rest periods.
- Encourage diet high in protein, iron, and vitamins.
- Assess for signs of constipation (commonly seen during iron therapy).
- Monitor laboratory findings—CBC, iron levels.

COMMUNITY AND SELF-CARE

Instruct client regarding:
- importance of medication regime and specifics of administration
- dietary modifications—high in iron.
- measures to prevent constipation if on iron replacement (high fiber diet, stool softener, increased fluids)
- importance of follow-up clinic appointments

(For more information, see pp. 1472–1474 of Black and Matassarin-Jacobs: *Medical-Surgical Nursing: Clinical Management for Continuity of Care,* 5th ed.)

Anemia, Pernicious

Overview

- Pernicious anemia is a type of megaloblastic anemia due to failure to absorb vitamin B_{12}.
- The principal cause of impaired vitamin B_{12} absorption is intrinsic factor deficiency. The small intestine cannot absorb vitamin B_{12} (the extrinsic factor) unless the intrinsic factor (a substance of internal origin) combines with it. A vitamin B_{12} deficiency impedes the formation of DNA precursors, which causes abnormal maturation of red blood cells (megaloblasts), leukocytes, and platelets. Lack of intrinsic factor, due to atrophy of the stomach's glandular mucosa, is the basic defect in pernicious anemia. Possible causes of mucosal atrophy and associated hypochlorhydria (deficiency of gastric hydrochloric acid) include: (1) heredity, (2) prolonged iron deficiency, and (3) autoimmunity. Causes of vitamin B_{12} deficiency include: (1) heredity (absence of the intrinsic factor), (2) gastric resection (loss of parietal cells that secrete intrinsic factor), and (3) dietary inadequacies—deficient in meat and dairy products.
- Pernicious anemia mainly strikes men and women 50–70 years of age.

CLINICAL MANIFESTATIONS

- weakness, fatigue
- dyspepsia; smooth, beefy tongue
- palpitations
- shortness of breath
- pallor
- sensitivity to cold
- anorexia, nausea, weight loss
- paresthesias of the hands and feet
- angina

ACUTE AND SUBACUTE CARE

Medical Management

- determination/treatment of underlying cause
- vitamin B_{12} therapy (lifelong therapy)
- iron replacement
- folic acid therapy (if history of poor nutrition)
- oxygen therapy
- dietary modifications

Nursing Management

- Administer replacement therapy as ordered.
- Monitor laboratory findings—CBC.
- Monitor response to activity and provide rest periods.

COMMUNITY AND SELF-CARE

Instruct client regarding:

- importance of lifelong therapy of monthly vitamin B_{12} injections
- importance of follow-up clinic appointments—clients with pernicious anemia are at risk for developing gastric carcinoma and should have a complete physical examination twice a year
- dietary modifications

(For more information, see pp. 1474–1476 of Black and Matassarin-Jacobs: *Medical-Surgical Nursing: Clinical Management for Continuity of Care,* 5th ed.)

Anemia, Sickle Cell

Overview

- Sickle cell anemia is a chronic, hereditary, hemolytic disorder. Sickle cell anemia primarily affects the world's black population.
- In sickle cell anemia, the red blood cells contain an abnormal hemoglobin; that is, hemoglobin S (HbS) instead of hemoglobin A (HbA). These abnormal cells assume a sickle, or crescent, shape when oxygen in the blood decreases. Once they "sickle,"

the red blood cells become rigid and may obstruct capillary blood flow, causing further hypoxia and, consequently, more sickling. The heavy concentration of misshapen cells during a sickling crisis makes the blood abnormally viscous, which results in sluggish circulation. The organs most vulnerable to infarction and necrosis are the brain and kidneys, because of their constant demand for oxygen, and the bone marrow and spleen, because of their normally sluggish circulation.

- Sickle cell *trait*, generally a relatively mild condition, may produce few or no symptoms. It is present in clients who are heterogeneous for sickle cell hemoglobin.
- Factors that result in hypoxia and may trigger a crisis include: climbing to high altitudes, flying in nonpressurized planes, exercising strenuously or undergoing anesthesia without proper oxygenation.
- Complications of sickle cell anemia include:
  — hemolytic anemia—secondary to destruction of sickle cells
  — cholelithiasis (gallstones)—due to elevated bilirubin from hemoglobin released during destruction of sickle cells
  — splenic infarction
  — renal medullary ischemia with diminished capacity to concentrate urine
  — pulmonary infarction
  — myocardial infarction
  — cerebrovascular accident
  — osteoporosis—secondary to proliferation of the bone marrow in an attempt to compensate for chronic anemia

CLINICAL MANIFESTATIONS

- jaundice or pallor
- bone or joint pain
- enlarged liver and spleen

Sickle Cell Crisis

- systolic murmur
- arrhythmias
- shortness of breath

- dyspnea, cyanosis
- signs/symptoms of increased intracranial pressure
- decreased urinary output
- edema

ACUTE AND SUBACUTE CARE

Medical Management

- bedrest
- oxygen therapy

increased ane-

Nursing Management

- Administer oxygen therapy.
- Administer analgesics.
- Encourage rest.
- Administer fluid and electrolyte therapy.
- Monitor intake and output.
- Daily weights.
- Assess all body systems for evidence of complications.

COMMUNITY AND SELF-CARE

Instruct client regarding:

- preventing a crisis:
  - — avoid high altitudes
  - — avoid flying in nonpressurized planes
  - — avoid becoming dehydrated
- signs/symptoms of complications and when to call the physician
- disease process
- need for genetic counseling
- need for follow-up laboratory and clinic visits

(For more information, see pp. 1512–1515 of Black and Matassarin-Jacobs: *Medical-Surgical Nursing: Clinical Management for Continuity of Care,* 5th ed.)

Aneurysm, Aortic—Ruptured or Dissecting

- An aneurysm is an outpouching of a vessel wall, usually due to arteriosclerotic changes or trauma involving the tunica media (muscular layer of the artery).
- The aneurysm may be saccular ("balloons out") or fusiform (encircles the vessel).
- Aortic aneurysms may involve the thoracic aorta or abdominal aorta.
- Abdominal aortic aneurysms occur in approximately 2 per cent of the population. Over 80 per cent of abdominal aortic aneurysms are asymptomatic and usually not treated as an emergency.
- In aortic dissection, blood separates the vessel layers and a larger portion of the vessel may be affected. In an expanding aneurysm, the aneurysm wall is still intact. Symptoms are caused by increased pressure on the surrounding structures.
- A rupture occurs when the vessel wall loses continuity.
- A ruptured or dissecting aneurysm is a surgical emergency.
- Assessment findings of a ruptured or dissecting aneurysm may include:
  - — severe abdominal and back pain if the aneurysm is leaking
  - — an enlarging abdominal girth with a palpable, pulsatile mass
  - — leg numbness, tingling, or loss of motor function
  - — mottled cyanosis below the level of the aneurysm
  - — profound hypotension
- Treatment is rapid surgical intervention.

NURSING MANAGEMENT

- Insert two to four large-bore intravenous lines.
- Monitor vital signs continuously.
- Monitor ECG.
- Administer antihypertensives to minimize extension of the dissection.

- Obtain blood for laboratory studies (including type and crossmatch for 10–20 units of whole blood).
- Ensure that necessary instruments are available if needed for cross-clamping the aorta.
- Transport the client to the operating room with resuscitative personnel in attendance and an emergency laparotomy tray on the stretcher.

Aneurysm (Intracranial) and Subarachnoid Hemorrhage

OVERVIEW

- Intracranial aneurysms are congenital, traumatic, arteriosclerotic, or septal weakenings or outpouchings in vessel walls. Ninety per cent of aneurysms are congenital. Eighty per cent occur on the circle of Willis.
- Aneurysms may weaken, leak, or rupture and cause bleeding into the subarachnoid space. This is called *subarachnoid hemorrhage* (SAH). The most common cause of spontaneous SAH is leaking or rupture of an intracranial aneurysm. The blood within the cerebrospinal fluid (CSF) causes irritation of the meninges. It also clots in the subarachnoid space and can obstruct CSF flow, leading to hydrocephalus and increased intracranial pressure (ICP). After an aneurysm ruptures, a clot forms at the site of hemorrhage. This reduces the risk of rebleeding for a few days. As the clot begins to dissolve, the possibility of rebleeding increases. The greatest risk of rebleeding is within the first 24 hours.
- SAH also may be caused by head trauma, blood dyscrasias, intracranial tumors, vascular anomalies, or central nervous system infection.
- Women are most often affected. Ruptures occur most frequently between the ages of 30 and 60 years; the peak incidence is in the fifth decade.

- Risk factors for SAH include: head trauma, hypertension, and cocaine use.

CLINICAL MANIFESTATIONS

An aneurysm is usually asymptomatic until it ruptures.

- sudden, severe headache with vomiting
- loss of consciousness, confusion, lethargy
- seizures
- stiff neck; leg and back pain
- motor weakness
- coma (within hours)

ACUTE AND SUBACUTE CARE

Medical Management

- use of albumin and vasopressors to induce hypertensive, hypervolemic hemodilution to minimize vasospasm and force blood through spastic vessels
- nifedipine (a calcium channel blocker) to inhibit vasospasm
- measures to decrease ICP (dexamethasone, head elevation, patent airway)

Surgical Management

- clipping of the aneurysm with a metal clip or suture through a craniotomy
- ventriculostomy—drainage of CSF to decrease ICP

Nursing Management

Medical

- Provide calm, quiet environment.
- Assess client's response to family visits and adjust visiting schedule accordingly.
- Administer vasoactive medications.
- Avoid sedation, which interferes with accurate neurologic assessment.
- Monitor BP closely.
- Maintain aneurysm precautions:
  — dim lights
  — elevate head of the bed 15–30 degrees, as ordered

— instruct client to avoid straining
— place needed items within easy reach
— assist with position changes
— instruct client not to tighten muscles during moving or turning
— instruct client not to rotate or flex the neck
— instruct client that no isometric or active exercises are permitted
— instruct client on avoidance of Valsalva's maneuver
— avoid rectal stimulation or straining at stool
— no enemas or rectal temperatures
— administer stool softeners and mild laxatives as ordered

- Monitor neurologic status.
- Monitor hemodynamic status.

Surgical

See care of the client after craniotomy, "Intracranial Tumors," p. 431.

(For more information, see pp. 812–816 of Black and Matassarin-Jacobs: *Medical-Surgical Nursing: Clinical Management for Continuity of Care,* 5th ed.)

Angina Pectoris

Overview

- Angina pectoris is a term used to describe chest pain resulting from myocardial ischemia (lack of blood supply). Myocardial ischemia develops if the blood supply through the coronary vessels or oxygen content of the blood is not adequate to meet metabolic demands. In some persons, the coronary arteries can supply adequate blood when the person is at rest; but when the person attempts activity or is taxed in some manner, angina develops.

- The major cause of angina pectoris is coronary artery disease (CAD). As vessels become lined and eventually occluded with atherosclerotic plaque, they lose their ability to dilate and supply the heart with blood. Angina occurs less commonly in clients with normal coronary arteries secondary to arterial spasm, causing increased resistance to blood flow.
- Conditions that cause angina fall into two categories:
  (1) conditions that decrease blood or oxygen supply to the heart or increase myocardial need for oxygen;
    — atherosclerosis
    — arterial spasm
    — hypotension
    — aortic stenosis or insufficiency
    — anemia and hypoxemia
    — polycythemia (increased blood viscosity slows blood flow through coronary arteries)
    — damage to the myocardium
    — hypertrophy of the myocardium
    — thyrotoxicosis
    — strong emotions
    — heavy exertion
  (2) conditions that increase demands on the myocardium;
    — exertion
    — emotion
    — digestion of a large meal
    — anemia
    — hyperthyroidism
- Myocardial ischemia occurs when either supply or demand is altered. In some clients the coronary arteries can supply adequate blood when the client is at rest, but with increased demand, angina develops. Myocardial cells become ischemic within 10 seconds of coronary artery occlusion. After several minutes of ischemia, the heart's pumping function is reduced. The reduction of pumping deprives the ischemic cells of much needed oxygen and glucose. The cells convert to anaerobic metabolism, which leaves lactic acid as a waste product. As lactic acid accumulates, pain develops. Angina pectoris is transient, lasting only 3–5

minutes. If blood flow is restored, no permanent myocardial damage occurs.

- Patterns of angina
  - — stable angina (classic angina)—chest pain triggered by a predictable degree of exertion or emotion
  - — unstable angina (crescendo angina)—chest pain triggered by an unpredictable degree of exertion or emotion, which may occur at night. Attacks characteristically increase in number, duration, and intensity over time.
  - — variant angina (Prinzmetal's angina)—chest pain similar to classic angina but of longer duration that may occur at rest and tends to occur in the early hours of the day; may result from coronary artery spasm
  - — nocturnal angina—occurs only during the night
  - — angina decubitus—chest pain that occurs when client reclines and lessens when client sits or stands up
  - — intractable angina—chronic, incapacitating angina unresponsive to intervention
  - — postinfarction angina—occurs after a myocardial infarction (MI), secondary to residual ischemia
- Factors that precipitate an anginal attack include exertion, emotion, and exposure to cold.

CLINICAL MANIFESTATIONS

- transient paroxysmal attacks of substernal or precordial pain with the following characteristics:
  - — description—squeezing, burning, choking, or pressing
  - — severity—mild to moderate in intensity
  - — location—retrosternal or slightly to the left of the sternum
  - — radiation—to the left shoulder and upper arm and travels down the inner aspect of the left arm to the elbow, wrist and fourth and fifth fingers. Pain may also radiate to right shoulder, neck, jaw, or epigastric region.
  - — duration—usually less than 5 minutes
  - — relief—quickly subsides with the administration of nitroglycerin and rest
- dyspnea

- pallor
- dizziness
- sweating
- faintness
- digestive disturbances
- palpitations

ACUTE AND SUBACUTE CARE

Medical Management

- vasodilators (nitrates/nitrites: nitroglycerin, isosorbide dinitrate [Isordil])—relax smooth muscle of coronary and peripheral blood vessels, decreasing workload of heart and promoting greater flow of blood and oxygen to heart muscle
- beta-blocking agents (propranolol [Inderal], atenolol [Tenormin], metoprolol [Lopressor])—decrease myocardial workload and oxygen demand by decreasing contractility, heart rate, and blood pressure
- calcium channel blockers (diltiazem [Cardizem], nifedipine [Procardia], verapamil [Calan])—reduce vascular smooth muscle tone by interfering with the ability of calcium ions to initiate muscular contraction (arterial vasodilating effect)
- antiplatelet medications (aspirin, dipyridamole [Persantine], sulfinpyrazone [Anturane])—decrease platelet aggregation and reduce thrombus formation
- analgesics—morphine sulfate is most commonly used, as it also reduces venous return (preload), thereby decreasing myocardial workload
- dietary modifications—low fat, low cholesterol, low calorie, high fiber (lowers triglyceride and cholesterol levels)
- hypertension therapy

Nursing Management

- Monitor cardiac rhythm.
- Provide restful environment.
- For episodes of angina:
  - — maintain bedrest
  - — assess pain characteristics and associated symptoms

— administer PRN nitroglycerin
— monitor vital signs
— administer PRN analgesic
— administer supplemental oxygen
— obtain 12-lead ECG
— monitor blood pressure during nitroglycerin administration
— notify physician for chest pain not relieved by three nitroglycerin tablets or ordered analgesic

COMMUNITY AND SELF-CARE

Instruct the client regarding:

- disease process and treatment regime
- management of anginal episodes
  — stop activity
  — lie or sit down
  — take nitroglycerin tablets sublingually 5 minutes apart
  — if pain not relieved after three nitroglycerin, the client should be taken to an emergency department
- modification of risk factors
  — hypertension management
  — dietary restrictions
  — weight control
  — smoking cessation
  — stress management
  — regular program of daily exercise
- avoiding activities or habits that precipitate angina, such as eating large meals, drinking coffee, excessive strenuous activity, and exposure to cold

(For more information, see pp. 1251–1258 of Black and Matassarin-Jacobs: *Medical-Surgical Nursing: Clinical Management for Continuity of Care,* 5th ed.)

Anorexia Nervosa

OVERVIEW

- Anorexia nervosa is a loss of 15-25 per cent of ideal body weight due to voluntary restriction of food intake.

- Clients with this disorder experience:
  - — severe weight loss
  - — physiologic changes associated with starvation
  - — distorted mental perceptions (weight phobia, alterations in body image, fear of being fat).
- The highest risk group is girls between the ages of 12 and 18 who have low self esteem.

CLINICAL MANIFESTATIONS

The changes seen are physiologic, but the real disorder is psychologic:

- weight loss (as above)
- amenorrhea
- cachexia
- constipation
- fine hair over the body
- dry, sandpaper-like skin
- bradycardia, hypotension, hypothermia
- facial puffiness (from parotid hypertrophy)
- bizarre rituals associated with food
- fluid and electrolyte imbalances
- excessive exercise

ACUTE AND SUBACUTE CARE

Medical Management

- improving the nutritional status through eating (if possible), tube feeding, or total parenteral nutrition
- improving self image through psychotherapy and behavior modification

Nursing Management

- Assist to select food from all food groups.
- Allow to refuse two to three foods.
- Remain with client for at least 1 hour after meals.
- Maintain accurate calorie count.
- Obtain weights at regular intervals.
- Monitor serum potassium and for signs/symptoms of hypokalemia.
- Assist to develop improved self esteem.
- Assist to find areas of self regard.

COMMUNITY AND SELF-CARE

- Instruct client regarding:
  — reinforcement of nutritional plan (as above)
  — signs/symptoms to report to physician
- Refer to outpatient therapy program.

(For more information, see pp. 1756–1758 of Black and Matassarin-Jacobs: *Medical-Surgical Nursing: Clinical Management for Continuity of Care,* 5th ed.)

Anterior Cruciate Ligament Injury

OVERVIEW

- The ligaments of the knee stabilize the joint and control motion. The anterior cruciate ligament (ACL) is the strongest and least compliant knee ligament. It functions to prevent anterior displacement of the tibia on the femur as well as to control the rotary stability of the knee joint. The ACL is the most frequent completely torn ligament of the knee.
- This type of injury commonly occurs when participating in football, skiing, basketball, or gymnastics.

CLINICAL MANIFESTATIONS

- snapping sensation at the time of injury
- tense, swollen, stiff, and painful knee
- knee gives way leading to falls

ACUTE AND SUBACUTE CARE

Surgical Management

- autograft or artificial ligament placement with application of leg brace

Nursing Management

In addition to routine postoperative care:
- collaborate with Physical Therapy for prescribed exercises and adaptive devices

- apply continuous motion machine (supports the limb and puts the knee through preset degrees of passive range of motion [ROM]) if ordered. Usually used at least 3 hours per day or until full ROM is achieved.

COMMUNITY AND SELF-CARE

Instruct client regarding:

- prescribed exercises
- use of long-leg limb brace (set at 40 degrees flexion)

(For more information, see p. 2166 of Black and Matassarin-Jacobs: *Medical-Surgical Nursing: Clinical Management for Continuity of Care,* 5th ed.)

Appendicitis

OVERVIEW

- Appendicitis is an inflammation of the vermiform appendix. It develops most commonly in adolescents and young adults.
- The appendix becomes obstructed, and the intraluminal pressure increases, leading to decreased venous drainage, thrombosis, edema, and bacterial invasion of the bowel wall. Perforation will result if untreated.

CLINICAL MANIFESTATIONS

- acute wavelike abdominal pain
- pain in epigastrium or periumbilical region
- pain eventually shifts to the right lower quadrant and becomes steady
- loss of appetite, vomiting, low-grade fever, coated tongue, bad breath
- older clients may have few clinical symptoms

ACUTE AND SUBACUTE CARE

Surgical Management

- appendectomy (removal of the appendix) within 24–48 hours of onset of the symptoms

- delay in treatment can result in rupture and peritonitis

NURSING MANAGEMENT

Medical

- Assess quality of pain.
- Monitor for signs/symptoms of ruptured appendix and notify physician immediately if these occur:
  — rigid boardlike abdomen
  — generalized abdominal pain.
- Administer pain medication as prescribed and assess effectiveness.
- *Never* give enemas, laxatives, or apply heat to the abdomen (may cause perforation).
- Monitor intake and output.
- Maintain nasogastric tube to suction.
- Monitor vital signs, assessing for increased temperature or a change in pulse or blood pressure (signifying a ruptured appendix).

Surgical

In addition to routine postoperative care:

- Maintain wound packing and patency of drain if appendix ruptured.
- Monitor vital signs, urine output and level of consciousness.
- Assess wound drainage.

COMMUNITY AND SELF-CARE

- Instruct client regarding:
  — resumption of normal activity in 2–4 weeks
  — signs/symptoms of infection
  — wound care if appendix ruptured—irrigation with sterile saline and sterile dressing change several times daily
- Assess need for home health care referral for assistance with wound care.

(For more information, see pp. 1791–1793 of Black and Matassarin-Jacobs: *Medical-Surgical Nursing: Clinical Management for Continuity of Care,* 5th ed.)

Arterial Ulcers

OVERVIEW

- The usual sites for arterial ulcers are the medial and lateral metatarsal heads and the tip of the heel.
- Arterial ulcers are very painful, which distinguishes them from venous stasis ulcers. Arterial ulcers have a "punched out" look, again in contrast to venous stasis ulcers, which are broad and flat.
- Once an arterial ulcer develops, it tends to heal poorly or not at all (especially in diabetics) because of damaged blood vessels and inadequate blood supply. Eventually, the client may be forced to undergo limb amputation.

CLINICAL MANIFESTATIONS

- painful skin lesion

ACUTE AND SUBACUTE CARE

Medical Management

- bedrest—reduces the oxygen needs of the impaired tissues
- debridement followed by application of wet-to-damp saline dressings
- whirlpool treatments

Surgical Management

- skin grafting
- arterial bypass grafting for revascularization

Nursing Management

Medical

- Maintain bedrest.
- Perform dressing changes as ordered.
- Initiate preventive measures for immobility.

Surgical

See "Peripheral Vascular Disease: Chronic Arterial," p. 556, for care following arterial bypass revascularization surgery.

(For more information, see p. 1424 of Black and Matassarin-Jacobs: *Medical-Surgical Nursing: Clinical Management for Continuity of Care,* 5th ed.)

Arteriovenous Malformation

- Arteriovenous malformations (AVMs) are congenital malformations consisting of tangles of thin-walled blood vessels without intervening capillaries located in the cerebrovascular system. Arterial and venous blood shunt together, and, hence, brain perfusion cannot occur through them.
- The vessels may leak small amounts of blood or rupture, causing hemorrhage into the subarachnoid space or brain.
- Bleeding vessels usually produce focal neurologic symptoms.
- Ruptured vessels produce clinical manifestations similar to those of subarachnoid hemorrhage. Aneurysm precautions may be prescribed (see "Aneurysm and Subarachnoid Hemorrhage," p. 54).
- About one-half of AVMs can be completely removed surgically. Other interventions that may be used to reduce the size of the aneurysm are:
  - — laser therapy
  - — radiation
  - — detachable balloon procedures
  - — artificially embolizing (clotting) the arteriovenous malformation
  - — ligating the feeding arteries of the arteriovenous malformation

(For more information, see p. 816 of Black and Matassarin-Jacobs: *Medical-Surgical Nursing: Clinical Management for Continuity of Care,* 5th ed.)

Ascites

OVERVIEW

- Ascites is the accumulation of fluid in the peritoneal cavity. It results from the interaction of several pathophysiologic changes: portal hypertension, lowered plasma colloidal osmotic pressure, and sodium retention. Specifically:
  - — Portal hypertension causes leaking of plasma directly from the liver capsule and portal vein into the peritoneal cavity. Plasma proteins are lost into the ascitic fluid, reducing oncotic pressure in the vascular compartment.
  - — Hepatocellular damage results in the liver's decreased ability to synthesize albumin. Decreased albumin synthesis results in lower plasma colloidal osmotic pressure and leakage of fluid into the peritoneal cavity.
  - — The circulating blood volume decreases from the loss of colloidal osmotic pressure. The secretion of aldosterone increases to stimulate the kidneys to retain sodium and water. As a result of hepatocellular damage, the liver cannot inactivate the aldosterone, so more fluid is retained and the volume of ascites grows.
- Diseases that may lead to these events include cirrhosis of the liver, right-sided heart failure, cancer, and complications of pancreatitis.

CLINICAL MANIFESTATIONS

- abdominal distention
- bulging flanks
- protruding, downward umbilicus
- shortness of breath, dyspnea

ACUTE AND SUBACUTE CARE

Medical Management

- correction of fluid and electrolyte imbalance
- discontinuation of medications that inhibit prostaglandin synthesis (such as aspirin and indomethacin) and that thus impair renal sodium excretion

- paracentesis—repeated, large-volume in combination with albumin to manage ascites from cirrhosis; small-volume (100ml) to relieve manifestations such as shortness of breath
- diuretics (especially Aldactone)
- intravenous albumin
- low-sodium diet with fluid restriction (protein in the diet is allowed, unless the client is encephalopathic)

Surgical Management

- insertion of a peritoneovenous shunt (such as a LeVeen or Denver shunt) for refractory and disabling chronic ascites—moves fluid from the peritoneal (abdominal) cavity into the venous blood of the superior vena cava.

Nursing Management

Medical

- Assess whether ascites is interfering with eating, sleeping, and breathing.
- Discuss diet and plan fluid restriction with the client.
- Measure abdominal girth daily or twice daily (mark spot on abdomen for consistency in measurements).
- Daily weights.
- Monitor intake and output.
- Discuss avoidance of aspirin and indomethacin.
- Monitor client after paracentesis:
  — check vital signs frequently
  — assess dressing over site for excessive fluid drainage
- Position in high-Fowler's to facilitate breathing.
- Assist to cough and deep breathe and use incentive spirometer hourly.
- Monitor respiratory status for development of atelectasis or pneumonia.
- Provide support for distended abdomen and good skin care.

See "Portal Hypertension," p. 582.

COMMUNITY AND SELF-CARE

- Instruct client regarding:
  - causes/treatment of ascites
  - need for dietary modifications and fluid restrictions
  - need to stop alcohol intake
  - measures to improve sleeping
  - measures to reduce gastric reflux
- Refer to chemical dependency programs or support groups such as Alcoholics Anonymous as appropriate.

Also see "Cirrhosis," p. 174, and "Portal Hypertension," p. 582.

(For more information, see pp. 1889–1891 of Black and Matassarin-Jacobs: *Medical-Surgical Nursing: Clinical Management for Continuity of Care,* 5th ed.)

Asthma

OVERVIEW

- Asthma is a disorder of the bronchial airways characterized by periods of bronchospasm. This disorder involves biochemical, immunologic, endocrine, infectious, and psychological factors. It involves a chronic inflammatory process that produces mucosal edema, mucus, secretions, and airway inflammation.
- Asthma affects 3–4 per cent of the U.S. population.
- Asthma is believed to be an inherited disorder that interacts with environmental factors to cause the disease.
- Extrinsic allergens include: dust, pollen, smoke, mold, medications, food, and respiratory infections.
- A severe, life-threatening complication of asthma is status asthmaticus. It is an acute episode of

bronchospasm that can increase the workload of breathing 5 to 10 times. Acute cor pulmonale can develop with a severe paradoxical pulse. Pneumothorax, cardiac arrest, or respiratory arrest can occur if untreated.

- Risk factors include viral infections, allergens, and pollutants.

CLINICAL MANIFESTATIONS

Asthma Attack

- marked respiratory effort, nasal flaring
- use of excessory muscles
- inspiratory and expiratory wheezing
- nonproductive coughing
- tachycardia, tachypnea

ACUTE AND SUBACUTE CARE

Medical Management

Emergency Management

- inhaled beta-adrenergics
- intravenous theophylline
- intravenous steroids
- oxygen, if needed

Status Asthmaticus

- intravenous corticosteroids
- inhaled beta-adrenergics
- oxygen, if needed
- intubation and mechanical ventilation, if needed

Nursing Management

- Assess respiratory status every hour during acute phase:
  - — lung sounds
  - — respiratory rate and depth
  - — presence and severity of wheezing
  - — breathing pattern
  - — presence of pursed lip breathing, nasal flaring, shortness of breath, sternal and intercostal retractions, prolonged expiratory phase
- Monitor arterial blood gases.
- Monitor results of pulmonary function tests.

- Monitor color, consistency, and amount of sputum production (client may have upper respiratory infection).
- Place client in Fowler's position.
- Encourage fluids to thin secretions.
- Reposition frequently.
- Administer oral care every 2–4 hours.
- Assess effectiveness of therapy.
- Monitor for side effects of bronchodilator therapy (tachycardia/tremors).
- Monitor for therapeutic levels of theophylline (8–20 μg/mL).

Community and Self-Care

Instruct client regarding:

- prescribed bronchodilators and steroids, including side effects
- importance of follow-up serum theophylline levels and signs/symptoms of theophylline toxicity
- use of inhalers and nebulizers
- early symptoms of asthma and when to seek medical attention
- avoidance of known allergens
- avoidance of stress; relaxation techniques
- avoidance of outdoor activities when pollen counts and pollution indexes high

(For more information, see pp. 1105–1111 of Black and Matassarin-Jacobs: *Medical-Surgical Nursing: Clinical Management for Continuity of Care,* 5th ed.)

Atelectasis

- Atelectasis is the collapse of lung tissue, which causes interference with lung expansion.
- Risk factors include: clients after upper abdominal or thoracic surgeries; the elderly; bedridden clients.
- Clinical manifestations include: dyspnea, tachycardia, cyanosis, decreased breath sounds or crackles, and fever. With severe atelectasis the client may have: tracheal shift toward the affected side,

decreased tactile fremitus, dull percussion, and decreased chest movement on the affected side.

- Medical management includes: (1) prevention, especially with high risk clients, (2) if atelectasis develops: oxygen, respiratory therapy, and bronchoscopy.
- Nursing management involves: identifying patients at risk; frequent position changes; deep breathing and coughing exercises; monitoring the progression; maintaining activity as tolerated; notifying the physician if respiratory distress occurs.

(For more information, see p. 1133 of Black and Matassarin-Jacobs: *Medical-Surgical Nursing: Clinical Management for Continuity of Care,* 5th ed.)

Atrophic (Senile) Vaginitis

- Atrophic vaginitis refers to thinning and atrophy of the vaginal mucosa that occurs in postmenopausal women. Vaginal secretions become more watery and alkaline.
- The vaginal mucosa is susceptible to infection due to the changes that occur.
- Clinical manifestations include: discharge that may be blood-flecked, a burning sensation, itching of the vagina and vulva, and dyspareunia.
- Treatment is short-term use of estrogen creams and antibiotic therapy if needed.

(For more information, see p. 2414 of Black and Matassarin-Jacobs: *Medical-Surgical Nursing: Clinical Management for Continuity of Care,* 5th ed.)

B

Balance Disorders

OVERVIEW

- Disorders of balance and coordination result from problems of the vestibular system and righting reflexes. Over 90 million Americans have experienced vertigo or a balance problem.
- Vertigo results from an imbalance of neural signals from the vestibular system in the ears.
- Dizziness is the feeling of disorientation in space.
- Causes of balance problems associated with vertigo and dizziness:
  - viral labyrinthitis—infection or inflammation of the cochlear and/or vestibular part of the ear, which affects hearing and balance. Balance usually is recovered within 1–2 weeks.
  - benign paroxysmal positional vertigo (BPPV)—short bursts of vertigo precipitated by quick head movement or sudden changes in position; no associated hearing loss.
  - presbyastasis—a balance disorder of aging.
  - Meniere's disease—recurring episodic, incapacitating bouts of vertigo, hearing loss, and tinnitus. It is thought that this disorder occurs from an abnormality in the formation or absorption of endolymph.
  - acoustic neuroma—tumor of the eighth cranial nerve. The client may experience tinnitis, hearing loss, and dizziness.
  - transient ischemic attack (TIA)—can also cause dizziness.
  - physiologic vertigo—disorders of motion sickness, space, and height.
  - orthostatic hypotension—low blood pressure on sitting or standing that leads to dizziness.

CLINICAL MANIFESTATIONS

- spinning vertigo

- sensation of falling
- imbalance
- staggering
- lightheadedness
- veering in one direction while walking
- faintness
- clumsiness
- feeling of floating
- nausea, vomiting

ACUTE AND SUBACUTE CARE

Medical Management

- vasodilators for chronic vertigo
- antivertigo agents
- antibiotics, steroids, diuretics, tranquilizers, and vitamins for specific disorders
- vestibular rehabilitation—head and total body exercises performed by the client to compensate for the disorder
- low sodium diet, diuretics, and balance exercises for Meniere's disease

Surgical Management

- endolymphatic sac procedures involving decompression and various forms of shunts to the central nervous system or mastoid cavity
- labyrinthectomy—removal of the membranous labyrinth
- vestibular nerve resection

Nursing Management

- Discuss ways to prevent injury when dizzy.
- Provide desired foods and fluids and small frequent meals if nausea and vomiting are present.
- Assist with ambulation.
- Discuss nature of disorder and planned tests.
- Encourage and assist with vestibular rehabilitation.

COMMUNITY AND SELF-CARE

Clients with vertigo usually are managed as outpatients.

(For more information, see pp. 1010–1016 of Black and Matassarin-Jacobs: *Medical-Surgical Nursing: Clinical Management for Continuity of Care,* 5th ed.)

Bell's Palsy

OVERVIEW

- Bell's palsy (facial paralysis) affects the motor aspects of the facial nerve, the seventh cranial nerve.
- Bell's palsy is the most common type of peripheral facial paralysis.
- Bell's palsy is an acute, unilateral paralysis of the facial muscles of expression with no evidence of a pathologic cause. Most clients recover from Bell's palsy within a few weeks without residual symptoms.
- Bell's palsy affects both women and men in all age groups. It is most common between the ages of 20 and 40 years.

CLINICAL MANIFESTATIONS

- upward movement of the eyeball on closing the eye (Bell's phenomenon)
- drooping of the mouth
- slight lag in closing the eye
- difficulty eating

ACUTE AND SUBACUTE CARE

Medical Management

No known cure—symptoms are treated with:
- analgesics
- corticosteroids to decrease nerve tissue edema
- physiotherapy—moist heat, gentle massage
- corneal protection—artificial tears, eye patch at night, sunglasses, etc.

Nursing Management

- Administer medications and assess effectiveness.

- Apply moist heat PRN to affected area of the face.
- Provide measures to protect cornea—patch, artificial tears, etc.

(For more information, see pp. 930–931 of Black and Matassarin-Jacobs: *Medical-Surgical Nursing: Clinical Management for Continuity of Care,* 5th ed.)

Benign Prostatic Hyperplasia

OVERVIEW

- Benign prostatic enlargement is an abnormal increase in the number of normal cells (hyperplasia) in the prostate rather than an increase in cell size (hypertrophy).
- Benign prostatic hyperplasia (BPH) is one of the most common disorders affecting men. The periurethral glands undergo hyperplasia and compress surrounding normal prostatic tissue, pushing it toward the gland periphery.
- Potential complications of prostatic enlargement include: (1) impeded urinary outflow and (2) urinary reflux because of decompensation of the uretero-vesical junction.
- By age 50, it is estimated that 50 per cent of men have some degree of benign prostatic hypertrophy (BPH); the incidence increases to more than 90 per cent in men over age 80.
- Aging is the major risk factor for the development of BPH, so few primary preventions exist.

CLINICAL MANIFESTATIONS

- frequent urination
- reduction in size and force of urinary stream
- hesitancy
- hematuria
- straining with urination
- urinary retention

ACUTE AND SUBACUTE CARE

Medical Management

- conservative interventions to treat symptoms—advise client to:
  - — void whenever the urge is present
  - — avoid taking large amounts of fluid over a short time
  - — avoid alcohol because of its diuretic effect
- antibiotic therapy for prostatitis, which may be associated with BPH
- pharmacologic agents:
  - — testosterone-ablating agents—decrease amount of circulating testosterone, leading to suppression of prostatic tissue growth—diethylstilbestrol (DES), flutamide (Eulexin)
  - — alpha-adrenergic blocking agents—block alpha receptors, improving urination by decreasing outlet obstruction—prozasin (Minipress), phenoxybenzamine (Dibenzylene)

Surgical Management

- Enlarged prostate tissue may be removed by various approaches, depending upon the size of the prostate and general health of the client. The term *prostatectomy* is really a misnomer. The procedure is actually an adenectomy of new tissue growth, and the true prostate and fibrous capsule are not removed. They include:
  - — transurethral resection of the prostate (TURP)—most widely used. Suitable for men with relatively small prostatic enlargement or who are poor surgical risks. TURP is performed by inserting a resectoscope through the urethra.
  - — suprapubic prostatectomy—approach made through lower abdominal incision into the bladder
  - — retropubic prostatectomy—lower abdominal incision approaching the prostate without entering the bladder
- Other newer surgical procedures:
  - — balloon dilation of the prostate
  - — microwave hyperthermia of the prostate
  - — transurethral laser incision

— insertion of prostatic stents

Nursing Management

Medical

- Monitor intake and output.
- Palpate bladder post-voiding to assess for urinary retention.
- Maintain a fluid intake of 2500–3000 ml/day unless otherwise contraindicated.

Surgical

In addition to routine postoperative care:

- Assess wound drains, wound packing, and catheter drainage for excessive bleeding.
- Avoid overdistention of the bladder because it can precipitate secondary hemorrhage—keep catheter from kinking or obstructing secondary to clot formation, mucous plug, sediment, etc.
- Maintain indwelling catheter (urethral or suprapubic) system:
  - — monitor continuous bladder irrigation (CBI) (closed irrigation permits constant or intermittent irrigation without breaking aseptic technique)
  - — frequently assess catheter patency
  - — maintain clear, slightly pink outflow
- Strict intake and output.
- Administer PRN antispasmodics to control bladder spasms.
- Administer stool softeners to prevent straining at stool, which could precipitate bleeding.
- Observe for local or systemic indications of infection.
- Assess for urinary retention (inability to pass urine and bladder overdistention) and urethral stricture (small urinary stream and dysuria) after urinary catheter removal.
- Monitor electrolytes and renal function tests.
- Encourage fluids.

COMMUNITY AND SELF-CARE

Instruct the client regarding:

- driving, activity, and weight-lifting restrictions

- need to avoid straining during defecation—use of stool softeners, juice, etc.
- perineal exercises to help client regain urinary sphincter control
- when to seek medical attention:
  - — bleeding
  - — signs of infection
  - — symptoms of obstructed urine flow
- need to maintain high fluid intake (2000-3000 ml/day)
- catheter care, if discharged with catheter in place

(For more information, see pp. 2350–2365 of Black and Matassarin-Jacobs: *Medical-Surgical Nursing: Clinical Management for Continuity of Care,* 5th ed.)

Biologic Response Modifiers

OVERVIEW

- Biologic response modifiers (BRMs) are agents that aim to boost immune system function or to attack tumor cells directly.
- BRMs are classified according to their mechanism of action, either to (1) restore, augment, or modulate the host's normal immune function, (2) have direct antitumor effects, (3) interfere with the tumor's ability to metastasize or promote cell differentiation.
- The classifications of BRMs include:
  - — interleukins—promote normal hematopoiesis; augment T-cell activities
  - — interferons—antiviral, immunomodulatory, and antiproliferative properties
  - — monoclonal antibodies
    - used diagnostically to identify surface markers on tumor cells or deliver radioisotopes to tumor site to aid tumor visualization
    - used therapeutically to deliver immunotoxins, such as chemotherapy, directly to tumor site
  - — colony-stimulating factors—naturally occurring growth factors that mediate hematopoiesis

- G-CSF (granulocyte colony-stimulating factor) or GM-CSF (granulocyte macrophage colony-stimulating factor) are being used for myeloid reconstitution after autologous BMT, in clients experiencing delayed bone marrow engraftment, and in chemotherapy-induced neutropenia
— erythropoietin—mediates red blood cell production

ACUTE AND SUBACUTE CARE

Nursing Management

- Administer ordered BRM therapy according to hospital protocol.
- Monitor for potential side effects:
  — interleukins
    - hypotension, pulmonary edema, and weight gain due to increased capillary permeability
    - generalized rash and pruritus
  — interferons
    - flu-like syndrome
  — monoclonal antibodies—to date clinical trials have shown limited success as a therapeutic option
  — colony-stimulating factors
    - bone pain in pelvis, sternum and long bones
    - skin rash
    - flu-like symptoms
  — erythropoietin
    - flu-like symptoms
    - hypertension
- Monitor laboratory findings—CBC, platelet count.

COMMUNITY AND SELF-CARE

- Instruct client regarding:
  — disease process and treatment regime
  — signs/symptoms to report to physician
  — care of venous access device
  — importance of follow-up clinic and laboratory appointments
- Refer to available community resources.

(For more information, see pp. 585–587 of Black and Matassarin-Jacobs: *Medical-Surgical Nursing: Clinical Management for Continuity of Care,* 5th ed.)

Bladder Neoplasms (Cancer)

OVERVIEW

- Bladder cancer occurs most frequently in the fifth to seventh decades of life. It occurs in men two to three times more often than in women.
- Common sites for metastasis include liver, bone, and lungs.
- Risk factors include:
  — cigarette smoking
  — industrial exposure to certain substances, such as aniline dyes, aromatic amines, and leather finishings. Processing petroleum products and industrial exposure to metal machinery also increase risk.
  — pelvic radiation
  — use of cyclophosphamide
  — chronic cystitis
  — bladder calculus disease
  — large phenacetin intake

CLINICAL MANIFESTATIONS

- painless, intermittent hematuria (early sign)
- bladder irritability, dysuria, frequency, gross hematuria, and obstruction

ACUTE AND SUBACUTE CARE

Medical Management

To determine the depth of penetration into the bladder wall and the degree of metastasis, staging is done before selection of treatment.

- intravesical installation of an alkylating chemotherapeutic agent, such as thiotepa, mitomycin, doxorubicin, or cyclophosphamide
- bacille Calmette-Guérin (BCG) as an intravesical agent, especially for carcinoma in situ and stage A tumors

- intracavity radiation—involves radiation to the bladder malignancy while adjacent tissues are protected—radium seeds are inserted through a cystoscope or through a suprapubic opening in the bladder and placed directly in the tumor
- external supervoltage radiation in combination with surgery or chemotherapy
- systemic chemotherapy with cisplatin, doxorubicin, methotrexate, cyclophosphamide, or pyridoxine

Surgical Management

- transurethral resection of the tumor and fulguration (destruction of tissue by electrical current through electrodes placed in direct contact with the growth)—for very early superficial tumors or for palliation of inoperable tumors
- segmental or partial cystectomy (removal of up to one-half the bladder). Over several months the bladder tissue regenerates, increasing its capacity to 200–400 ml.
- total or radical cystectomy with urinary diversion for advanced potentially curable disease:
  - total cystectomy involves removal of the bladder and urethra in women and the bladder, urethra, prostate, and seminal vesicles in men
  - radical cystectomy includes the above plus dissection of the pelvic lymph nodes and possibly the uterus, fallopian tubes, and ovaries in women
- permanent urinary diversion is necessary after total or radical cystectomy:
  - cutaneous ureterostomy—the ureter is brought to the surface of the abdomen where urine flows into a drainage appliance.
  - nephrostomy (temporary or permanent)—insertion of catheters into the renal pelvis by surgical incision or a percutaneous puncture procedure. The catheters are attached to an external drainage system.
  - ileal conduit (also called ureteroileostomy or Bricker's procedure)—the most common urinary diversion. A segment of the intestine is used as a conduit with the proximal end being closed and the distal end being brought out

through a hole in the abdominal wall. It is sutured to the skin to form a stoma. The ureters are implanted into the ileal segment and urine flows by peristalsis out through the stoma into an appliance the client wears.

— Kock pouch (continent internal ileal reservoir)—a reservoir made from a segment of ileum. Ureters are implanted into the side of the reservoir. A nipple valve is used to attach the reservoir to the skin. The client uses a catheter to drain the pouch rather than wearing a permanent drainage bag.

— Indiana pouch—a new procedure, similar to the Kock pouch, but a larger reservoir is created from the ascending colon and terminal ileum. Clients use a catheter to drain the pouch every 4-6 hours.

Nursing Management

Medical

- Radiation therapy
  - — Administer antispasmodics as prescribed.
  - — Encourage fluid intake.
  - — Administer urinary tract antiseptics for cystitis as prescribed.
  - — For patients with proctitis, instruct on low-residue diet and administer agents to decrease intestinal motility.
  - — See also, "Radiation Therapy," p. 605.
- Chemotherapy
  - — See "Chemotherapy," p. 149.

Surgical

- TUR

In addition to routine postoperative care:
  - — Maintain urethral catheter and bladder irrigation as appropriate.
  - — See "Benign Prostatic Hyperplasia," p. 76.
- Segmental/partial cystectomy

In addition to routine postoperative care:
  - — Maintain continuous urinary drainage from the urethral and suprapubic catheters to prevent any strain on the suture line due to bladder distention.

- Instruct the client on care of the suprapubic catheter (it is usually left in place for 2 weeks).

- Kock or Indiana pouch

In addition to routine postoperative care:

- Maintain Medena tube to continuously drain the urine (catheter will be removed 3-4 weeks after surgery).
- Irrigate the catheter with normal saline as needed.
- Instruct the client on the self-catheterization procedure (will be done after the Medena catheter is removed).

- Urinary diversion
  - Preoperative care

    In addition to routine preoperative care:
    - Instruct that diversion results in elimination of urine through the skin or stoma and not through the urethral meatus.
    - Instruct on/perform bowel preparation: low-residue diet; bowel cleansing with cathartics or enemas; sterilization of the bowel with neomycin.
    - Instruct on role of the enterostomal therapist.
    - Instruct on selection of the stoma site by enterostomal therapist.
    - Provide emotional support and allow to verbalize feelings concerning change in body image.
  - Postoperative care

    In addition to routine postoperative care:
    - Measure urine output every hour for the first 24 hours and then at least every 8 hours. Monitor for blocking of ureteral catheters (urine will contain mucous from the bowel).
    - Keep drainage tubing patent, if nephrostomy tubes were placed.
    - Assess stoma site every hour for the first 24 hours postoperatively. Note the stoma's size, shape, and color. An edematous stoma is expected in the immediate postoperative period. A dusky or cyanotic color of the stoma may indicate an insufficient blood supply or the onset of necrosis—this is an

emergency. Other complications may include prolapse or retraction into the skin.
  - Assess for signs/symptoms of peritonitis, bleeding, and urinary tract infection.
  - Maintain nasogastric tube to prevent paralytic ileus.
  - Assess skin integrity.
  - Ensure proper fit of appliance as stoma shrinks.

COMMUNITY AND SELF-CARE

- Instruct client regarding:
  - — suprapubic catheter or Medena tube, if present
  - — catheterization procedure for Kock or Indiana pouch once Medena tube is removed
  - — adequate fluid intake
  - — signs/symptoms to report to physician
  - — need for follow-up to ensure cancer has not recurred
- In males, refer to support groups as appropriate for impotence, which may develop after radical cystectomy.

Ileal Conduit/Urinary Diversion

- Instruct client regarding
  - — stoma skin care
  - — how to apply, remove, and empty the system appliance and attach it to the night drainage system
  - — control of odor
  - — need for fluid intake of 2000 ml/daily
  - — selection of clothing that will not constrict the pouch
  - — signs/symptoms to report to physician:
    - changes in color or quantity of urine output
    - cloudy or foul-smelling urine
    - stoma color changes
- Discuss concerns regarding work/leisure/sexual activity.

(For more information, see pp. 1582–1595 of Black and Matassarin-Jacobs: *Medical-Surgical Nursing: Clinical Management for Continuity of Care,* 5th ed.)

Bladder Trauma

OVERVIEW

- Bladder trauma is a blunt or penetrating injury to the bladder that may or may not cause bladder rupture.
- This injury may occur from a seat belt in an automobile accident; a fractured pelvis; bullet or knife wounds; or internal instruments, such as a catheter or cystoscope.

CLINICAL MANIFESTATIONS

- abdominal pain, which may be referred to the shoulder
- hematuria
- difficulty voiding

ACUTE AND SUBACUTE CARE

Medical Management

- placement of a Foley or suprapubic catheter unless blood is coming from the urethral meatus

Surgical Management

- repair of the bladder wall and drainage of extravasated urine in the perivesical space

Nursing Management

Medical

- Monitor intake and output.
- Monitor for hematuria.
- Report anuria to physician immediately.

Surgical

In addition to routine postoperative care:

- Maintain patent urinary drainage system to prevent tension on the sutures in the bladder.
- Change dressings around Penrose drain as needed.

COMMUNITY AND SELF-CARE

- Instruct client regarding:
  — care of suprapubic or indwelling catheter as appropriate
  — signs/symptoms of urinary tract infection.
- Assess need for follow-up by home health care agency.

(For more information, see pp. 1619–1620 of Black and Matassarin-Jacobs: *Medical-Surgical Nursing: Clinical Management for Continuity of Care,* 5th ed.)

Blepharoplasty

- Blepharoplasty is the surgical removal of excess tissue from the upper or lower eyelid. It may be cosmetic, or, if eyelid tissue is obstructing vision, reconstructive.
- Excess eyelid tissue may occur due to aging, heredity, allergic reaction, or as a result of cardiovascular or thyroid disease.
- Blepharoplasty usually is performed on a day-surgery basis with local or general anesthesia.
- Postoperatively, the nurse instructs the client to:
  — apply cold compresses to the eyes, usually for 24–48 hours after surgery
  — sleep supine with the head elevated for the first 48 hours
  — avoid bending over from the waist for 48 hours
  — avoid vigorous activity for 1 month
  — report changing vision or eye pain not relieved by prescribed analgesics to the surgeon
  — wear sunglasses, if desired, to cover initial bruising and swelling around the eyes

(For more information, see pp. 2272–2273 of Black and Matassarin-Jacobs: *Medical-Surgical Nursing: Clinical Management for Continuity of Care,* 5th ed.)

Blood Component Transfusion

OVERVIEW

- Blood component transfusion may be required for the following conditions:
  - — hematologic disorders
  - — hematologic diseases requiring aggressive ablative therapy
  - — chronic or acute blood loss
- Two alternatives to homologous (random) blood transfusion should be considered:
  (1) Autologous donation
  - — clients who do not have leukemia or bacteremia may donate their own blood before a scheduled surgical procedure
    - donations may be made every 3 days if the donor's hemoglobin remains at or above 11 g/dl
  - — intraoperative, postoperative or post-traumatic blood salvage
    - suctioning of blood from body cavities, joint spaces and other closed operative or trauma sites for reinfusion

  (2) Directed (designated) donation
  - — transfusion recipients designate their donors
- Irradiated blood components—clients with Hodgkin's or non-Hodgkin's lymphoma, acute leukemia or congenital immunodeficiency disorders and bone marrow transplant recipients may develop post-transfusion graft vs. host disease (GVHD) if lymphocytes containing cellular components engraft and divide. A small dose of radiation delivered to the unit renders the lymphocytes incapable of division.

ACUTE AND SUBACUTE CARE

Nursing Management

Pretransfusion

- Ensure that informed consent has been obtained (not required in all institutions).

- Obtain blood sample for type and crossmatch if central line is in place.
- Obtain venous access with large-bore cannula.
- Flush IV set-up with normal saline (no solution other than normal saline should be added to blood components).
- Obtain and record vital signs.
  - Fever may be a cause for delaying the transfusion—in addition to masking an acute transfusion reaction, fever can compromise the efficacy of platelet transfusions.
- Premedicate before transfusion as prescribed for the client who has a history of adverse reactions:
  - acetaminophen or diphenhydramine hydrochloride (Benadryl) to help prevent febrile reactions
  - steroids to avoid fever, rigors, and chills that accompany granulocyte transfusions
  - antihistamines for a history of allergic reactions

Beginning the Transfusion

- Confirm product compatibility and verify client identity.
- Inspect the unit for leaks, abnormal color, clots, excessive air and bubbles.
- Administer blood component through administration set as outlined in institutional policy.
  - A filter is used to trap fibrin, clots, and other debris that accumulate during blood storage.
  - Blood warmers may be used to prevent hypothermia, which can be induced by rapid infusion of large volumes of refrigerated blood.

During Transfusion

- Initiate transfusion at a rate to infuse 50 ml over 10–15 minutes.
  - The first 10–15 minutes of any transfusion are the most critical. If a major ABO incompatibility exists or a severe allergic reaction (such as anaphylaxis) occurs, it is usually evident within the first 50 ml of the transfusion.
- Increase flow to prescribed rate if no reaction is noted in the first 15 minutes.

- Instruct client to report anything unusual immediately.
- Obtain and record vital signs per institutional policy.
- Ensure the infusion is completed within 4 hours (to avoid septicemia).
- Monitor for signs/symptoms of a transfusion reaction:
  - — allergic reaction
    - urticaria
    - flushing
    - itching
    - no fever
  - — febrile, nonhemolytic reaction
    - sudden chills and fever
    - headache
    - flushing
    - anxiety
    - muscle pain
  - — acute hemolytic reaction (ABO incompatibility)
    - chills
    - fever
    - low back pain
    - flushing
    - tachycardia
    - hemoglobinuria
    - hypotension
    - shock
    - cardiac arrest
  - — anaphylactic reaction
    - anxiety
    - urticaria
    - wheezing
    - cyanosis
    - shock
  - — circulatory overload (due to pretransfusion cardiac status or too rapid infusion)
    - cough
    - dyspnea
    - pulmonary congestion
    - hypertension
    - tachycardia
    - distended neck veins
  - — septicemia (contaminated blood component)

- rapid onset of chills
  - high fever
  - vomiting
  - diarrhea
  - hypotension (marked)
  - shock
- Stop the transfusion and keep the line open with normal saline if a reaction is suspected (remove blood infusion tubing and infuse normal saline through separate infusion set).
- Follow institution's standard procedure for suspected blood reaction.
- Administer prescribed therapies if reaction occurs.

COMMUNITY AND SELF-CARE

Instruct client regarding:

- signs/symptoms of delayed transfusion reactions (3 days to several months following a transfusion):
  - — fever
  - — mild jaundice
- signs/symptoms of iron overload (may occur in clients receiving more than 100 units over a period of time):
  - — congestive heart failure (shortness of breath, ankle edema)
  - — palpitations
- signs/symptoms of post-transfusion graft-vs.-host disease:
  - — fever
  - — rash
  - — diarrhea
  - — signs/symptoms of hepatitis
- signs/symptoms of hepatitis:
  - — anorexia
  - — malaise
  - — nausea and vomiting
  - — dark urine
  - — jaundice

(For more information, see pp. 1518–1530 of Black and Matassarin-Jacobs: *Medical-Surgical Nursing: Clinical Management for Continuity of Care,* 5th ed.)

Bone Marrow Transplantation

Overview

- In the last 25 years, bone marrow transplantation (BMT) has progressed from a treatment of last resort to a viable therapeutic modality for a variety of hematologic, malignant, and nonmalignant disorders. BMT allows the client to receive lethal and potentially more effective doses of chemotherapy and radiation therapy without regard to hematopoietic toxicity. The damaged bone marrow is replaced by healthy marrow.
- Indications for bone marrow transplant include:
  — aplastic anemia
  — leukemia (certain types of acute and chronic)
  — lymphoma
  — multiple myeloma
  — neuroblastoma
  — selected solid tumors (breast cancer, poor-risk germ cell tumors, ovarian cancer)
  — thalassemia, sickle cell anemia

Bone Marrow Harvesting

- There are three classifications of bone marrow donors:
  (1) allogeneic:
    — obtained from a relative or unrelated donor having a close HLA type (HLA system antigens are a complex set of protein structures found on the surface membrane of all human nucleated cells, solid tissues, and circulating blood cells except red cells. This genetically inherited mixture of antigens is considered representative of the tissue type of each client.)
    — siblings have a one in four chance of having identical sets of HLA antigens and would provide the optimal match. Nonrelated clients have less than a 1 in 5000 chance of matching.
      - newer methods use the cord blood of a newborn

- has the highest rate of morbidity and mortality because of complications of incompatibility

(2) syngeneic:
- — donated by identical twin
- — perfect HLA match, eliminating the risk of rejection, but the risk of leukemic relapse is higher than when an allogeneic donor is used since graft vs. host disease (GVHD) is considered to have an antileukemic effect

(3) autologous:
- — removed from the intended recipient during a remission phase
- — eliminates risk of rejection, but relapse is frequent and may be due to contamination of harvested marrow cells by malignant cells or failure of pretransplant chemotherapy to completely eradicate tumor cells
- — used for solid tumors that include breast, ovarian, testicular, neuroblastoma, and lung (small and nonsmall cell) and hematologic malignancies such as Hodgkins's and non-Hodgkin's lymphoma, myeloma, and acute and chronic leukemia
- — another type of autologous BMT is peripheral blood stem cell transplant (PBSC).The peripheral stem cells are harvested by leukopheresis and stored. After the client receives lethal doses of chemotherapy and radiation therapy, the stem cells are reinfused.

Donor Preparation

- extensive work-up to insure compatibility and mental and physical well-being
- syngeneic and allogenic donors are required to donate autologous blood before the procedure because of the significant loss of red blood cells during the harvesting process

Marrow Collection

- general or spinal anesthesia is used
- marrow is obtained in 2–5 ml aliquots by aspirating from the marrow spaces of the posterior and, occasionally, anterior iliac crests and sternum

- numerous skin punctures are required; the aspiration needle is redirected to various marrow spaces without being withdrawn
- a total of 400–800 ml is obtained
- blood is placed in heparinized tissue culture media and filtered for removal of fat and bone particles
- marrow can be infused immediately or frozen

Recipient Preparation

- physical and psychological work-up
- central line placement
  - receives immunoablative therapy before transplant to: (1) destroy malignant cells, (2) inactivate the immune system, thereby reducing the risk of rejection, and (3) empty the marrow cavities to provide space for transfused stem cells
  - common protocols combine total body irradiation with high doses of chemotherapy

Bone Marrow Infusion

- marrow is usually infused 48–72 hours after the last dose of chemotherapy or radiation therapy
- marrow is infused from a large blood infusion bag through a standard blood filter
- potential immediate adverse reactions are allergic (urticaria, chills, fever), volume overload, and pulmonary complications secondary to fat emboli
- period immediately after transplant is critical as multisystem failure related to ablative therapy is common, as are immune reactions caused by transplanted cells
- delayed reaction—GVHD
  - may occur acutely 7–30 days after infusion
  - probable cause—T lymphocytes from donor attack and destroy vulnerable host cells
  - staged according to organ system affected:
    - Stage I
      - maculopapular rash
      - moderate manifestations of liver dysfunction
      - mild gastrointestinal symptoms

    - a majority of allogeneic transplants develop Stage I GVHD
  - Stage II to IV
    - increasing degrees of erythema and desquamation, hepatic coma, and diarrhea
    - prognosis and treatment depend on severity of syndrome
- — chronic GVHD
  - less acute symptoms
  - may occur even if the client has not experienced acute GVHD
  - appears approximately 100 days after transplant
  - may affect the liver, gastrointestinal system, oral mucosa, and skin

ACUTE AND SUBACUTE CARE

Nursing Management

Pretransplant

- Administer ablative chemotherapy as ordered. See "Chemotherapy," p. 149. See "Radiation Therapy," p. 605.
- Maintain protective isolation precautions.
- Assess for any signs/symptoms of infection.
- Monitor temperature.
- Monitor laboratory findings—CBC, platelet count, culture reports.
- Assess for any signs of bleeding and institute appropriate safety measures.
- Monitor vital signs for indication of altered tissue perfusion.
- Encourage well-balanced diet (no raw fruits or vegetables).
- Provide emotional support to client, family, and donor (if present).

Transplant

- Infuse marrow per hospital procedure.
- Monitor for immediate adverse reaction:
  - — allergic
  - — volume overload

— pulmonary complications (secondary to fat emboli)

Post-transplant

In allogeneic or syngeneic transplants, the pre-engraftment period lasts for 2–4 weeks, during which time the marrow cannot produce any cells. In autologous transplants, there is a period of 1–2 weeks of limited marrow development before engraftment occurs. During this time, the client is at high risk of bleeding and infection.

- Maintain protective isolation and bleeding precautions.
- Assess for signs of GVHD.
- Monitor laboratory findings—indication of successful engraftment is an increase in platelets and red blood cells in the peripheral blood count.
- Assess for any signs of bleeding or infection.

COMMUNITY AND SELF-CARE

- Instruct client regarding:
  - — treatment regime
  - — measures to prevent infection:
    - good personal hygiene
    - avoidance of crowds and people with infectious disease
    - need to wear a mask in public
    - no raw fruits or vegetables, no raw meat
  - — measures to prevent bleeding:
    - soft toothbrush
    - electric razor
    - care when doing yardwork
    - safety precautions
  - — signs/symptoms to report to physician
  - — signs/symptoms of GVHD
  - — importance of balancing activity and rest
  - — importance of a well-balanced diet
  - — central line care
  - — see "Chemotherapy," p. 149, and "Radiation Therapy," p. 605.
  - — importance of follow-up clinic and laboratory visits
- Refer to available community resources.

(For more information, see pp. 1495–1497 of Black and Matassarin-Jacobs: *Medical-Surgical Nursing: Clinical Management for Continuity of Care,* 5th ed.)

Bone Tumors, Metastatic

Overview

- Sketetal metastases are the most common form of malignant bone tumor, and virtually every malignant tumor can metastasize to bone.
- Metastases seem to develop from tumor seed cells that travel through the lymphatic system, blood vessels, and other surrounding tissues.
- Primary lesions of the prostate, the breasts, the kidney, the thyroid, and the lung most commonly metastasize to bone.
- The femur, the pelvis, the ribs, and the vertebrae are the most commonly affected bone sites.
- Pathologic fractures are common, especially in the acetabulum and proximal femur.

CLINICAL MANIFESTATIONS

- bone pain
- local swelling
- guarded or restricted movement
- fracture pain
- low-grade temperature
- elevated alkaline phosphatase
- elevated calcium and erythrocyte sedimentation rate (ESR)

ACUTE AND SUBACUTE CARE

Medical Management

- pain management
- radiation and chemotherapy followed by radical surgery

Surgical Management

- radical excision of the tumor

- fracture repair
- bone grafts after resection to fill defect

NURSING MANAGEMENT

Medical

- Administer analgesics as prescribed.
- Administer chemotherapy as prescribed and monitor/intervene for side effects. See "Chemotherapy," p. 149.
- See "Radiation Therapy," p. 605.
- Offer emotional support and facilitate referrals.

Surgical

Nursing management is dependent upon type of procedure performed.

In addition to routine postoperative care:

- Immobilize and elevate the limb.
- Administer PRN analgesics.
- Monitor for signs/symptoms of infection, DVT, and nonunion of the bone grafts.
- Consult Physical Therapy for assistive devices.
- Initiate progressive ambulation program.

COMMUNITY AND SELF-CARE

- Instruct client regarding:
  - — disease process and treatment regime
  - — management of chemotherapy and radiation therapy side effects (See "Chemotherapy," p. 149 and "Radiation Therapy," p. 605)
  - — use of PRN analgesics
  - — postoperative incision care and use of assistive devices
  - — cast care (if fracture repaired)
  - — progressive ambulation program
  - — signs/symptoms to report
  - — importance of follow-up visits
- Refer to available community resources.

(For more information, see pp. 2122–2123 of Black and Matassarin-Jacobs: *Medical-Surgical Nursing: Clinical Management for Continuity of Care*, 5th ed.)

Bone Tumors, Primary

OVERVIEW

- Primary bone tumors (originating in bone) may be benign or malignant.
- Benign tumors are characterized by their uniform density and well-defined margins.
- Malignant bone tumors are characterized by borders that extend into surrounding tissues.
- Types of primary bone tumors:
  - Chondrogenic tumors (from cartilage)—benign
    - Osteochondroma
      - most common benign tumor
      - about 10 per cent become sarcomas
      - femur and tibia are most common sites
    - Chondroma
      - frequently cause pathologic fractures
  - Osteogenic tumor (from bone)—benign
    - Osteoid osteoma
      - small lesion
      - occurs in the femur, tibia, wrist, or foot
      - often causes night pain
    - Osteoblastoma
      - grows more rapidly and is larger than osteoid osteoma
      - occurs in the vertebrae, femur, hands, and long bones
    - Giant cell tumor
      - aggressive and extensive lesion
      - occurs in the femur, tibia, radius, sacrum, and humerus
  - Malignant osteogenic osteosarcoma
    - most common primary malignant bone tumor
    - occurs in femur, tibia, humerus
  - Ewing's sarcoma - malignant
    - common in young adults
    - occurs in the pelvis and lower extremities
    - metastasizes quickly to the lungs and other bones
  - Chondosarcoma—malignant
    - occurs in pelvis, ribs, femur, and humerus
  - Fibrosarcoma—malignant

– rare tumor of the femur or tibia

Clinical Manifestations

- may be asymptomatic
- bone pain
- swelling
- fracture pain
- low-grade fever

ACUTE AND SUBACUTE CARE

Medical Management

- pain management
- chemotherapy
- radiation therapy

Surgical Management

- repair of fracture
- removal of tumor (usually involves bone grafting to fill the defect left after tumor removed)

Nursing Management

Medical

- Administer analgesics as ordered.
- See "Chemotherapy," p. 149 and "Radiation Therapy," p. 605.

Surgical

Postoperative care is dependent upon size and location of tumor.

In addition to routine postoperative care:

- Immobilize and elevate the limb.
- Administer PRN analgesics.
- Monitor for signs/symptoms of infection, DVT, and nonunion of the bone graft.
- Consult Physical Therapy for assistive devices.
- Initiate a progressive ambulation program.

COMMUNITY AND SELF-CARE

- Instruct client regarding:
  — use of PRN analgesics
  — care of the incision

— cast care (if fracture repaired)
— use of assistive devices
— progressive activity program
— signs/symptoms to report
— See "Chemotherapy," p. 149 and "Radiation Therapy," p. 605.

- Refer to available community resources.

(For more information, see pp. 2122–2123 of Black and Matassarin-Jacobs: *Medical-Surgical Nursing: Clinical Management for Continuity of Care,* 5th ed.)

Brain Abscess

OVERVIEW

- A brain abscess is a collection of either encapsulated or free pus within brain tissue arising from a primary focus elsewhere (e.g., ear, mastoid sinuses, nasal sinuses, heart, lungs, etc.). Brain abscesses may follow penetrating head trauma or intracranial surgery. *Staphylococcus* is the most common organism in trauma-related cases, whereas *Toxoplasma* is the usual agent found in clients with human immunodeficiency virus (HIV) infection.
- Brain abscesses vary in size. A large abscess may involve most of one cerebral hemisphere. Other abscesses may be microscopic.
- Brain abscesses are relatively rare. They may occur at any age, but are more common in persons under age 30. The current mortality rate is 5–15 per cent, depending on the location of the abscess and pre-existing condition.

CLINICAL MANIFESTATIONS

- drowsiness
- transient focal neurologic disorders (e.g., weakness on one side, loss of speech)
- depressed mental status
- headache and lethargy
- fever and chills

- focal or generalized seizures

ACUTE AND SUBACUTE CARE

Medical Management

- antibiotic therapy—penicillin
- corticosteroids

Surgical Management

- needle aspiration by guided CT imaging

Nursing Management

- Monitor temperature and initiate antipyretic measures.
- Administer antibiotics and steroids as ordered.
- Initiate appropriate safety measures.
- Monitor for signs of increasing ICP.

COMMUNITY AND SELF-CARE

Instruct the client regarding:

- disease process and treatment regime
- importance of completing medication regime
- signs/symptoms to report.
- importance of follow-up visits.

(For more information, see pp. 857–858 of Black and Matassarin-Jacobs: *Medical-Surgical Nursing: Clinical Management for Continuity of Care,* 5th ed.)

Breast Cancer

Overview

- One in every eight women is expected to develop breast cancer. Early detection and new treatment modalities have improved the 5-year survival rate. Breast cancer is the second leading cause of cancer deaths in women. Breast cancer in men is rare.
- Histopathologic types of breast cancer include:
  — intraductal carcinoma
    - a precancerous lesion

- axillary metastases are uncommon
- if untreated, will develop into infiltrating ductal carcinoma
- prognosis is excellent

— infiltrating ductal carcinoma
- found in 70–80 per cent of breast cancers
- palpated as stony, hard lump
- axillary metastases are common
- has the poorest prognosis

— medullary carcinoma
- 5–7 per cent of breast cancers
- often reaches a large size but prognosis is better than for many other types of breast cancer

— mucinous (colloid) carcinoma
- frequently occurs with other types of breast cancer
- good prognosis

— tubular carcinoma
- frequently occurs with other types of cancer
- axillary metastases are uncommon

— lobular carcinoma in situ
- a precancerous marker that indicates a higher risk for invasive breast cancer
- usually an incidental finding with removal of a benign breast lesion

— infiltrating lobular carcinoma
- found in 5–10 per cent of breast cancers
- presents as an area of ill-defined thickening
- axillary lymph node metastasis is frequently present

— inflammatory breast cancer
- characterized by skin redness and induration
- palpable axillary and supraclavicular nodes with distant metastasis
- poor prognosis

— Paget's disease
- 1-4 per cent of breast cancers
- crusting, scaling, burning, itching, or bleeding at the nipple

• Staging of breast cancer is based on the (1) size of the primary lesion, (2) extent of the cancer's spread to regional lymph nodes, and (3) presence or absence of metastases.

- Risk factors for development of breast cancer include (1) advancing age, (2) female gender, (3) mother or sister with history of breast cancer, (4) North America or Northern Europe as country of birth, (5) high socioeconomic status, (6) previous radiation to the chest, and (7) early menarche and late menopause, (8) first pregnancy after the age of 30, (9) genetic predisposition may be involved.

CLINICAL MANIFESTATIONS

- unilateral, single mass or thickening most often in a breast's upper outer quadrant
- mass is usually painless, nontender, hard, irregular in shape, and nonmobile
- nipple discharge, retraction, edema with *peaud 'orange* skin, and dimpling may be present

ACUTE AND SUBACUTE CARE

Medical Management

- radiation therapy
  - — to the breast and chest wall alone for women who are poor surgical candidates
  - — to the breast and chest wall after lumpectomy or quadrantectomy for local control
  - — to the chest wall if chest wall is involved, or after mastectomy with positive margins
  - — to the axilla in women at high risk for metastases or if disease was left behind following surgery
  - — to the supraclavicular areas for management of metastatic disease of the brain, bone, or skin
  - — interstitial implant therapy using iridium (^{192}Ir)
- adjuvant chemotherapy (given after surgical removal of any measurable cancer)—cyclophosphamide (Cytoxan), fluorouracil (CMF regimen), and methotrexate. Doxorubicin, thiotepa, paclitaxel, and vincristine are some of the other medications used for treatment.
- high-dose chemotherapy with autologous bone marrow transplantation
- neoadjuvant chemotherapy (given before surgical removal of breast lesion to shrink local disease

and reduce the risk of systemic spread)—methotrexate, 5-FU, cyclophosphamide, doxorubicin
- systemic therapy for metastatic breast cancer—cisplatin, cyclophosphamide, 5-FU, doxorubicin, methotrexate, mitomycin, paclitaxel, thiotepa, vinblastine, vincristine
- hormonal therapy (breast cancer with a high level of estrogen receptor-positive (ER+) or progesterone receptor-positive (PR+) cells may respond to hormonal therapy)—tamoxifen, estrogen, androgen, progestin, Aminoglutethimide

Surgical Management

- lumpectomy—removal of cancerous mass and some normal tissue for clean margins
- quadrantectomy—removal of the quadrant of the breast where tumor is located; a greater portion of normal tissue surrounding the cancer with some overlying skin and underlying muscular fascia is removed to provide a clean margin
- modified radical mastectomy—removal of the breast, axillary lymph nodes, and overlying skin—most commonly performed mastectomy
- axillary node dissection—removal of ipsilateral lymph nodes
  - dissection is not done to treat the disease but to stage the disease and determine the need for chemotherapy
- total (simple) mastectomy—resection of breast tissue and some skin from clavicle to costal margin and from midline to the latissimus dorsi
  - rarely used to treat diagnosed cancer, more frequently done to prevent breast cancer in women at high risk
  - axillary nodes are not removed
- standard radical mastectomy—removal of the breast, overlying skin, pectoral muscles, and axillary nodes
- extended radical mastectomy—removal of internal mammary nodes in addition to structures removed during a standard radical mastectomy
- surgical hormonal manipulation—removal of the ovaries (bilateral oophorectomy) in premenopausal women with advanced breast cancer

- breast reconstruction—option for postmastectomy clients, with use of tissue expanders, implants, or autografts of latissimus dorsi muscle, transverse rectus abdominal muscle, or gluteus maximus muscle. See "Breast Reconstruction (Post Mastectomy)," p. 109.

Nursing Management

Medical

- Administer chemotherapy or hormonal agents as prescribed and monitor side effects. See "Chemotherapy," p. 149.
- Monitor for side effects of radiation therapy. See "Radiation Therapy," p. 605.
- Provide emotional support to client and family.

Surgical (Modified Radical Mastectomy)

Preoperatively:

- Recognize that this is a very stressful time for the client and the need for support.
- Address concerns regarding knowledge, coping, self-concept, and sexuality.
- Make sure the client and family are fully informed about the treatment options.

Postoperatively:

In addition to routine postoperative care:

- Monitor incisional dressing and surgical drains.
- Monitor for lymphedema, infection, hematoma, and cellulitis.
- Elevate the arm on the affected side to promote drainage and prevent infection.
- Within the first 24 hours, perform hand and wrist movements with flexion and extension of the elbow.
- Encourage arm exercises as prescribed.
- Ensure that no blood pressure readings, injections, intravenous lines, or blood draws are done on the arm of the operative side.
- Encourage self-care activities (e.g., feeding, combing hair, washing face) and other activities that use the arm, with care taken not to abduct the arm or

raise the arm or elbow above shoulder height until the drains are removed.
- Begin teaching wound care at the first dressing change; prepare the client to look at the incision.
- Facilitate Reach for Recovery consult if authorized by physician.
- Begin progressive full range of motion of upper arm after drains are removed.
- Administer pain medication as needed to allow exercise without pain hindrance.
- Prepare client for adjuvant chemotherapy, radiation therapy, or hormonal therapy.
- Facilitate/provide counsel and support regarding the issues of body image change, self esteem, fear of death, coping strategies, and fear of metastases.

COMMUNITY AND SELF-CARE

- Instruct the client regarding:
  - — wound management
  - — surgical drain management
  - — arm exercises
  - — precautions after axillary lymph node dissection (the affected arm may swell and is less able to fight infection)
    - avoid any kind of trauma to the arm
    - avoid sunburn or insect bites
    - use an electric razor for underarm shaving
    - assess arm regularly for redness, soreness, pus, or other signs of infection
    - avoid strong detergents, harsh chemicals, and abrasive compounds
    - avoid injections, vaccinations, blood samples, and blood pressure measurements on the affected arm whenever possible
    - wear a medical alert identification that cautions no injections or blood pressure readings on affected arm
    - carry handbag and other heavy objects on the other arm
    - avoid elastic cuffs on blouses and nightgowns
    - elevate arm on pillow when lying or sitting
  - — possibility of phantom breast pain
  - — side effects of chemotherapy and radiation

- delayed grieving, which commonly occurs 2–3 months after mastectomy
- available temporary and permanent prosthetic devices
- monthly self breast examination.
- annual mammogram and breast examination by a physician after the age of 50
- importance of laboratory and clinic visit follow-up

- Refer to available community resources.

(For more information, see pp. 2431–2450 of Black and Matassarin-Jacobs: *Medical-Surgical Nursing: Clinical Management for Continuity of Care,* 5th ed.)

Breast Cancer, Metastatic

OVERVIEW

- Breast cancer metastases usually develop in one or more of the following sites: lymph nodes, skin, remaining breast tissue, bones, lung, pleura, peritoneum, liver, and central nervous system. Women with metastases to the liver or central nervous system have a poorer prognosis.
- Metastases have been known to occur up to 25 years after initial diagnosis of breast cancer.

CLINICAL MANIFESTATIONS

- dependent upon site of metastasis

ACUTE AND SUBACUTE CARE

Medical Management

- radiation therapy
- hormonal therapy
- chemotherapy
- autologous bone marrow transplant
- management of hypercalcemia (common complication of metastatic breast cancer due to bone involvement or hormonal therapy)
  - hydration

— diuretics
— mithramycin (calcium binder) or gallium citrate

Surgical Management

- dependent upon site of metastasis

Nursing Management

- Administer chemotherapy and hormonal therapy. Assess for side effects and institute appropriate interventions. See "Chemotherapy," p. 149.
- Assess for side effects of radiation therapy and institute interventions. See "Radiation Therapy," p. 605.
- Assess for signs of hypercalcemia (muscle weakness, increased heart rate and blood pressure, disorientation, anorexia, and abdominal cramping).
- Administer diuretics, fluid, and calcium binders and monitor response.
- Provide emotional support.

COMMUNITY AND SELF-CARE

Instruct the client regarding:

- chemotherapy, hormonal therapy, or radiation therapy regime
- signs/symptoms of hypercalcemia
- importance of follow-up laboratory and clinic visits

(For more information, see pp. 2450–2451 of Black and Matassarin-Jacobs: *Medical-Surgical Nursing: Clinical Management for Continuity of Care,* 5th ed.)

Breast Reconstruction (Post Mastectomy)

- Breast reconstruction may be performed immediately after mastectomy (during the same operation) or many years later.

- Several approaches are available:
  - — insertion of a tissue expander. A tissue expander is inserted under the chest tissues and expanded slowly via percutaneous fluid injection. Eventually the expander is removed and an implant inserted.
  - — rotation of the latissimus dorsi muscle and formation of a breast mound on the chest. An implant then is inserted.
  - — transrectus abdominal musculocutaneous (TRAM) flap—breast reconstruction using abdominal muscle and skin
  - — free flap—tissue is harvested from one area of the body to reconstruct the breast
- The nipple-areola area can be reconstructed by using tissue from the contralateral nipple, labial tissue, or a local flap from breast skin. A projectile nipple can be created from ear cartilage. An areola can be tattooed or grafted on the breast mound.
- In addition to routine postoperative nursing care:
  - — Assess the breast or flap area including color, temperature, and capillary refill.
  - — Assess the nipple-areolar area—report to physician any dusky, deep-red, purple, or black-edged color, as this indicates circulatory impairment.
  - — Monitor effect of analgesics—if epidural analgesia is used, assess the respiratory rate, presence of numbness or paralysis in lower extremities and degree of pain relief.
  - — Instruct the client that the implant will feel very firm and high initially. It will soften and drop with time.
  - — Discuss with client that psychosocial adjustment to breast reconstruction may not occur until 3–4 months after surgery.
  - — Reinforce that the reconstructed breast will not exactly match the opposite breast.

(For more information, see pp. 2284–2285 of Black and Matassarin-Jacobs: *Medical-Surgical Nursing: Clinical Management for Continuity of Care,* 5th ed.)

Bulimia Nervosa

Overview

- Bulimia nervosa is an eating disorder characterized by compulsive eating of large quantities of food followed by purging through vomiting or laxative use. It may overlap with anorexia nervosa. Clients binge after some psychological-emotional event, such as depression, anxiety, anger, or boredom.
- Weight is essentially maintained but may be less than average for the client's age and height.
- Bulimia is a common problem among young women during late adolescence and early adulthood.
- Clients generally have a history of poor family relationships with low self esteem and poor impulse control.

CLINICAL MANIFESTATIONS

- history of repeated binge-eating (rapid consumption of a large amount of food in 2 hours or less) followed by purging
- awareness of abnormality of eating patterns, with fear of being unable to stop eating
- depressed mood, self-deprecating thoughts following the eating binge
- inconspicuous eating
- frequent weight fluctuations of 10 pounds or more
- use of amphetamines, diuretics, laxatives, fasting, and excessive exercise to avoid gaining weight
- psychological symptoms:
  - — impaired impulse control
  - — fear of obesity
  - — low self esteem
  - — depression, gloom, suicidal thoughts, irritability, impaired concentration
- rectal bleeding (from laxative abuse)
- irritation of the throat and esophagus, swelling of the salivary glands, fluid and electrolyte imbalances, and erosion of tooth enamel from chronic vomiting

ACUTE AND SUBACUTE CARE

Medical Management

- psychotherapy and self-help groups
- aversion therapy
- family therapy
- pharmacotherapy (a monoamine oxidase inhibitor may be used to decrease the urge to binge)—serotonin blockers are also used

All interventions attempt to help the clients gain control of their eating habits and to change attitudes toward food, eating, body size, and self.

Nursing Management

- Instruct on healthy diet with correct portions.
- Encourage to eat slowly.
- Assist to develop a regular exercise pattern.
- Provide emotional support for stressful periods.
- Monitor weight.
- Monitor serum potassium and for signs/symptoms of hypokalemia.
- Assist to develop improved self esteem.
- Assist to find areas of self regard.
- Assist to find ways to deal with stress, boredom, and anxiety other than bingeing-purging.

COMMUNITY AND SELF-CARE

- Instruct client regarding:
  — reinforcement of diet/exercise as above
  — signs/symptoms to report to physician
- Refer to outpatient therapy program.

(For more information, see pp. 1759–1760 of Black and Matassarin-Jacobs: *Medical-Surgical Nursing: Clinical Management for Continuity of Care,* 5th ed.)

Burn Injury

OVERVIEW

- Burns are injuries that result from direct contact or exposure to any thermal, chemical, electrical, or radiation source.

(1) Thermal burns are caused by exposure to or contact with flames, hot liquids, steam, semi-solids (e.g., tar), or hot objects.
(2) Chemical burns are caused by tissue contact with strong acids, alkalis, or organic compounds. Tissue damage results from heat energy that is generated.
(3) Electrical burns are caused by heat that is generated by electrical energy as it passes through the body. Injury may result from contact with exposed or faulty electrical wiring or from being struck by lightning.
(4) Radiation burns are caused by exposure to radiation sources in industry or medicine. A sunburn also is considered a radiation injury.

- 1.4 million people in the United States suffer burn injuries each year; of these, 54,000 are hospitalized with severe injuries and 5,000 die each year.
- Seventy five per cent of all burn injuies result from the actions of the victim.
- Inhalation injury can result from exposure to smoke and asphyxiants. Clinical manifestations include: facial burns, erythema, swelling of the oropharynx or nasopharynx, singed nasal hairs, aggitation, anxiety, tachypnea, flaring nostrils, stridor, wheezing, dyspnea, hoarse voice, sooty sputum, and cough.
- Measures to prevent burn injuries in the home include:
  — turning pot handles toward the back of the stove
  — purchasing a stove with controls on the front or side to reduce the likelihood of clothing ignition as one reaches across the hot elements
  — placing a screen around any heating appliance as a barrier
  — setting the thermostat on water heaters to a temperature of 130° F. (54.5° C) or lower
- Measures to prevent residential fires include:
  — routine cleaning and checking of heating units and chimneys
  — treatment of wood-shingled roofs with a fire retardant coating
  — installation of residential sprinkler systems
  — presence of an operable smoke detector and fire extinguisher

— careful attention to the use of fuels for wood burning stoves

- Factors that determine the severity of the burn are:
  (1)burn depth
  — partial-thickness (first and second degree)—epithelium and into the dermis
  — full-thickness (third and fourth degree)—epidermis, dermis, and possibly subcutaneous tissue; produces eschar (devitalized tissue)—fourth degree may involve subcutaneous fat, fascia, muscle, or bone
  (2)burn size—determined by rule of nines (body divided into anatomic sections, each representing 9 per cent or a multiple of nine) or Lund and Browder method (modifies percentage according to age and is more accurate)
  (3)burn location
  (4)age
  (5)general health
  (6)mechanism of injury

ACUTE AND SUBACUTE CARE

Medical Management

Major Burns

Emergent Phase—begins at the time of injury and ends with restoration of capillary permeability (usually at 48–72 hours following injury).

With the exception of chemical burns, the burn wound should not take precedence over other life-threatening trauma or complications.

- ensurance of adequate airway, breathing, and circulation
- treatment of any associated trauma
- initiation of fluid resuscitation
- placement of an indwelling urinary catheter
- placement of a nasogastric tube
- vital signs
- pain management
- tetanus prophylaxis
- wound care
- psychological support

Acute Phase—begins when the client is hemodynamically stable, capillary permeability is restored and diuresis has begun (usually at 48–72 hours after the time of injury)

- control of infection
- wound care (e.g., hydrotherapy, debridement)
- specialized wound coverings
- autografting (surgical removal of a thin layer of the client's own unburned skin and application of it to the excised burn wound)
- nutritional support
- pain management
- physical therapy

Nursing Management

Emergent Phase (time of injury until 48–72 hours following injury)

- Assess for signs/symptoms of hypovolemia every hour for 36 hours.
- Monitor and document hourly intake and output.
- Daily weights.
- Administer intravenous fluid and electrolyte replacement as prescribed.
- Monitor serum electrolytes and hematocrit.
- Maintain nasogastric tube to low suction (ileus may occur with burn injury).
- Monitor amount, color, heme content, and pH of gastric output.
- Ensure patency of urinary catheter.
- Monitor urine color (urine is red or dark brown when hemachromagens are present due to deep burn or crushing injury).
- Send urine samples for urine myoglobin/hemoglobin levels per physician order.
- Assess for signs/symptoms of respiratory distress (secondary to carbon monoxide poisoning, smoke poisoning, or heat damage to the lungs).
- Monitor arterial blood gas and carboxyhemoglobin levels.
- Monitor SaO_2 levels continuously and oxygen as prescribed.
- Elevate head of bed.
- Assist with turning, coughing, deep breathing every 1–2 hours for 24 hours, then every 2–4 hours while awake.
- Instruct on use of incentive spirometer.

- Perform endo- or nasotracheal suctioning PRN.
- Monitor need for ventilatory support and endotracheal intubation.

Emergent and Acute Phase

- Prior to family's/significant other's initial visit, communicate extent of burn and changes in appearance.
- Explain basis of burn care, rationale, and interventions.
- Discuss fluid resuscitation, wound care, physical therapy, and nutritional needs.
- Maintain normothermia:
  — Monitor rectal or core temperature.
  — Limit the amount of body surface area exposed during wound care.
  — Limit hydrotherapy treatment sessions to 30 minutes or less with water temperature 98° to 102° F.
  — Maintain appropriate environmental temperature.
  — Use external sources of heat to maintain body temperature.
- Promote adequate tissue perfusion:
  — Remove all constricting jewelry and clothing.
  — Limit use of blood pressure cuffs on affected extremity.
  — Monitor strength of arterial pulses (by doppler if needed).
  — Assess capillary refill of unburned skin.
  — Elevate affected extremities above the level of the heart.
  — Assist with active range of motion exercises.
  — Anticipate and prepare client for escharotomy.
- Prevent gastric ulcer development:
  — Monitor gastric pH values and administer antacids as prescribed.
  — Administer antacids and/or hydrogen receptor antagonists as prescribed.
  — Hematest all stools and nasogastric drainage.
- Provide pain control:
  — Medicate prior to painful procedures.
  — Explore nonpharmacologic pain management techniques: relaxation techniques, music

therapy, guided imagery, distraction, and hypnosis.
  - Document response to pain management techniques.
- Prevent infection:
  - Administer tetanus prophylaxis as prescribed.
  - Instruct family on infection control measures.
  - Use strict, aseptic technique for all procedures.
  - Assess for and report any signs/symptoms of infection.
  - Debride wound of loose, nonviable tissue.
  - Shave or cut body hair in and around wound margins.
  - Administer systemic and/or topical antibiotics as prescribed.
- Provide adequate nutrition:
  - Consult dietician for assessment of caloric and protein needs.
  - Provide oral hygiene every shift and PRN.
  - Administer oral, enteral, and/or parenteral nutrition as prescribed.
  - If a feeding tube is in place, use twill tape tied around the head and above the ears to secure the tube. Ensure that it does not rub the ears.
  - For clients taking an oral diet:
    - Determine food/fluid preferences.
    - Schedule treatments to provide for uninterrupted mealtimes.
    - Allow rest periods before meals.
- Prevent impaired physical mobility:
  - Assess range of motion and muscle strength every day.
  - Maintain burned areas in functional position within limits imposed by associated injuries, grafting, etc.
  - Consult physical and occupational therapy for an individualized rehabilitation schedule.
  - If client is susceptible to neck contractures, sleeping with a pillow is contraindicated.
  - Encourage active range of motion every 2–4 hours unless contraindicated due to a recent grafting procedure.
  - Provide passive exercise and stretching if client is unable to participate.
  - Splints may be used for extremities.

- Provide emotional support and assist with coping strategies.
  — Be consistent with treatment schedule.
  — Arrange for client to talk with others who have had similar injuries.
  — Assess effective coping strategies used in the past.
  — Explore coping strategies.
  — Provide emotional support.
  — Facilitate consults with psychologist, psychiatrist, or social worker.
  — Encourage client/significant other attendance at support group meetings.

Acute and Rehabilitation Phases

- Promote independence in self care.
  — Assess ability to provide self care in grooming, bathing, eating ,and elimination.
  — Obtain consult to occupational therapy for assistive devices.
  — Encourage client participation in self-care tasks and provide positive reinforcement for efforts.
- Assist to accept changes in body image.
  — Explain and reinforce projected appearance of burns and grafts during the various phases.
  — Encourage realistic perceptions of changes in body image.
  — Allow to progress at own pace through stages of denial, grief, and acceptance of injury and recovery.
  — Provide encouragement by discussing progress made.
  — Assist with coping strategies and help prepare for social interactions after discharge.

COMMUNITY AND SELF-CARE

Care after discharge will vary greatly depending upon many factors. In general:

- Arrange for transfer to long-term care facility and ensure continuity of care.
- If client returns home, make home health care referrals as needed to assist with needed therapy, further teaching, and care requirements.

(For more information, see pp. 2233–2263 of Black and Matassarin-Jacobs: *Medical-Surgical Nursing: Clinical Management for Continuity of Care,* 5th ed.)

C

Candidiasis, Oral (Moniliasis, Thrush)

OVERVIEW

- Candidiasis is an overgrowth of the normal flora, candida albicans, in the oral cavity.
- It commonly is seen in clients who are immunosuppressed, such as those receiving chemotherapy or those infected with human immunodeficiency virus (HIV). There is also a higher incidence in clients who are pregnant, under stress, on high doses of prolonged antibiotics, on prolonged tube feedings, or who have diabetes mellitus.
- Major risk factors include immunosuppression and the prolonged use of antibiotics.

CLINICAL MANIFESTATIONS

- white patches on the tongue, palate, and buccal mucosa (often described as "milk curds")
- subjective complaints of lesions as dry and hot

ACUTE AND SUBACUTE CARE

Medical Management

- oral nystatin swish and swallow

Nursing Management

- Administer oral analgesics, topical agents, or swishes to relieve pain.
- Provide soft, pureed, or liquid bland diet. Avoid spicy, citrus, or hot foods.
- Provide solution of 1:1 warm water and hydrogen peroxide for oral rinses (avoid commercial mouthwashes because of their high alcohol content).
- Provide gauze pads or foam toothettes for oral care.
- Administer antifungals as prescribed.

- Administer oral antibiotics as prescribed to prevent secondary infection.

COMMUNITY AND SELF-CARE

Instruct client regarding:

- oral hygiene regimen
- diet
- medications
- signs/symptoms of complications and to report to physician

(For more information, see pp. 1725–1726 of Black and Matassarin-Jacobs: *Medical-Surgical Nursing: Clinical Management for Continuity of Care,* 5th ed.)

Carcinoma of the Gallbladder

OVERVIEW

- Cancer of the gallbladder accounts for only 5 per cent of all cancers.
- At least 70 per cent of these clients have gallstones.
- Of all clients who develop this malignancy, 91 per cent are over the age of 50 years and the incidence in women is four times that of men.
- The prognosis of gallbladder cancer is poor. About 88 per cent die within the first year, and only about 5 per cent are alive at 5 years.

CLINICAL MANIFESTATIONS

- unrelenting right upper quadrant pain
- weight loss
- jaundice
- right upper quadrant mass

ACUTE AND SUBACUTE CARE

Medical Management

Treatment modalities are widely debated and are generally palliative.

- chemotherapy
- radiation therapy

Surgical Management

- measures to relieve duct obstruction
- radical resection of the gallbladder—widely debated

Nursing Management

- See "Chemotherapy," p. 149.
- See "Radiation Therapy," p. 605.

COMMUNITY AND SELF-CARE

See references in Nursing Management as listed above.

(For more information, see pp. 1920–1921 of Black and Matassarin-Jacobs: *Medical-Surgical Nursing: Clinical Management for Continuity of Care,* 5th ed.)

Cardiac Surgery

OVERVIEW

- There are three types of cardiac surgery: reparative, reconstructive, and substitutional.
  - *Reparative surgeries* are likely to produce cure or prolonged improvement. These operations include closure of a patent ductus arteriosus; atrial septal defect and ventricular septal defect, repair of mitral stenosis; and simple repair of tetralogy of Fallot.
  - *Reconstructive procedures* are not always curative and reoperation may be needed. These procedures include coronary artery bypass graft and reconstruction of an incompetent mitral, tricuspid, or aortic valve.
  - *Substitutional surgeries* are not curative because of the preoperative condition of the client. Examples include valve replacement, cardiac transplant, ventricular replacement or assistance, and cardiac replacement by a mechanical device.

- Types of heart surgery
  (1) Valvular surgery:
    - valve commissurotomy (reconstruction)—performed if valve is still pliable. May include the use of a flexible ring that is sewn into the valve for stabilization.
    - balloon aortic valvuloplasty—use of a catheter with a balloon to dilate the valve orifice
    - valve replacement—mechanical and tissue prosthetic valves are currently available

  (2) Heart transplantation:
    - used in end-stage cardiac disease
    - orthotopic technique—retains a large portion of the right and left atrium in the recipient and implants the donor heart to the atria
    - heterotopic technique—donor heart is placed parallel to the recipient heart. The right side of the heart continues to function while the dysfunctional left side is bypassed.
    - 80 per cent of heart transplant patients survive 1 year, 75 per cent survive 3 years, and approximately 70 per cent survive 10 years.

  (3) Assisted circulation and mechanical hearts:
    - intra-aortic balloon counterpulsation (pump) IABP—increases coronary artery perfusion during diastole and reduces afterload
    - external centrifugal and roller pumps
    - external pulsatile ventricular assist devices
    - implantable left ventricular assist systems
    - orthotopic biventricular replacement prosthesis (artificial heart)

Many of these devices offer a bridge to transplantation when the client's heart is failing and a donor heart is not available.

ACUTE AND SUBACUTE CARE

Nursing Management

Postoperative Care

In addition to routine postoperative care:

- Monitor cardiovascular function and tissue perfusion by assessing vital signs, pulses, arterial blood pressures, venous and left heart filling pressures, and cardiac rhythm.

- Assess heart sounds for presence of pericardial rubs, murmurs, or gallops, indicating possible complications.
- Monitor ECG rhythm for heart block, ventricular tachycardia, and atrial fibrillation, which commonly complicate open heart surgery.
  - Temporary pacing wires often are implanted during surgery and can be connected to an external pacemaker should bradycardia or heart block occur.
- Assess respiratory status: rate, depth, effort, presence of rales or rhonchi, skin color, and sputum production.
  - Ventilator and supplemental oxygen adjustments are determined by physical assessment and arterial blood gas analysis.
  - Sedate as needed for maximal ventilator benefit.
  - Encourage to cough, deep breathe, and use incentive spirometer every 1-2 hours after extubation.
  - Suction PRN to maintain patent airway.
- Assess for presence of pain and medicate as needed.
- Measure and observe chest/mediastinal tube drainage.
- Assess incision, monitor drainage.
- Strict intake and output.
- Daily weights.
- Monitor laboratory values—electrolytes, hemoglobin, hematocrit, prothrombin time, and renal function.
- Assess neurologic response: level of consciousness, orientation, ability to move extremities, and pupil size and reaction.
- Administer anticoagulant therapy (valvular surgery).
- Administer antibiotics as ordered.
- Administer anti-rejection medications (cardiac transplantation).
- Monitor for cardiac tamponade: sudden cessation of chest drainage, dyspnea, paradoxical pulse greater than 10 mm Hg, distant heart sounds, distended neck veins, hypotension, narrowed pulse pressure.

- Initiate progressive activity schedule per cardiac rehab and monitor cardiopulmonary response.
- Monitor for signs of rejection (heart transplant)—decrease in oxygenation, fever, malaise, anxiety.

COMMUNITY AND SELF-CARE

- Instruct the client regarding:
  — medication regime
  — activity/rest schedule
  — weight-lifting restrictions
  — driving restrictions
  — dietary restrictions
  — need to monitor pulse daily for rate and regularity and when to call physician
  — how to assess response to exercise and activity
  — incision care
  — notification of physician for:
    - signs and symptoms of infection
    - palpitations, tachycardia, or irregular pulse
    - dizziness or increased fatigue
    - sudden weight gain or peripheral edema
    - shortness of breath
  — need for lifelong anticoagulant therapy following valve replacement
    - bleeding precautions
  — need for anti-rejection therapy (cardiac transplant)
  — importance of follow-up visits
- Refer to cardiac rehabilitation program.

(For more information, see pp. 1350–1363 of Black and Matassarin-Jacobs: *Medical-Surgical Nursing: Clinical Management for Continuity of Care,* 5th ed.)

Cardiac Tamponade

OVERVIEW

- Cardiac tamponade is a life-threatening complication. It exists when fluid or air accumulates in the pericardial sac. The fluid can be blood or pus that accumulates fast enough and in sufficient quantity to compress the heart and restrict blood flow in and out of the ventricles.

- Large or rapidly accumulating effusions raise the intrapericardial pressure to a point at which venous blood cannot flow into the heart, which decreases ventricular filling. As a result, venous pressure rises, and cardiac output and arterial blood pressure falls.

CLINICAL MANIFESTATIONS

- narrowing pulse pressure
- tachycardia
- hypotension
- jugular venous distention
- cyanosis of lips and nails
- dyspnea
- muffled heart sounds
- diaphoresis
- paradoxical pulse greater than 10 mm Hg
- feeling of impending doom

ACUTE AND SUBACUTE CARE

Medical Management

- pericardiocentesis—needle aspiration of fluid or air from the pericardial sac

(For more information, see pp. 1337–1338 of Black and Matassarin-Jacobs: *Medical-Surgical Nursing: Clinical Management for Continuity of Care,* 5th ed.)

Cardiomyopathy

OVERVIEW

- Cardiomyopathy is a heart muscle disorder of unknown etiology (idiopathic). The dominant feature is the involvement of the heart muscle itself.
- The three major classes are:

  (1) dilated cardiomyopathy

  — characterized by cardiac enlargement

— ventricular enlargement is followed by contractile dysfunction that eventually leads to heart failure
— many patients die within 5 years after the onset
— results in diffuse degeneration of myocardial fibers

(2)hypertrophic cardiomyopathy (also known as idiopathic hypertrophic subaortic stenosis [IHSS])—disproportionate thickening of the interventricular septum compared to the free wall of the ventricle
— the overgrowth of the wall leads to rigidity and increases resistance to blood flow from the left atrium and left ventricle
— appears to be a genetically transmitted disease of the heart muscle
— it appears most often in young adults, both men and women

(3)restrictive cardiomyopathy
— excessively rigid ventricular walls
— is the least common of the three cardiomyopathies
— the rigid walls impair filling during diastole; however, contractility with systole is usually normal. Eventually, cardiac failure and mild ventricular hypertrophy occur.
— any infiltrative process of the heart that results in thickening and fibrosis can cause restrictive pericarditis. The most frequently associated diseases are amyloidosis, hemochromatosis, and sarcoidosis.

- Four conditions lower the threshold for the development of cardiomyopathy
  — chronic alcohol ingestion
  — pregnancy
  — systemic hypertension
  — a variety of infections

CLINICAL MANIFESTATIONS

Symptoms usually develop gradually.

- Dilated cardiomyopathy
  — fatigue and weakness
  — chest pain

— blood pressure is usually normal or low
— symptoms of right-sided failure (dyspnea, orthopnea, tachycardia, peripheral edema)
— S_3, S_4, and murmurs

- Hypertrophic cardiomyopathy
  — sudden death may be first clinical manifestation
  — dyspnea, angina pectoris, fatigue, and syncope
  — dizzy spells
  — cardiac dysrhythmias
  — exertion tends to worsen symptoms
- Restrictive cardiomyopathy
  — exercise intolerance, fatigue
  — shortness of breath
  — neck vein distention, peripheral edema, and ascites

ACUTE AND SUBACUTE CARE

Medical Management

- Dilated cardiomyopathy
  — digitalis preparations, vasodilators, diuretics, and sodium-restricted diet
  — antiarrhythmic agents to suppress ventricular irritability
  — anticoagulants to prevent clots and emboli from pooled blood in the heart
  — prescribed rest and activity limitations
- Hypertrophic cardiomyopathy:
  — beta-adrenergic blocking agents to decrease myocardial contractility and heart rate (reduces myocardial workload)
  — calcium-channel blocking agents to improve activity tolerance
- Restrictive cardiomyopathy
  There are no specific interventions for restrictive cardiomyopathy. Interventions aim at decreasing congestive heart failure.
  — diuretics, vasodilators, and salt restriction

Surgical Management

- excision of a portion of the hypertrophied septum (myotomy or myectomy) in hypertrophic cardiomyopathy

- excision of fibrotic endocardium (restrictive cardiomyopathy)
- cardiac transplantation is becoming increasingly common surgery for dilated cardiomyopathy

NURSING MANAGEMENT

Medical

- Assess for signs/symptoms of increasing congestive heart failure.
- Maintain strict intake and output.
- Restrict fluids as ordered.
- Monitor BUN and creatinine.
- Daily weights.
- Monitor for signs/symptoms of decreasing cardiac output.
- Encourage adequate rest periods.
- Monitor pulses, respirations, color, and ECG during activity.

COMMUNITY AND SELF-CARE

Instruct client regarding:

- need to avoid strenuous physical exercise or competitive sports, as syncope or sudden death may follow exertion
- prophylactic antibiotics before and after dental or surgical procedures due to high risk of infective endocarditis
- need to abstain from alcohol, which depresses myocardial contractility
- importance of adequate rest
- avoidance of emotional stress that may exacerbate the symptoms
- importance of CPR instruction for household members
- need for follow-up clinic appointments

(For more information, see pp. 1338–1342 of Black and Matassarin-Jacobs: *Medical-Surgical Nursing: Clinical Management for Continuity of Care,* 5th ed.)

Carpal Tunnel Syndrome

OVERVIEW

- Carpal tunnel syndrome (CTS) is an entrapment neuropathy that occurs when the median nerve is compressed as it passes through the wrist along a pathway (carpal tunnel) to the hand.
- CTS may develop spontaneously or may result from disease or injury. The most commonly reported cause is repetitive motion of the wrist, with the wrist in constant flexion.
- A higher incidence of CTS is reported among:
  — homemakers
  — factory workers
  — cashiers
  — musicians
  — secretaries
  — computer operators

CLINICAL MANIFESTATIONS

- sensory and motor changes in the thumb, index, and middle fingers and radial aspect of the ring finger
- presence of Tinel's sign (tingling or shocklike pain elicited by light percussion over the median nerve)
- presence of Phalen's sign (hand tingling with acute wrist flexion)
- positive wrist compression test—paresthesias develop after manual application of pressure over the flexor retinaculum

ACUTE AND SUBACUTE CARE

Medical Management

- pain management
- wrist immobilization

Surgical Management

- decompression of median nerve by transecting the transverse carpal ligament

Nursing Management

Medical

- Administer analgesics.

Surgical

- Routine postoperative care.

COMMUNITY AND SELF-CARE

Instruct client regarding:

Medical

- use of a wrist splint
- pain management

Surgical

- use of PRN analgesics
- signs/symptoms to report
- use of a wrist splint
- weight lifting restrictions
- incisional care

(For more information, see pp. 927–928 of Black and Matassarin-Jacobs: *Medical-Surgical Nursing: Clinical Management for Continuity of Care,* 5th ed.)

Casts

OVERVIEW

- Casts are temporary devices of plaster or fiberglass that immobilize a body part, usually an extremity. Before the cast is applied, the skin is cleansed thoroughly and covered with stockinette, padding, or webroll.
- Casts are used for (1) immobilization, (2) prevention or correction of deformity, (3) maintenance, support, and protection to realign bone, and (4) promotion of healing, which allows early weight bearing.

- Types of casts include:
  - — arm or leg casts
  - — cast brace—consists of two parts, one above and one below the knee, with a hinge at the knee to allow range of motion (used for distal femur fractures)
  - — hip spica cast—extends from mid-trunk to one foot or both feet with hips abducted with an abductor bar; used to treat fractures of the hip and to immobilize the hip
- Windowing casts is the cutting of windows into a dried cast to allow visualization of certain areas, to assess a pulse, to remove drains, care for wounds, or to relieve pressure.
- Bivalving a cast means splitting it along both sides to (1) allow for tissue swelling, (2) allow removal of one-half of the cast to facilitate care and x-rays, (3) make a half-cast for use as an intermittent splint, and (4) to allow removal and reapplication while the client is learning to adjust to being without a cast.

ACUTE AND SUBACUTE CARE

Nursing Management

- Assess the following in the casted extremity: color, warmth, sensation, swelling, pulses distal to cast, and movement of distal fingers or toes.
- Promote the circulation of warm, dry air around the cast to speed the drying process.
- Cover noncasted areas to provide adequate warmth (the client may feel cold while the cast is drying).
- Instruct the client that there may be a sensation of heat under the cast during its early setting.
- Turn the client in a new cast periodically to expose more of the cast to air (unless contraindicated).
- If a hair dryer is used to hasten drying, do not hold it in one spot too long.
- Do not touch the cast without gloves until it is dry.
- Do not lay casted areas on drainage pads (such as blue pads) because the plastic will adhere to the cast.
- Place new plaster casts on pillows protected by plastic until they are dry.

- Monitor for signs/symptoms of complications:
  (1)Impaired blood flow
    — Assess for:
      - pulselessness, diminished capillary refill
      - skin pallor, prolonged blanching time, cyanosis, coolness
      - paresthesias, numbness

  (2)Nerve damage from pressure where a nerve passes over a bony prominence
      - increasing, persistent, localized pain
      - diminished sensitivity, numbness, motor weakness or paralysis not previously present

  (3)Infection, necrosis due to skin breakdown
      - musty, unpleasant odor
      - drainage
      - "hot spot" on cast
      - fever

  (4)Compartment syndrome (which compromises circulation, viability, and function of tissues within the compartment)
      - painful edema peripheral to the cast
      - paresthesias, numbness
      - loss of movement or sensation
      - pain with passive motion
      - pulselessness
      - skin pallor, blanching, cyanosis, or coolness

  (5)Cast syndrome—may occur with body casts; is caused by compression of the duodenum between the superior mesenteric artery anteriorly and the aorta and vertebral bodies posteriorly
      - prolonged nausea and vomiting
      - abdominal distention and pain
      - bloated feeling
- Assess the cast surface for wound drainage or bleeding. Assess for wet spots, which may indicate drainage beneath the cast.
- Prevent swelling by elevating the casted extremity above the level of the heart (especially in the first 24–48 hours), exercising fingers or toes, and placing ice bags around the cast.
- Ensure that the foot is supported in a 90-degree flexion angle to prevent foot drop if a leg is casted.

- Encourage the client to exercise joints above and below the cast to prevent complications of disuse (especially the shoulder if the arm is casted).
- Instruct client on isometric exercises for the casted extremity.
- Instruct on gluteal sitting, abdominal tightening, and deep breathing if client is confined to bed.
- Encourage dietary fiber and fluids to maintain normal elimination.

If the client is in a hip spica cast:

- Position the client carefully on a fracture bedpan for elimination.
- After elimination, wash and dry area thoroughly and keep the cast dry.
- Instruct client to avoid gas-forming foods to prevent abdominal distention.

COMMUNITY AND SELF-CARE

Instruct client/significant other regarding:

- skin care and how to prevent skin damage
- how to assess skin condition
- signs/symptoms of infection to report
- assessment and reporting of: swelling or discoloration of the extremity distal to the cast; areas of friction; skin irritation; and change in movement or sensation of the distal extremity
- avoidance of inserting anything under a cast to "scratch," as skin injury or damage to the padding can result
- reporting loose, cracked, molded, soft, or broken casts to physician
- follow-up with physical therapy
- when to return for cast removal

(For more information, see pp. 2146–2153 of Black and Matassarin-Jacobs: *Medical-Surgical Nursing: Clinical Management for Continuity of Care,* 5th ed.)

Cataracts

OVERVIEW

- A cataract is an opacity of the lens of the eye.
- The cumulative exposure to ultraviolet light over the lifespan is the single most important risk factor in the development of cataracts.
- Cataract formation is characterized by a reduction in oxygen uptake and an initial increase in water content followed by dehydration of the lens. Sodium and calcium contents are increased. The protein in the lens undergoes numerous changes, including yellowing.
- Some degree of cataract formation is to be expected in most people over age 70. Over one million cataract operations are performed annually in the United States.
- Types of cataracts:
  - — age-related (senile)
    - most common
    - onset usually around the age of 50
  - — related to other disorders, such as:
    - diabetes
    - tetany
    - Down's syndrome
    - myotonic dystrophy
    - retinitis
    - retinal detachment
    - blunt trauma
    - chronic corticosteroid use
    - exposure to infrared light

CLINICAL MANIFESTATIONS

- blurred vision
- monocular diplopia
- photophobia and glare
- ability to see better in low-lighted conditions when the pupil is dilated, which allows vision around a central opacity
- cloudy lens
- absence of pain

ACUTE AND SUBACUTE CARE

Medical Management

No measures can prevent or reduce cataract formation.

Surgical Management

Objective is to remove the opacified lens.

- cataract extraction—excision of the lens
- phasoemulsification—use of ultrasound vibrations to break up the lens into particles that are then removed by suction
- intraocular lens implementation—following cataract extraction, a new lens is inserted (or the client may be left without a lens and corrected by use of eyeglasses or contact lenses)

Nursing Management

Surgical

Preoperative

- Administer preoperative eye drops—tropicamide (Mydriacyl)—to dilate the pupil, and cycloplegic (Cyclogyl) to paralyze ciliary muscles.

Postoperative

In addition to routine postoperative care:

- Maintain eye patch in place.
- Monitor for signs of increased intraocular pressure (pain, nausea).
- Assist with ambulation and activities of daily living.
- Instruct not to lie on operative side.
- Instruct on measures to prevent increased intraocular pressure (see Focused Discharge Care).

COMMUNITY AND SELF-CARE

Instruct client regarding:

- measures to avoid increasing intraocular pressure:
  - — no lifting heavy objects
  - — no bending from the waist
  - — no straining with stool
  - — avoidance of coughing and vomiting
  - — no sleeping on the operative side

- eye care
- technique for instilling eye drops, antibiotics, and/or corticosteroids
- signs/symptoms of increased intraocular pressure (pain, decreased vision, nausea)
- signs/symptoms of infection (redness, swelling, drainage, blurred vision, or pain)
- need to wear eye protection (shield or glasses)
- importance of clinic follow-up visits

(For more information, see pp. 958–961 of Black and Matassarin-Jacobs: *Medical-Surgical Nursing: Clinical Management for Continuity of Care,* 5th ed.)

Cellulitis and Erysipelas

- Cellulitis is a suppurative inflammation of the dermis and subcutaneous tissues that spreads widely through tissue spaces. The skin is erythematous, edematous, tender, and sometimes nodular. The areas of inflammation are without sharp, indurated borders. Lymphangitis may occur. If untreated, gangrene, metastatic abscesses, and sepsis may result. Streptococcus pyogenes is the most common causative organism.
- Erysipelas is an acute, superficial, rapidly spreading inflammation of the dermis and lymphatics. The usual causative organism is beta-hemolytic streptococcus group A.
- With erysipelas, the organism enters tissue via a wound or abrasion. The skin is elevated, beginning with a small, bright red area. The involved area spreads peripherally to become a plaque with sharp, indurated borders. Lesions are common on the face and extremities.
- Clients at risk for cellulitis and erysipelas include the elderly and clients with lowered resistance due to diabetes, malnutrition, steroid therapy, or the presence of wounds or ulcers. There is a tendency for recurrence.

- Medical treatment is with oral or intravenous antibiotics that cover *Streptococcus* and *Staphylococcus Aureus.*

ACUTE AND SUBACUTE CARE

Nursing Management

- Monitor client's temperature and administer antipyretics as prescribed.
- Provide warm soaks as prescribed.
- Monitor for and report signs/symptoms of sepsis: high fever, tachycardia, confusion, or hypotension.
- Instruct client on careful handwashing and careful disposal of linen, clothing, and dressings to prevent spread of infection.
- Monitor infected areas for signs/symptoms of worsening infection, such as increasing redness or increasing edema.

(For more information, see pp. 2222–2223 of Black and Matassarin-Jacobs: *Medical-Surgical Nursing: Clinical Management for Continuity of Care,* 5th ed.)

Cerebrovascular Accident (CVA)

OVERVIEW

- A cerebrovascular accident (CVA) or stroke is a term used to describe neurologic changes brought on by an interruption in blood supply to the brain (ischemia).
- The two major causes of ischemia are:
  (1) Occlusion
    — thrombosis—this is the most common cause and is usually due to atherosclerosis
    — embolism—a cerebral vessel is occluded by emboli (fragments of clotted blood, tumor, fat, bacteria or air)
  (2) Hemorrhage

— intracerebral hemorrhage—rupture of a cerebral vessel that causes bleeding into the brain tissue. Intracerebral hemorrhage is most often secondary to hypertension. These hemorrhages produce extensive residual functional loss and have the slowest recovery time.

- Other causes include;
  — cerebral arterial spasm—usually due to some irritation of the outer part of the arterial wall, it reduces blood flow to the area of brain supplied by the vessel.
  — compression of cerebral vessels due to tumor, large blood clot, or swollen brain tissue.
  — aneurysm rupture
- The brain is very sensitive to loss of blood supply. Unlike other body tissues, the brain cannot resort to anaerobic metabolism in the absence of oxygen and glucose. The brain is perfused at the expense of other less vital organs. Short-term ischemia leads to temporary or transient ischemic attacks (TIAs). Long-term ischemia leads to permanent infarction (death) of cerebral cells. The extent of the infarction depends on the location and size of the occluded vessel, and the adequacy of collateral circulation.
- Cerebrovascular disorders are the third most common cause of death in the United States, preceded only by heart disease and cancer. Approximately 3 million Americans are living with varying degrees of disability from stroke.
- Risk factors related to stroke are:
  — prior ischemic episodes
  — cardiac disease
  — diabetes mellitus
  — atherosclerotic disease of intracranial and extracranial vessels
  — hypertension
  — polycythemia
  — hypercholesterolemia
  — smoking
  — oral contraceptive use
  — emotional stress
  — obesity

— family history of stroke
— age (incidence increases with age)

CLINICAL MANIFESTATIONS

Warning signs that may precede CVA:

Thrombolytic Stroke

- paresthesias involving one-half of the body
- transient hemiparesis
- transient loss of speech

These manifestations are called transient ischemic attacks (TIAs) and should not be ignored.

Cerebral Hemorrhage

- severe occipital or nuchal headaches
- vertigo (dizziness) or syncope (fainting)
- paresthesias
- transient paralysis
- epistaxis (nosebleed)
- retinal hemorrhage

Embolic Stroke

Unfortunately, there are no warning signs.

- General findings for all types:
  - vomiting
  - seizures
  - mental changes (including coma)
  - fever
  - ECG changes

Specific deficits that may occur after CVA:

Deficits depend upon the area of the brain damaged as well as the side of the brain, i.e., dominant vs. nondominant. Manifestations of deficit must persist longer than 24 hours to be diagnostic of a CVA.

- hemiplegia (paralysis) or hemiparesis (weakness) —on one side of the body. Complete hemiplegia involves one-half of the face and tongue as well as the arm and leg of the same side).
- aphasia—a defect in using and interpreting the symbols of language; it may involve any or all aspects of language use (reading, writing, speaking, or understanding spoken language). Aphasia

may be sensory or motor (usually is a combination of both).

— sensory aphasia (also called receptive aphasia)—loss of the ability to comprehend written, spoken, or printed words

— motor aphasia (also called expressive aphasia)—loss of the ability to write, make signs, or speak (i.e., words may be recalled, but the client cannot combine speech sounds into words and syllables)

- apraxia—a condition in which a client can move the affected part but cannot use it for specific purposeful actions (walking, speaking, or dressing)
- homonymous hemianopia—defective vision or visual loss in the same half of the visual field of each eye (i.e., the client may see clearly on one side of the midline, but nothing on the other side)
- agnosia—a disturbance in interpreting visual, tactile, or other sensory information. The client is unable to recognize objects.
- dysarthria—imperfect articulation that causes difficulty in speaking (client understands language, but has difficulty pronouncing and enunciating words)
- dysphagia—difficulty swallowing
- kinesthesia—alterations in sensation—may include:
  - paresthesia (feelings of numbness, tingling, heaviness)
  - hemianesthesia (loss of sensation)
  - loss of muscle-joint sense-proprioception (ability to perceive the relationship of body parts to the external environment)
- incontinence—bowel/bladder
- shoulder pain
- Horner's syndrome—paralysis of the sympathetic nerves to the eye, causing sinking of the eyeball, ptosis of the upper eyelid, lack of tearing in the eye, and slight elevation of the lower lid
- unilateral neglect—failure to attend to one side of the body, failure to report or respond to stimuli on one side of the body; or failure to use one extremity
- other problems with memory, spatial perception, and loss of direction

Emotional or Behavioral Reactions

- severe mood swings
- confusion
- forgetfulness
- depression
- social withdrawal
- inappropriate sexual behavior
- outbursts of frustration/anger
- regression to earlier behavior

ACUTE AND SUBACUTE CARE

Medical Management

- supportive care
- prevention of further emboli for embolic stroke
- management of increased intracranial pressure and hyperthermia with hemorrhagic stroke
- bedrest with head of the bed elevated 30 degrees (hemorrhagic stroke), or kept flat (ischemic stroke)
- external ventriculostomy drainage—may be used to reduce pressure from cerebrospinal fluid accumulation
- blood pressure management—prevent excessively high blood pressure but maintain adequate cerebral perfusion
- ventilatory support
- fluid volume management—avoidance of fluid volume excess
- tissue plasminogen activator (tPA) to dissolve the clot (once hemorrhage is ruled out)
- steroids or osmotic diuretics to reduce intracranial pressure
- antihypertensives and diuretics to control hypertension
- anticoagulants (for embolic or thrombotic stroke)
- mild analgesics (codeine and acetaminophen) to treat headache and neck stiffness, yet prevent sedation which would make neurologic assessment inaccurate
- antiplatelet therapy—inhibits platelet function, decreasing the risk of thrombus formation (aspirin, dipyridamole[Persantine], ticlopidine [Ticlid])
- phenytoin or phenobarbital, if the client develops seizures

Surgical Management

- rapid evacuation of the hematoma for select clients with hemorrhagic stroke
- intracranial aneurysm repair
- carotid endarterectomy to reduce the risk of CVA

Nursing Management

- Monitor intracranial pressure hourly, if intracranial pressure monitor is placed.
- Perform neurologic assessments hourly using the Glasgow Coma scale. Monitor for changes in level of consciousness and for signs/symptoms of increased intracranial pressure.
- Prevent any increases in intracranial pressure:
  - — Suction minimally.
  - — Keep head of the bed elevated.
  - — Prevent excessive coughing, straining with stool, vomiting, lifting, or use of arms to change position.
  - — Administer laxatives or stool softeners as ordered.
  - — Treat fever with antipyretics and cooling blanket (avoid inducing shivering).
  - — Avoid restraints, which may increase agitation.
- Initiate aspiration precautions.
- Monitor intake and output.
- Monitor lab values—PT/PTT, electrolytes, renal profile.
- Facilitate Physical/Occupational Therapy referrals.
- Change hemiplegic client's position every 2 hours (keep mainly on unaffected side).
- Avoid long periods of sitting (may contribute to hip flexion deformity).
- No pillows under the knee when client supine (contributes to flexion deformity and thrombus formation).
- Do not flex the upper thigh acutely when turning to side (contributes to hip flexion deformity).
- Position prone for 15–30 minutes several times daily with pillow under pelvis to hyperextend hip joints.
- Use footboard and high-top tennis shoes to prevent footdrop and heel cord shortening.

- Use trochanter roll (from crest of ilium to mid-thigh) to prevent external hip rotation.
- Prevent adduction of the affected shoulder by placing a pillow in the axilla between the upper arm and chest wall to keep the arm abducted 60 degrees.
- Place the hand in a splint or hand roll to prevent finger flexion and thumb adduction. The preferred position is slight supination with fingers slightly flexed and the thumb in opposition.
- Discuss exercises the client can do in bed (gluteal setting, quadriceps setting).
- Perform passive range of motion exercises four times daily and encourage active range of motion if client is able.
- Assist with progressive activity as prescribed (transferring to chair, wheelchair).
- Assist with progressive self-care activities (washing, eating, grooming), encouraging use of paralyzed limb and instructing client to avoid tendency to do everything with the unaffected limb.
- If eye is paralyzed, irrigate with physiologic saline, instill artificial tears, and cover with eye patch as ordered.
- Keep bed side-rails raised.
- Remind client to walk slowly, rest adequately between intervals of walking, and to look ahead while walking.
- Inspect skin for any injury or breakdown—provide protective devices as needed.
- Inspect oral mucosa for any injuries (especially affected side of tongue and mouth). Provide oral care three to four times daily.
- Assess total intake and facilitate referral to dietician as needed.
- Monitor hemoglobin, lymphocytes, and nutritional panel.
- Provide supplemental snacks or high calorie liquid supplements.
- Place patient in most upright position for meals.
- Assist with specific difficulties in feeding process as needed: mouth opening, mouth closing, sucking, tongue movement, swallowing, or inadequate salivation.

- Facilitate referral to speech therapy—reinforce lessons as appropriate.
- Repeat simple directions until they are understood.
- Do not shout—patient can hear.
- When a client cannot identify objects by name, give practice in receiving word images (point to an object and state its name).
- When a client has difficulty with verbal expression, give practice in repeating words after you.
- When talking to a client with receptive difficulty, stand within six feet and face the client directly.
- Assist family with communication techniques.
- Reorient the client and position a calendar and clock where the client can see them.
- If visual impairment is present, approach the side that is not visually impaired. Position needed items on that side.
- Minimize environmental stimuli if patient has perceptual defects.
- For clients with unilateral neglect, initially adapt environment by positioning items on unaffected side. Gradually move personal items, etc. to affected side. Encourage the client to groom the affected side first. Cue the client to scan the entire environment.
- Provide emotional support to the client and family and assist to identify coping strategies to deal with loss of function, powerlessness, self-esteem disturbance, and social isolation. Make referrals as necessary.
- Encourage attempts at independence and praise all successes.
- Assist to become as independent as possible in activities of daily living.
- Reinforce techniques taught by physical therapy/occupational therapy.

COMMUNITY AND SELF-CARE

- If client returns home:
  — Instruct client/significant other regarding:
    - disease process and treatment regime
    - ways to prevent recurrence: dietary modification, stress reduction, smoking cessation

- medication regime
- exercise program
- residual deficits and balancing realistic expectations while allowing maximal independence
- skin care
- providing a safe home environment
- equipment needed at home
- bleeding precautions if on anticoagulant therapy
- special methods of feeding or enteral feedings
- signs/symptoms to report

- Make home health care referrals as appropriate.
- Provide continuity of care and emotional support to client and family if client is placed in a nursing home or rehabilitation facility.

(For more information, see pp. 784–808 of Black and Matassarin-Jacobs: *Medical-Surgical Nursing: Clinical Management for Continuity of Care,* 5th ed.)

Cervical Cancer

OVERVIEW

- Cervical cancer is the second most fatal cancer of the reproductive system, although death rates have dropped 50 per cent over the last 20 years.
- The cause is unknown, but seems to have a strong relationship with chronic irritation and human papillomavirus (HPV).
- All women with carcinoma in situ potentially can be cured. Ninety per cent of women with nonmetastatic disease can be cured.
- The Pap smear is the primary diagnostic tool for cervical cancer.
- Spread occurs by direct extension to the vaginal mucosa, lower uterine segment, parametrium, pelvic wall, bladder, and bowel. Distant metastasis may be to the liver, lungs, or bone.

- Risk factors include:
  - — age 25–40 years (for carcinoma in situ)
  - — age 40–60 years (for invasive cancer)
  - — lower socioeconomic class
  - — prostitutes
  - — blacks, native Americans
  - — multiparity
  - — early age of and frequent intercourse with multiple partners
  - — early first pregnancy
  - — untreated, chronic cervicitis
  - — sexually transmitted disease
  - — women whose partners have a history of penile or prostate cancer
  - —infection with HPV

CLINICAL MANIFESTATIONS

There are no early indications of carcinoma in situ or early cervical cancer.

Late assessment findings include:

- vaginal discharge and bleeding
- metrorrhagia (uterine bleeding between normal menses)
- postmenopausal bleeding
- polymenorrhea (increased frequency of menstrual bleeding)

If metastasis is present:

- pressure on the bowel or bladder
- bladder irritation
- rectal discharge
- heavy, aching abdominal pain

ACUTE AND SUBACUTE CARE

Medical Management

- irradiation (usually curative but induces menopause)

Surgical Management

- cryosurgery for local stage 0 tumors (involves the local freezing of abnormal cells and tissues with volatile gases, such as nitrous oxide, Freon or carbon dioxide—the dead tissue sloughs off)

- conization for local stage 0 tumors (involves the removal of a small cone of tissue with a sharp instrument)
- total abdominal hysterectomy (removal of the uterus and cervix) for carcinoma in situ, if the client is finished with childbearing
- total abdominal hysterectomy with bilateral salpingo-oophorectomy (TAH-BSO)—removal of the uterus, cervix, fallopian tubes, and ovaries
- radical hysterectomy for invasive cancer (same as a TAH-BSO plus removal of the lymph nodes, upper one-third of the vagina, and parametrium)
- pelvic exenteration (removal of all pelvic organs including the uterus, fallopian tubes, ovaries, vagina, bladder, rectum, colon) for invasive cancer. An ileostomy or ileal conduit also are formed.

Nursing Management

Cryosurgery or Laser Therapy

- Discuss that the procedure is performed with a vaginal speculum in place, much like a routine pelvic examination.
- Discuss that headaches, dizziness, flushing, and some cramping may be felt during the procedure.
- Discuss use of slow deep breathing during the procedure and postoperatively.

For other nursing management:

- See "Uterine Tumors, Benign," p. 743, for care of the client after a hysterectomy.
- See "Radiation Therapy," p. 605, for care of the client with a radiation implant.
- See "Bladder Neoplasms (Cancer)," p. 81, for care of the client with an ileal conduit.
- See "Ulcerative Colitis," p. 725, for care of the client with an ileostomy.

COMMUNITY AND SELF-CARE

Instruct client regarding:

- need for regular Pap smears and pelvic examinations to detect for recurrence as directed by physician

Cryosurgery/Laser Therapy

- use of mild analgesics for pain that may continue for several days
- presence of clear, watery drainage initially, which will change into a discharge containing dead cells that may be malodorous
- reporting discharge lasting longer than 8 weeks to physician
- meticulous perineal hygiene
- use of showers or sponge baths, avoidance of tub or sitz baths

Irradiation

- need for vaginal penetration to minimize vaginal adhesions and stenosis (may be accomplished by client's own fingers, a vaginal dilator, or sexual partner's fingers or penis)
- need for vaginal lubrication

Post Hysterectomy

- See "Uterine Tumors, Benign," p. 743, for discharge teaching following hysterectomy
- If client had ovaries removed, see "Uterine Tumors, Benign," p. 743, for instructions on surgical menopause

Also see sections listed under "Nursing Management" for discharge care for other procedures.

(For more information, see pp. 2406–2409 of Black and Matassarin-Jacobs: *Medical-Surgical Nursing: Clinical Management for Continuity of Care,* 5th ed.)

Chemotherapy

OVERVIEW

- Chemotherapy is the administration of cytotoxic drugs to kill or suppress tumor activity. Chemotherapy is a systemic intervention and is appropriate when disease is widespread or when risk of undetectable disease is high.

- The objective of cancer chemotherapy is to destroy all malignant tumor cells without excessive destruction of normal cells.
- Cancer cells reproduce in the same manner as normal cells. However, growth occurs in an uncontrolled manner. In general, cells that are actively dividing are the most sensitive to chemotherapy. Chemotherapy directly or indirectly disrupts reproduction of cells by altering essential biochemical processes.
- Chemotherapy may be used as three types of treatment modalities:
  — primary treatment modality
    - chemotherapy is the only treatment used and leads to cure
  — adjuvant treatment modality—after initial treatment with either surgery or radiation therapy, chemotherapy is used to eliminate remaining cancer cells.
    - in conjunction with surgery
    - in conjunction with radiation therapy
  — palliative treatment modality—used to control tumor growth when cure is not possible
    - to relieve pain or obstruction
- The desired outcome of chemotherapy is control or eradication of all malignant cells. Most types of chemotherapy do not kill all cancer cells during one exposure. According to the cell kill hypothesis, only a percentage of cancer cells will be killed with each course of chemotherapy. Repeated doses, therefore, must be used.
- Combination chemotherapy has been consistently superior to single-agent therapy. When combined, medications destroy malignant cells more effectively and produce fewer side effects.
- Chemotherapeutic agents are classified according to pharmacologic action and effect on cell generation cycle.
- Chemotherapy administration routes:

Intravenous Routes

  — peripheral access
    - large veins in the forearm are the preferred sites

- areas of impaired lymphatic drainage, phlebitis, impaired venous circulation, joints and sites distal to a recent venipuncture site need to be avoided
- avoid veins on the dorsal aspect of the hand or over an area of flexion, such as a wrist or elbow

— vascular access devices (VADs)
- a catheter is inserted into one of the major veins of the upper chest and the distal tip advanced to the level of the superior vena cava at or above the junction of the right atrium
- types of vascular access devices:
  - tunneled (Hickman, Groshong)
  - totally implanted ports (Port-A-Cath)
  - peripherally inserted central catheters (PICC)

Intra-arterial Routes

— major organs or tumor sites receive maximal exposure to the chemotherapy with limited serum levels, resulting in decreased systemic side effects

— chemotherapy is administered into an artery of an involved organ (i.e., hepatic artery infusion for liver cancer)

Intrathecal Routes

— many systemic chemotherapy agents cannot cross the blood-brain barrier

— instillation of chemotherapy into the central nervous system through a reservoir placed in the ventricle of the brain (Ommaya reservoir) or via a lumbar puncture

Intracavitary Routes

— allows for higher concentration of chemotherapy to the tumor site with minimal exposure of healthy tissue

— instillation of chemotherapy directly into areas such as the abdomen, bladder, or pleural space

Topical

— application of creams or ointments to affected areas

- Antineoplastic agents are capable of damaging not only malignant cells but also certain normal cells. Normal cells most vulnerable are those that divide and proliferate rapidly, specifically cells of the bone marrow, hair, and mucosa. In addition, these agents may exert organ specific toxicities resulting in cardiac, renal, hepatic, reproductive, and neurologic dysfunction. Side effects may be acute or delayed.

Nursing Management

- Check complete blood count and platelet count results before administration of chemotherapy and periodically after drug administration.
- Administer premedications (antiemetics, sedatives) and hydration as prescribed.
- Administer chemotherapy according to institutional policy and safe handling guidelines.
- Monitor IV site for edema, redness, and presence of a blood return at frequency outlined in institutional policy before, during, and after infusion:
  - — institutional guidelines for management of extravasation should be readily available
- Take precautions to ensure client safety when administering antineoplastics with anaphylactic potential (L-asparaginase, cisplatin, bleomycin).
  - — review allergy history
  - — obtain baseline vital signs
  - — administer test dose as ordered
  - — stay with client the entire time the drug is administered
  - — have emergency drugs and equipment available
  - — establish a free-flowing IV line for administration of emergency drugs should the need arise
- Monitor for toxic effects of chemotherapy and implement appropriate intervention.

Gastrointestinal Effects

- nausea and vomiting
- anorexia
- stomatitis, esophagitis
- taste alterations
- diarrhea
- weight loss
- constipation

Management

- Administer PRN antiemetics.

- Monitor laboratory findings—nutritional panel, electrolytes.
- Monitor intake and output.
- Daily weights.
- Perform frequent oral care and apply moisturizers and topical anesthetics.
- Encourage frequent, small, high-calorie, high-protein meals.
- Maintain calorie count.
- Administer PRN anti-diarrheals.

INTEGUMENTARY EFFECTS

- skin reactions—depend on drug administered
  - red patches (erythema) or hives (urticaria) at the site or on other body parts
    - generally disappear within hours
  - hyperpigmentation—darkening of the skin in nailbeds, mouth, gums, and along the veins used for administration
    - occurs 2–3 weeks after administration and continues for 10–12 weeks
  - photosensitivity (sensitivity to sunlight)
    - disappears once chemotherapy is stopped
  - radiation recall—chemotherapy given several weeks or months after radiation therapy causes skin changes at the site of the radiation treatment
    - skin is permanently darkened after healing has occurred
- alopecia

Management

- Provide meticulous skin/perineal care.
- Prepare the client for hair loss, if anticipated, and encourage the use of wigs, scarves, hats, or turbans.

HEMATOPOIETIC EFFECTS

- anemia
- thrombocytopenia
- neutropenia

Management

- Monitor temperature (often the only sign of infection, as these clients are not able to produce an adequate inflammatory response).
- Obtain cultures as ordered.
- Maintain protective isolation, if indicated.
- Administer antibiotics as ordered.

- Administer granulocyte colony-stimulating factor (G-CSF) or granulocyte macrophage colony-stimulating factor (GM-CSF); reduced duration and severity of neutropenia.
- Institute bleeding precautions.
- Hematest urine, stool, and NG contents.
- Assess for changes in level of consciousness—may be an early indication of intracranial hemorrhage.
- Do not administer rectal suppositories, enemas, or perform rectal temperatures.
- Provide adequate rest.
- Administer blood component replacement therapy. See "Blood Component Transfusion," p. 88.
- Monitor laboratory findings—WBC, RBC, platelet count, culture reports, and absolute granulocyte count.
- Determine nadir (predicted time after chemotherapy that WBC and platelets are at the lowest value) to predict when client is at greatest risk for infection and bleeding. For most agents, the nadir occurs 7–14 days after drug administration.

GENITOURINARY EFFECTS

- nephrotoxicity
- hemorrhagic cystitis

Management

- Monitor intake and output
- Hematest urine output
- Monitor laboratory findings—BUN, creatinine, renal profile
- Encourage fluids

HEPATIC EFFECTS

- hepatotoxicity
- cirrhosis
- portal hypertension

Management

- Monitor laboratory findings—liver function tests.
- Assess for signs of liver failure—ascites, jaundice, abdominal pain, hepatomegaly, etc.

CARDIAC EFFECTS

- ECG changes
- dysrhythmias
- congestive heart failure
- tachycardia

Management

- Monitor rhythm strip and/or 12-lead ECG for changes.
- Auscultate heart sounds.
- Assess for signs of heart failure—peripheral edema, dyspnea on exertion, presence of S_3, etc.

PULMONARY EFFECTS

- pneumonitis
- pulmonary fibrosis

Management

- Monitor arterial blood gas results and oxygen saturations.
- Assess lung sounds.
- Monitor response to activity.

NEUROLOGIC/SENSORY-PERCEPTUAL EFFECTS

- ototoxicity
- peripheral neuropathy
- cranial nerve neuropathy

Management

- Perform neurologic assessment.

REPRODUCTIVE EFFECTS

- azoospermia, oligospermia, and sterility in males
- amenorrhea, menopausal manifestations, and sterility in females

COMMUNITY AND SELF-CARE

- Instruct client regarding:
  - — disease process and treatment regime
  - — importance of clinic and laboratory follow-up
  - — signs/symptoms to report to physician
  - — care of venous access device, if in place
  - — measures to protect against infection
    - maintain adequate nutrition and fluid intake
    - avoidance of crowds, people with infections and those who have been recently vaccinated with live or attenuated vaccines
    - avoid raw or uncooked foods
    - avoidance of contact with animal excrement
    - report fever over 100° F., cough, sore throat, chills, or painful urination immediately
    - maintain personal hygiene
    - obtain adequate rest and exercise
    - avoid indiscriminate use of antipyretics because they can mask fever

— measures to reduce the risk of bleeding:
  - soft toothbrush
  - electric razor
  - guard against falls
  - report bleeding gums, increased bruising or petechiae, tarry stools, blood in urine, coffee-ground emesis, hemoptysis, epistaxis, heavy menses, headaches, or blurred vision immediately

— oral hygiene measures

— use of PRN antiemetics and analgesics

- Refer to available community resources (cancer support groups).

(For more information, see pp. 573–584 of Black and Matassarin-Jacobs: *Medical-Surgical Nursing: Clinical Management for Continuity of Care,* 5th ed.)

Chest Trauma

- Chest injuries can result from falls, the use of certain types of machinery, or the employment of lethal weapons (guns, knives). Motor vehicle accidents are also a common cause.
- Chest injuries may be penetrating or nonpenetrating.
  — Penetrating injuries are caused by bullets, knives, or impaled objects. They may cause an open chest wound and permit air to enter the pleural space.
  — Nonpenetrating injuries are caused by falls, blows to the chest, or by deceleration injuries in motor vehicle accidents.
- General management includes:
  — initial assessment and treatment of life-threatening conditions
  — maintenance of airway, breathing, and circulation
  — thorough assessment and physical examination after initial emergencies are addressed
  — use of oxygen or mechanical ventilation
  — monitoring of respiratory status and arterial blood gases

- — frequent vital signs
  - — monitoring for dysrhythmias
  - — thoracentesis, chest tube insertion, bronchoscopic aspiration, or thoracotomy as indicated
  - — fluid replacement with blood, blood products, or crystalloid intravenous solutions
  - — monitoring for signs/symptoms of shock
  - — use of analgesics to reduce pain and maximize effective breathing
- Possible complications of chest trauma include:
  - — pneumothorax
  - — tension pneumothorax and mediastinal shift
  - — open pneumothorax and mediastinal flutter
  - — hemothorax
  - — fractured ribs
  - — fractured sternum
  - — flail chest
  - — cardiac tamponade
  - — myocardial contusion

These items are discussed individually—see index.

(For more information, see pp. 2522–2524 of Black and Matassarin-Jacobs: *Medical-Surgical Nursing: Clinical Management for Continuity of Care,* 5th ed.)

Chlamydial Infections

OVERVIEW

- Chlamydia trachomatis, the causative organism, is a gram-negative bacterium.
- Chlamydial infections are the most common sexually transmitted disease (STD) in the United States today. The incidence is three times that of gonorrhea.
- The disease is always transmitted by intimate sexual contact, never casual contact.
- Infection does not cross the placenta, but exposure during delivery can cause conjunctivitis and pneumonia in newborns.
- The infection primarily affects the urethra, cervix, and rectum.

- In men, the infection can cause epididymitis, and produce sterility. In women, salpingitis with subsequent infertililty or high risk of ectopic pregnancy can occur. Secondary extension to the female peritoneum can cause a pelvic inflammatory disease (PID).

CLINICAL MANIFESTATIONS

- Female
  - — may be asymptomatic
  - — yellow, mucopurulent vaginal discharge
  - — friable, edematous cervix
  - — spotting at menstrual mid-cycle or with sexual intercourse
  - — dysuria
  - — pharyngitis
- Male
  - — may be asymptomatic
  - — dysuria
  - — clear to mucopurulent urethral discharge
  - — pharyngitis

ACUTE AND SUBACUTE CARE

Medical Management

All sexual contacts within 30 days before diagnosis should be treated.

- doxycycline for 7 days or one dose of azithromycin (Zithromax)
- repeat culture after therapy completed

Nursing Management

- Administer antibiotics as prescribed.
- Monitor temperature.

COMMUNITY AND SELF-CARE

Instruct client regarding:

- importance of completing the course of antibiotics and follow-up culture
- information about the disease, mode of transmission, and treatment regime
- the increased risk of infection with multiple sex partners

- importance of identifying and treating sex partners
- importance of avoiding all sexual activity until cured
- importance of the use of condoms thereafter to prevent reinfection
- medication administration:
  — take medication 1–2 hours after meals
  — avoid iron, dairy products, and antacids

(For more information, see pp. 2469–2470 of Black and Matassarin-Jacobs: *Medical-Surgical Nursing: Clinical Management for Continuity of Care,* 5th ed.)

Cholangitis

OVERVIEW

- Cholangitis is inflammation of the bile duct.
- Cholangitis is frequently associated with choledocholithiasis (stones in the common bile duct).

CLINICAL MANIFESTATIONS

- chills and fever
- frequently recurring attacks of severe right upper quadrant pain
- elevation of serum bilirubin and alkaline phosphatase
- history of jaundice

ACUTE AND SUBACUTE CARE

Medical Management

- antibiotic therapy
- antipyretic therapy
- parenteral hydration

Surgical Management

None

Nursing Management

- Administer antibiotics as prescribed.
- Monitor temperature and administer PRN antipyretics.
- Monitor intake and output.
- Monitor laboratory findings—WBC, bilirubin, electrolytes

COMMUNITY AND SELF-CARE

Instruct client regarding:

- importance of antibiotic therapy

(For more information, see pp. 1918–1920 of Black and Matassarin-Jacobs: *Medical-Surgical Nursing: Clinical Management for Continuity of Care,* 5th ed.)

Cholecystitis, Acute

OVERVIEW

- Acute cholecystitis refers to acute inflammation of the gallbladder wall.
- Gallstones are the major cause of acute cholecystitis. Stones obstruct the cystic duct, causing distention of the gallbladder. Subsequently, (1) venous and lymphatic drainage is impaired; (2) proliferation of bacteria occurs; (3) localized cellular irritation and/or infiltration takes place; and (4) areas of ischemia may develop. The inflamed gallbladder wall is edematous and thickened and may have areas of gangrene or necrosis.
- There is an increased incidence in clients who are overweight, especially those with sedentary lifestyles.

CLINICAL MANIFESTATIONS

- tenderness in right upper quadrant, epigastrium, or both
- pain of sudden onset that steadily increases and reaches a peak in 30 minutes, located in epigastric,

subscapular, or right upper quadrant areas, sometimes referred to the right scapula
- positive Murphy's sign—while palpating the gallbladder, the client is asked to take a deep breath and experiences extreme tenderness and stops breathing on inspiration
- nausea and vomiting
- fever
- elevated white blood cell count
- mild jaundice

ACUTE AND SUBACUTE CARE

Medical Management

- antibiotic therapy
- analgesics
- parenteral hydration
- nasogastric tube placement
- retrograde endoscopy, endoscopic papillotomy for stone removal. See "Cholelithiasis," p. 164.

Surgical Management

- cholecystectomy (removal of the gallbladder). See "Cholelithiasis," p. 164.

Nursing Management

Medical

- same as nursing management of clients with cholelithiasis except that these clients will receive a course of antibiotics. See "Cholelithiasis," p. 164.

Surgical

- same as nursing management for cholecystectomy. See "Cholelithiasis," p. 164.

COMMUNITY AND SELF-CARE

See "Cholelithiasis," p. 164.

(For more information, see pp. 1915–1918 of Black and Matassarin-Jacobs: *Medical-Surgical Nursing: Clinical Management for Continuity of Care,* 5th ed.)

Cholecystitis, Chronic

OVERVIEW

- Chronic cholecystitis refers to chronic inflammation of the gallbladder wall.
- Chronic cholecystitis sometimes arises as a sequelae to acute cholecystitis; however, it typically develops independently of acute cholecystitis and is almost always associated with gallstones.
- It affects middle-aged and older, obese women. The female-to-male ratio is 3:1.

CLINICAL MANIFESTATIONS

- right upper quadrant tenderness
- elevated temperature
- pain in epigastric, subscapular, or right upper quadrant areas
- dyspepsia, dietary fat intolerance, flatulence
- elevated white blood cell count

ACUTE AND SUBACUTE CARE

Medical Management

- low fat diet
- weight reduction
- anticholinergics
- antacids
- analgesics

Surgical Management

- cholecystectomy—excision of the gallbladder (performed if medical management is ineffective)
  See "Cholelithiasis," p. 164.

Nursing Management

Medical

- Administer medications as prescribed and assess effectiveness.
- Maintain low-fat diet.

Surgical

- See "Cholelithiasis," p. 164.

COMMUNITY AND SELF-CARE

Instruct client regarding:
- medication regime
- dietary restrictions
- postoperative care for cholecystectomy, see "Cholelithiasis," p. 164.

(For more information, see p. 1918 of Black and Matassarin-Jacobs: *Medical-Surgical Nursing: Clinical Management for Continuity of Care,* 5th ed.)

Choledocholithiasis

OVERVIEW

- Choledocholithiasis is defined as stones in the common bile duct.
- Common bile duct calculi can arise from the gallbladder or hepatic ducts. Thus, common duct stones can occur in the absence of a gallbladder.
- Common duct stones are found in 10–15 per cent of clients with cholelithiasis (presence of gallstones in the gallbladder).
- The pathophysiology is essentially the same as for cholelithiasis. The majority of bile duct stones are cholesterol or mixed stones. They form in the gallbladder and move into the biliary tree through the cystic duct.

CLINICAL MANIFESTATIONS

- may be asymptomatic
- mild to severe upper midline or right quadrant pain sometimes referred to right scapula
- jaundice—may be intermittent, if obstruction is intermittent, but may be progressive, if stones become impacted

ACUTE AND SUBACUTE CARE

Medical Management

- analgesics
- parenteral hydration

Surgical Management

- endoscopic sphincterotomy—endoscope is passed orally and the sphincter enlarged to allow stone passage
- extracorporeal shock wave therapy—external application of shock waves to the area of stones to fragment them (used if stones are too large to extract by endoscope)
- choledochostomy—opening the common bile duct surgically, removing stones and inserting a T-tube for drainage to prevent bile from spilling into the peritoneal cavity and to maintain patency of the duct during healing. The T-tube is attached to a gravity drainage system.

Nursing Management

- Same as for client with cholelithiasis, see "Cholelithiasis," p. 164.

COMMUNITY AND SELF-CARE

- Same as for client with cholelithiasis, see "Cholelithiasis," p. 164.

(For more information, see pp. 1918–1920 of Black and Matassarin-Jacobs: *Medical-Surgical Nursing: Clinical Management for Continuity of Care,* 5th ed.)

Cholelithiasis (Gallstones)

OVERVIEW

- Cholelithiasis is the presence of gallstones in the biliary system, which is composed of the gallbladder, bile ducts, and the cystic duct.

- Most gallstones form in the gallbladder but may also form in the common duct and hepatic ducts of the liver. Gallstones are divided into three groups: (1) cholesterol stones—the most common, (2) pigment stones—contain an excess of unconjugated bilirubin, and (3) mixed stones—a combination of cholesterol and pigment stones or either of these stones with another substance, i.e., calcium carbonate, phosphate, bile salts.
- It is estimated that 20 million people in the United States have gallstones. The incidence increases with age. Women account for nearly 70 per cent of those treated.
- Risk factors include:
  - — diabetes mellitus
  - — multiple pregnancies
  - — vagotomy (removal of a section of the vagus nerve)—results in decreased gallbladder motility
  - — long-term parenteral nutrition—decreases gallbladder motility
  - — cirrhosis of the liver
  - — obesity
  - — pancreatitis

CLINICAL MANIFESTATIONS

- may be asymptomatic
- pain or biliary colic—starts in upper midline area, may radiate around to back and right shoulder blade or to the back and substernal area
- jaundice—when common bile obstruction is present
- nausea and vomiting
- bloating, dyspepsia
- intolerance to fatty foods

ACUTE AND SUBACUTE CARE

Medical Management

- analgesics
- antiemetics, antacids
- nasogastric tube placement
- intravenous therapy to maintain fluid and electrolyte balance

- retrograde endoscopy for stone removal—endoscope is passed orally into the duodenum, where a wire snare is passed into the common bile duct through the ampulla of Vater to secure and remove the stone
- endoscopic papillotomy—endoscope is passed orally and the ampulla of Vater is enlarged for easier stone passage
- oral administration of dissolution agents—chenodeoxycholic acid (chenodiol), urodeoxycholic acid (ursodiol)
- dietary management—avoidance of foods that precipitate biliary colic

Surgical Management

- cholecystectomy—excision of the gallbladder from the posterior liver wall and ligation of the cystic duct, vein, and artery. The approach is usually through a right upper paramedian or upper midline incision. Common bile duct exploration may also be performed with dilation of the common duct and stone removal by passing a fine instrument into the duct. Following exploration of the common duct, a T-tube is usually inserted to ensure adequate bile drainage during duct healing. It also provides a route for postoperative cholangiography or stone dissolution. The T-tube is attached to a gravity drainage system.
- laparoscopic cholecystectomy—using general anesthesia, a pneumoperitoneum is created by injecting carbon dioxide through a needle inserted near the umbilicus. An endoscope is then inserted through a small incision near the umbilicus to view the gallbladder. Three other small incisions are made, one for grasping the gallbladder, one for suction and irrigation, and another for the dissection instrument and clips. This is the treatment of choice.
- extracorporeal shock wave lithotripsy—external application of shock waves to the area of stones to fragment them
- percutaneous cholecystolithotomy—use of cystoscopes, stone baskets, and instruments designed for nephrolithotomy. General anesthesia is not used.

NURSING MANAGEMENT

Medical

- Administer analgesics as ordered and monitor effectiveness (Demerol is the medication most frequently ordered. Morphine is contraindicated because it may increase spasm of the sphincter of Oddi.).
- Administer oral dissolution agents.
- Provide a quiet, restful environment.
- Assess client for signs of dehydration—dry mucous membranes, decreased skin turgor, decreased urinary output.
- Maintain nasogastric tube—relieves distention and vomiting and removes gastric juices that stimulate cholecystokinin, which causes painful contractions of the gallbladder.
- Administer IV fluids as ordered.
- Monitor intake and output.
- Assess for return of gag reflex before allowing oral intake following a retrograde endoscopy (a local anesthetic is sprayed on the throat).

Surgical (Post Cholecystectomy)

POSTOPERATIVE CARE

In addition to routine postoperative care:

- Assess lung status closely and encourage pulmonary hygiene measures (location of incision may make this painful).
- Monitor intake and output.
- Monitor electrolyte laboratory values.
- Maintain nasogastric tube.
- Provide frequent oral hygiene.
- Assess and monitor amount of T-tube drainage if placed during surgery.

COMMUNITY AND SELF-CARE

Instruct the client regarding:

MEDICAL

- importance of medication regime—analgesics and oral dissolution agents

- dietary restrictions—low fat, avoidance of greasy foods

SURGICAL

- wound care
- signs/symptoms of infection
- signs/symptoms to report—jaundice, dark-colored urine, pale-colored stools, and pruritus
- care of the T-tube (if in place)
- activity restrictions
- dietary restrictions

(For more information, see pp. 1907–1915 of Black and Matassarin-Jacobs: *Medical-Surgical Nursing: Clinical Management for Continuity of Care,* 5th ed.)

Chronic Airflow Limitations (CAL) or Chronic Obstructive Pulmonary Disease (COPD) (includes Chronic Obstructive Bronchitis, Emphysema)

OVERVIEW

- *Chronic airflow limitation* (CAL) is a term that encompasses the disorders of obstructive bronchitis, emphysema, and asthma. Although the term *COPD* (chronic obstructive pulmonary disease) or *COLD* (chronic obstructive lung disease) is used commonly for this group of disorders, pulmonary specialists use the term CAL because it is more completely accurate.
- Chronic obstructive bronchitis and emphysema will be discussed in this section. Asthma is discussed under its own heading (p. 69).
- COPD affects one in every 10 Americans.
- *Chronic obstructive bronchitis* is inflammation of the bronchi, which causes increased mucous production and chronic cough. Thicker, more tenacious mucus and impaired ciliary function is

present. The airways collapse, and air is trapped in the distal part of the lung. This obstruction leads to reduced alveolar ventilation, hypoxia, and acidosis. There is poor tissue oxygenation, a fall in PaO_2, and a rise in $PaCO_2$.

- Emphysema is a disorder in which the alveolar walls are destroyed, which leads to permanent overdistention of the air spaces. Air passages are obstructed due to these changes, rather than from mucous production, as in chronic bronchitis. Expiration is difficult due to the destruction of the walls between the alveoli, partial airway collapse, and loss of elastic recoil. As the walls collapse, pockets of air form between the alveolar spaces (called blebs) and within the lung parenchyma (bullae). There is increased ventilatory dead space.
- Cigarette smoking is the leading risk factor for this disorder. Chronic respiratory infections, aging, hereditary and genetic predisposition also may play a role.

CLINICAL MANIFESTATIONS

Chronic Bronchitis

- productive cough
- decreased exercise tolerance
- wheezing
- shortness of breath
- prolonged expiration
- elevated hematocrit, polycythemia
- cyanosis and peripheral edema—"blue bloater"
- signs/symptoms of cor pulmonale—right-sided heart failure
- pulmonary infection is common

Emphysema

- dyspnea on exertion that progresses eventually to dyspnea at rest
- tachypnea with prolonged expiration
- use of accessory muscles
- enlarged anteroposterior diameter of the chest
- characteristic sitting position of leaning forward with arms braced on knees to support the shoulders and chest for breathing

- thinness
- pink color (normal arterial oxygen levels) and dyspnea ("pink puffer")
- cor pulmonale (right-sided congestive heart failure)

ACUTE AND SUBACUTE CARE

Medical Management

Chronic Bronchitis and Emphysema

- bronchodilators, antihistamines
- steroids, antibiotics, expectorants
- mast cell membrane stabilizers
- oxygen for severe exertional or at-rest hypoxemia
- nebulized bronchodilators
- positive-pressure airflow or positive end-expiratory pressure devices
- postural drainage and chest physiotherapy
- diuretics and digitalis for edema and cor pulmonale
- phlebotomy for elevations in hematocrit (>60%)
- pneumovax and flu vaccine

Surgical Management

- rare, but bullectomy may be performed for clients with repeated spontaneous pneumothorax
- lung volume reduction surgery—removal of portions of diffusely emphysematous lungs

Nursing Management

- Assess respiratory status and report changes to physician:
  - — respiratory rate, pattern, use of accessory muscles
  - — arterial blood gas results
  - — skin color
  - — signs/symptoms of hypoxia/hypercapnia
- Maintain high-Fowler's position.
- Administer low flow oxygen—remember that the normal respiratory drive is obliterated by long-standing hypercapnia. Use caution as excessive oxygen may diminish respiratory drive.

- Monitor effectiveness of bronchodilators and assess for side effects.
- Monitor for therapeutic levels of bronchodilators.
- Encourage 8–10 glasses of fluid daily, if not contraindicated.
- Use caution when administering narcotics, sedatives, and tranquilizers, which are respiratory depressants.
- Instruct on:
  - — proper coughing techniques
  - — pursed lip breathing (performed during exhalation to prevent early airway collapse and to help the lungs empty more completely)
    - encourage the client to relax and breathe in through the nose
    - next, instruct the client to exhale slowly and completely through pursed lips for a comfortable length of time. Expiration should take twice as long as inspiration.
  - — diaphragmatic breathing (abdominal breathing)—a technique that involves using the diaphragm more effectively, thereby reducing the use of accessory muscles for breathing
    - instruct the client to assume a comfortable semi-Fowler's position with the knees bent
    - when performed properly, diaphragmatic breathing causes the abdomen to rise visibly during deep inhalation and contract during exhalation
  - — program of progressive walking
  - — avoidance of conditions that increase oxygen demand, such as smoking, temperature extremes, high altitudes, excess weight, and stress
  - — pacing activities throughout the day and energy conservation techniques
  - — performing active exercise after respiratory therapy or medication
- Assess for any changes in vital signs during activity and instruct client to stop if these occur.
- Remain with the client during acute episodes of dyspnea.
- During acute episodes, open doors and curtains and limit number of people in the room.
- Promote adequate nutrition:
  - — encourage high-calorie liquid supplements

- assist with oral care before meals
- encourage six small meals per day
- instruct to avoid gas-producing foods (may cause abdominal bloating, distention, and impair ventilation)
- instruct to use oxygen via nasal cannula during mealtimes
- monitor food intake, weight, serum hemoglobin, and albumin levels

- Use/encourage relaxation techniques (massage, music, warm bath, warm beverage) to promote sleep.
  - suggest patient sleep in recliner chair when dyspnea is severe
  - avoid caffeine and exercise in the evening
- Provide emotional support to the family and client for coping with long-term illness.
- Facilitate discussion of changes in sexual function—suggest alternative positions, alternative forms of sexual expression (hugging, cuddling), and use of bronchodilators before sexual activity.

COMMUNITY AND SELF-CARE

- Instruct client/significant other regarding:
  - smoking cessation programs; use of nicotine patch
  - avoidance of known allergens, smoke, dust, mold, pollution, and high altitudes
  - use of inhalers
  - prescribed medications, side effects, and symptoms of toxicity and to report these to physician
  - importance of follow-up laboratory tests, arterial blood gases, and pulmonary function tests
  - hazards of infection and ways to avoid (obtain immunizations against influenza and pneumococcal organisms, avoid crowds, cleanse respiratory equipment well)
  - signs/symptoms of impending respiratory problems (increased confusion, drowsiness) and right-sided heart failure (peripheral edema, distended neck veins) and to report these to physician
  - above information in "Nursing Management"

- Make arrangements for home oxygen therapy and instructions on use.
- Refer to Meals on Wheels if help with nutrition is needed.
- Encourage use of self-help or support groups, such as Better Breathers Club, sponsored by the American Lung Association.
- Refer to a professional skilled in sexuality, if appropriate.

(For more information, see pp. 1111–1124 of Black and Matassarin-Jacobs: *Medical-Surgical Nursing: Clinical Management for Continuity of Care,* 5th ed.)

Chronic Venous Insufficiency

- Chronic venous insufficiency, also known as postphlebotic syndrome, is characterized by (1) chronically swollen limbs, (2) thick, coarse, brownish skin around the ankles (referred to as the "gaiter" area), and (3) venous stasis ulceration.
- Chronic venous insufficiency results from dysfunctional valves that reduce venous return, which increases venous pressure, causing venous stasis.
- Chronic venous insufficiency follows most severe cases of deep vein thrombosis (DVT) but may take as long as 5–10 years to manifest. Therefore, clients with a history of DVT must be monitored periodically throughout their lives.
- Instruct the client regarding:
  - — elevation of the legs above the heart level whenever possible when sitting or lying
  - — not crossing legs
  - — not using chairs that are too high for feet to touch the floor and thus apply pressure to the popliteal area
  - — avoiding constrictive clothing
  - — use of elastic stockings
  - — avoiding standing or sitting for prolonged periods of time
  - — importance of daily skin inspection for signs of skin cracking or ulceration

(For more information, see p. 1436 of Black and Matassarin-Jacobs: *Medical-Surgical Nursing: Clinical Management for Continuity of Care,* 5th ed.)

Cirrhosis

OVERVIEW

- Cirrhosis of the liver is the disorganization of the liver architecture by widespread fibrosis and nodule formation. It occurs when the normal flow of blood, bile, and hepatic metabolites is altered by fibrosis and changes in the hepatocytes, bile ductules, vascular channels, and reticular cells.
- There are four major types of cirrhosis:
  (1) Laennec's (alcoholic)—most commonly found in clients who chronically abuse alcohol.
  (2) Postnecrotic—usually follows acute viral hepatitis.
  (3) Biliary—occurs secondary to chronic biliary inflammation or obstruction.
  (4) Cardiac—ocurs secondary to congestive heart failure with prolonged venous hepatic congestion.
- The cirrhotic liver usually has a nodular consistency, with bands of fibrosis (scar tissue) and small areas of regenerating tissue. There is extensive destruction of the hepatocytes. This alteration in the architecture of the liver alters the flow in the vascular system and lymphatic bile duct channels. Periodic exacerbations are marked by bile stasis, precipitating jaundice.
- Risk factors include: alcohol abuse, viral hepatitis, biliary disorders, genetic predisposition with a familial tendency, congestive heart failure, and exposure to industrial or chemical compounds.
- Progression of the cirrhotic process usually results in death due to hepatic encephalopathy, bacterial infection, peritonitis, liver tumor, or complications of portal hypertension.
- Forty-five per cent of all cirrhosis cases are related to alcohol. Cirrhosis is the fourth leading cause of death in clients between 35 and 54 years of age. It

is the tenth leading cause of death overall in the United States.

CLINICAL MANIFESTATIONS

Laennec's Cirrhosis

- may have no symptoms for long periods
- weakness, fatigue
- anorexia, weight loss
- nausea and vomiting
- abdominal pain
- jaundice
- ascites
- spider angiomas

Postnecrotic Cirrhosis

- similar to Laennec's except less muscle wasting and more jaundice

Biliary Cirrhosis

- generalized pruritis
- dark urine, pale stools
- jaundice
- steatorrhea

Cardiac Cirrhosis

- slight jaundice
- enlarged liver
- ascites
- right upper quadrant pain
- cachexia
- fluid retention

Advanced Stages

- ascites
- prominent abdominal wall veins
- gastrointestinal bleeding (from esophageal varices)
- muscle wasting
- splenomegaly
- leg edema
- jaundice
- gynecomastia
- palmar erythema

- encephalopathy
- spider angiomata

ACUTE AND SUBACUTE CARE

Medical Management

Essentially the same for the four types of cirrhosis.

- adequate rest, nutritious diet high in protein (if not encephalopathic) and measures to prevent infection
- corticosteroids
- B vitamins and fat-soluble vitamins (vitamins A, D, E, and K)
- control of complications (ascites, bleeding esophageal varices, and hepatic encephalopathy)

Nursing Management

- Monitor for ascites and hepatic encephalopathy.
- Provide diet high in carbohydrates and calories with some protein, but not enough to precipitate hepatic encephalopathy.
- Maintain calorie count.
- Monitor nutritional panel and liver function tests.
- Restrict sodium and fluids as prescribed if ascites or edema present. (These may be admitted intravenously, in severe malabsorption.)
- Obtain daily weights.
- Measure abdominal girth daily.
- Monitor intake and output every shift.
- Provide small, frequent meals if anorexia is present.
- Administer oral fat soluble vitamins (vitamins A, D, E, and K) if fat absorption present.
- Be aware that medications metabolized by the liver may require dosage adjustment or discontinuation.
- Ensure adequate rest to reduce metabolic demands on the liver.
- Assist client to plan reasonable activity with rest periods.
- Avoid administering sedatives and opiates.
- Monitor for signs/symptoms of bleeding:
  - — bleeding gums
  - — melena
  - — purpura

— hematuria
— hematemesis.

- Prevent bleeding:
  — maintain safety precautions
  — avoid intramuscular and subcutaneous injections, but, if unavoidable, use small gauge needle
  — instruct the client to avoid vigorous nose blowing and straining with bowel movements
  — discuss use of soft toothbrush or foam toothettes for oral care

COMMUNITY AND SELF-CARE

- Instruct client/significant other regarding:
  — avoidance of ingesting hepatotoxins, especially alcohol
  — prevention of and signs/symptoms of bleeding
  — need for nutritious diet high in calories, carbohydrates, and protein (unless encephalopathy is present)
  — low-sodium diet and fluid restriction, if needed due to edema or ascites
  — need for potassium supplements if on a thiazide diuretic
  — signs/symptoms of fluid retention
  — signs/symptoms of progressive liver failure or complications (such as encephalopathy or bleeding varices) and when to call physician
- Refer to a substance abuse program or support groups such as Alcoholics Anonymous for assistance with abstinence from alcohol.
- Discuss importance of follow-up at regular intervals to follow progression of the disease.

Also see "Portal Hypertension," p. 585, "Ascites," p. 67, and "Hepatic Encephalopathy," p. 337 for further information.

(For more information, see pp. 1872–1884 of Black and Matassarin-Jacobs: *Medical-Surgical Nursing: Clinical Management for Continuity of Care,* 5th ed.)

Closed Chest Drainage

OVERVIEW

- Closed chest drainage is the use of a chest drainage system (closed to atmospheric pressure) connected to a chest catheter for the purpose of removing air or fluid from the pleural space.
- Closed chest drainage commonly is used after chest surgery and to treat pneumothorax or empyema.
- Closed chest drainage may be accomplished by glass bottle water-seal set-ups or with disposable single units (e.g., Pleur-evac). Most health care facilities now use the disposable single units.
- Three principles are used in all closed drainage systems: gravity, water seal, and suction.
  (1) gravity—air and fluid flow from a higher level to a lower level.
  (2) water seal—a water seal provides a barrier between atmospheric pressure (pressure on the outside of the body) and subatmospheric (negative) intrapleural pressure. On expiration, air and fluid from the pleural space travel through the drainage tubing into the first compartment. The air bubbles up through the chamber and enters atmospheric air. On inspiration, the water seal prevents atmospheric air from being sucked back into the pleural space.
  (3) suction—air or fluid moves from higher to lower pressure. A suction of 20 cm H_2O creates a subatmospheric pressure of 746 mm Hg.
- In a Pleur-evac system, the first chamber collects drainage from the pleural cavity, the second chamber acts as the water seal and the third chamber acts as the suction control.

ACUTE AND SUBACUTE CARE

Nursing Management

- Monitor the amount and type of chest tube drainage. Report abnormally large amounts of grossly bloody drainage. (Following surgery, 500–1000 ml may drain in the first 24 hours. Grossly bloody drainage is normal for the first few hours following surgery.)

- Monitor respiratory status and lung sounds.
- Encourage frequent coughing, deep breathing, and incentive spirometry.
- Observe the water seal for tidaling (fluid in the water-seal compartment rises with inspiration and falls with expiration). If this is not present, the tubes may not be patent. (Tidaling may not occur or may be minimal in systems using suction.) If no tidaling is present:
  - — check to be sure the tube is not kinked or compressed
  - — milk or strip the tube (as prescribed)
  - — change the client's position
  - — ask the client to cough and deep breathe
- Observe for bubbling in the water-seal compartment (intermittent bubbling is normal, but constant bubbling represents an air leak and must be immediately reported to the physician).
- Maintain prescribed amount of suction and ensure continuous bubbling in suction control compartment.
- Check for air leaks in the system if the bubbling in the suction control chamber stops.
- Ensure that all connections of the system are tight.
- Maintain patent tubing and ensure the tubing is correctly positioned, not kinked, and has no dependent loops.
- Keep the drainage apparatus about 2–3 feet below the client's chest (if the apparatus is above the level of the client's chest, fluid from the drainage chamber is siphoned back into the pleural cavity).
- Position the client as prescribed. If turning to the side with chest tube catheters, be sure they are not compressed.
- Check the patency of drainage tubing and chest catheters frequently.
- "Milk" or "strip" chest tubes only as prescribed (routine milking or stripping is not performed because it creates excessive negative pressure).
  - — To "strip" a chest drainage tube—gently compress the tube and slide the hand over the tubing in a direction away from the client's chest and toward the drainage system.

— To "milk" a chest drainage tube—clasp one hand around the tube as close to the chest as possible and squeeze the tube against the palm of the hand. Then proceed similarly, hand-over-hand, toward the drainage apparatus.

- Maintain a clean, dry, and intact dressing over the chest catheter site (a petroleum gauze pad should be placed directly over the insertion site).
- Encourage activity as prescribed, always keeping the drainage system 2–3 feet below the chest.
- Always keep rubber-shod clamps at the bedside—never clamp the catheter unless prescribed.
- Contact the surgeon immediately if the drainage system is accidently elevated above the client's chest.
- If a chest tube is accidently removed, cover the insertion site with sterile petroleum gauze and notify the surgeon.

(For more information, see pp. 1157–1166 of Black and Matassarin-Jacobs: *Medical-Surgical Nursing: Clinical Management for Continuity of Care,* 5th ed.)

Colon Cancer

OVERVIEW

- Cancer of the colon is the second most frequent cause of death from cancer in the United States.
- Some researchers propose that bulk in the stool and the rate of transit of fecal matter may influence the development of colon cancer. They theorize that metabolic and bacterial end products are carcinogenic and that constipation allows a longer contact with the bowel wall, thus increasing the probability of cancer developing.
- Early detection includes yearly digital rectal exam at age 40; stool guaiac examinations and rectal exam at age 50; flexible sigmoidoscopy every 3-5 years after two yearly negative exams after age 50.
- Risk factors include:
  —family history of colon cancer
  — previous colon cancer

- — over age 40
- — ulcerative colitis
- — high-fat, low-residue diet that is high in refined foods
- — familial polyposis
- — adenomatous polyps
- — living in highly industrialized, urban societies
- — slow bowel transit time

CLINICAL MANIFESTATIONS

- rectal bleeding
- change in bowel habits
- tenesmus
- intestinal obstruction
- abdominal pain
- weight loss
- anorexia
- nausea and vomiting
- anemia
- palpable mass

ACUTE AND SUBACUTE CARE

Medical Management

The primary treatment for colon cancer is surgery, but medical treatment is used as an adjunct to improve survival, when the tumor cannot be completely removed.

- radiation therapy prior to surgery
- implantation of isotopes into the tumor area after surgery
- electrocoagulation after surgery
- chemotherapy to reduce metastasis and control symptoms of metastasis

Surgical Management

Intervention depends upon the type of tumor, its location and stage, and on the client's general condition. A variety of surgical procedures may be performed.

- colon resection with end-to-end anastomosis:
  - — removal of the tumor with several inches of colon on either side of the tumor excised—the two remaining ends are rejoined
- colon resection with a temporary or permanent colostomy

- abdominal-perineal resection with a permanent or end colostomy—removal of the entire rectum and affected colon and closure of the anus (performed for rectal tumors)

Nursing Management

Preoperative Care

In addition to routine preoperative care:

- Encourage diet high in calories, protein, and carbohydrates but low in residue.
- Administer total parenteral nutrition as ordered.
- Perform bowel preparation as ordered:
  - — low-residue or liquid diet
  - — administer cathartics for 12-24 hours preoperatively
  - — administer antibiotics for 12–48 hours preoperatively
  - — administer enemas
  - — administer blood transfusions to correct anemia.
- Consult and discuss role of enterostomal therapist and reinforce teaching done by enterostomal therapist:
  - — enterostomal therapist selects site
  - — enterostomal therapist instructs on ostomy care.

Postoperative Care

In addition to routine postoperative care:

Colon Resection with Temporary or Permanent Colostomy

- Monitor colostomy output.
- Use care to keep fecal contents away from the incisional site.
- Assess the stoma for ischemia. If the stoma becomes dark or dusky, notify the physician immediately.
- Ensure that the colostomy pouch is not applying any pressure to the stoma, interfering with its blood supply.
- Assess for return of bowel sounds.

- Maintain nasogastric suction.
- Assess for abdominal cramps or abdominal distention. Report to physician (a rectal tube may be needed).
- Provide emotional support and encourage discussion of feelings and concerns.
- Encourage participation in care.
- Instruct on ostomy care:
  — application of pouch
  — emptying pouch
  — stoma care
  — colostomy irrigation (if end colostomy was performed)
  — stoma dilation to prevent strictures.
- Encourage discussion of concerns regarding sexuality.

Abdominal-Perineal Resection

- Maintain perineal drains and assess the character, volume, and odor of the drainage.
- Change rectal dressings as needed.
- Provide sitz baths 3 to 4 times daily.
- Provide adequate pain medication.
- Encourage side-lying position.
- Prevent postoperative phlebitis (increased risk due to the high lithotomy position used during surgery).
  — Assess for Homan's sign.
  — Assess for any redness, swelling, or cords in calf area.
  — Administer subcutaneous Heparin as ordered.
  — Assist with leg exercises.
  — Apply sequential pressure boots as prescribed.
  — Maintain thigh high antiembolism stockings.

COMMUNITY AND SELF-CARE

- Instruct client regarding:
  — dressing change
  — signs/symptoms of infection to report to physician
  — dietary or activity restrictions
  — signs/symptoms of intestinal obstruction and perforation

- colostomy care (if applicable) including:
- management of diarrhea
  - medications to control
  - prevention of electrolyte imbalance
  - prevention of skin breakdown
- management of constipation
- management of flatus
  - holding purse, jacket, arm over colostomy
  - use of odor proof pouches or charcoal filter discs
  - avoidance of gas causing foods

- Also see items listed in Nursing Management, Preoperative Care
- Assess need for home health referral.
- Discuss need for follow-up with enterostomal therapist.
- Refer to ostomy support groups/American Cancer Society.

(For more information, see pp. 1808–1816 of Black and Matassarin-Jacobs: *Medical-Surgical Nursing: Clinical Management for Continuity of Care,* 5th ed.)

Comatose State

OVERVIEW

- Coma is a state of sustained unconsciousness. The client in a coma does not respond to verbal stimuli, has varying responses to painful stimuli, may not move voluntarily, has altered respiratory patterns, may exhibit altered pupillary responses to light, and does not blink. In general, the longer the state of unconsciousness lasts, the more likely it is due to a permanent disorder in the structure of the brain (and irreversible), rather than a temporary alteration in function (and reversible).
- To produce unconsciousness, a disorder must (1) disrupt the ascending reticular activating system that is found in the center of the brain stem and thalamus; (2) significantly disrupt the function of both cerebral hemispheres; or (3) metabolically depress the cerebrum or reticular activity system.

- Three kinds of disorders produce sustained unconsciousness. They are:
  (1) structural lesions in the brain that place pressure on the brain stem or in the posterior fossa — brain tumors, concussion, head trauma, and cerebral hemorrhage
  (2) metabolic disorders, which impair the usual functions of the cerebrum by decreasing the oxygen supply or by allowing waste products to accumulate. Common causes include hypoxia, blood loss, high altitudes, carbon monoxide poisoning, drug overdose, ischemia, disorders of the liver, lungs and kidneys, poisons, hypoglycemia, fever, infection, fluid, electrolyte or acid-base imbalance.
  (3) psychogenic causes, in which the client looks comatose but self-awareness is usually intact, such as seen in catatonia.
- Some clients in a coma awaken slowly and begin to respond normally. They may require physical and speech therapy to regain previous levels of function. Irreversible coma, also called cerebral death, is due to damage to the cerebral hemispheres, leaving the client unable to respond to the environment. The brain stem and cerebellum remain intact, and vital functions, such as heart, lung, and gastrointestinal functions, exist. Clients may remain in irreversible coma for years.

CLINICAL MANIFESTATIONS

- no motor or verbal response to the environment or any stimuli, even deep pain or suctioning
- change in respiratory rate or rhythm
  — Cheyne-Stokes—respirations that become faster and deeper than normal, then slower, alternating with periods of apnea
  — central neurogenic hyperventilation—sustained, regular, rapid respirations with forced inspiration and expiration
  — apneustic breathing—prolonged, gasping inspirations followed by extremely short, inefficient expirations
  — cluster breathing— clusters of irregular respirations alternating with longer periods of apnea

  - ataxic breathing—completely irregular pattern with random deep and shallow respirations
- impaired eye movement
  - dysconjugate gaze (conjugate deviation)—eyes do not track together
  - doll's eye test—doll's eyes are present if the eyes move to the right when the head is rotated to the left and vice versa
  - abnormal caloric test—failure to produce nystagmus (involuntary oscillation of the eyes) when water is instilled in the ear canal
  - eyes appear to be slowly jumping up and down or roving (eyes slowly wander or move around)
- pupillary changes
  - fixed and dilated
  - pinpoint
  - unequal
- posturing (brain loses the ability to inhibit muscle contraction)
  - decorticate—abnormal flexion of arms, wrists, and fingers with arms adducted, legs fully extended and internally rotated, with feet in plantar flexion
  - decerebrate—arms are extended and adducted, hands are hyperpronated, legs are extended abnormally
- impaired motor function
  - primitive sucking or snout reflexes
  - strong reflexic hand grasp
  - restlessness
  - resistance to passive movement
  - hemiplegia
  - hemiparesis
  - seizures
  - flaccidity
- decreased pulse
- widened pulse pressure (the difference between systolic and diastolic pressure readings)
- abnormal deep tendon reflexes
- loss of corneal reflex (client does not blink when sterile gauze or cotton is touched to the sclera)

ACUTE AND SUBACUTE CARE

Medical Management

The goal of medical management is to remove or correct the cause. In the interim, the brain must be protected from further injury.

- respiratory support—airway, intubation, ventilation
- circulatory support—blood pressure monitor
- diazepam (Valium) to control seizures
- parenteral therapy to correct fluid, acid-base, or electrolyte imbalances
- osmotic diuretics or corticosteroids to relieve cerebral edema
  - overhydration and IV fluids with glucose are avoided because cerebral edema may follow
- antibiotic therapy (encephalitis)
- drug antidotes and gastric lavage for drug overdose
- nutritional support
- prevention of complications—heparin administration, pulmonary hygiene, etc.

Surgical Management

- may be indicated in the presence of tumor or intracranial hemorrhage

Nursing Management

- Perform complete neurologic and mental status assessments; compare with previous assessments and note trends.
  - Glasgow coma scale (GCS) is the most common neurologic assessment tool. The scale provides objective measurements of three essential components—level of consciousness, pupil reaction, and motor activity. The three scores are totalled and range from 3–15. The client who is unresponsive to painful stimuli, does not open the eyes, and is flaccid has a score of 3. A score of 7 or less is equal to coma.
- Monitor for signs of airway obstruction, abnormal lung sounds, cyanosis, unequal lung expansion, and stridor.

- Maintain respiratory support—oral airway, intubation, tracheostomy.
- Position patient in a lateral or semi-prone position with head elevated 30 degrees to facilitate drainage of secretions and to prevent tongue from obstructing the airway.
- Perform tracheobronchial suctioning as needed. Suctioning should be gentle and the catheter should not remain in the airway for longer than 10 seconds to prevent increased ICP.
- Institute aspiration precautions.
- Monitor arterial blood gases and oxygen saturation results.
- Maintain NPO status.
- Reposition every 2 hours.
- Monitor for signs of increased ICP—seizure activity, bradycardia, posturing, hypertension with widened pulse pressure.
- Administer diuretics and steroids.
- Frequent oral care.
- Monitor skin for areas of breakdown and implement preventive measures—foam mattress, low air loss bed, meticulous hygiene.
- Prevent corneal abrasion and irritation with moisturizing eye drops and eye shields.
- Maintain extremities in functional positions.
- Perform passive range of motion exercises.
- Daily weights.
- Monitor intake and output.
- Monitor laboratory results—hemoglobin, electrolytes, nutritional panel, white blood count.
- Administer nasogastric feedings. Monitor residual amounts and ensure correct placement.
- Institute appropriate safety measures.
- Monitor for signs of complications—deep vein thrombosis, pulmonary embolism, constipation.
- Offer support to significant others.

FOCUSED DISCHARGE CARE

The site for discharge placement is totally dependent upon the condition of the client and the cause of the coma. If the client is still in a coma and recovery is expected, placement in a rehabilitation center is planned. If client is in a coma but not expected to awaken, placement in a skilled nursing center is common.

(For more information, see pp. 743–763 of Black and Matassarin-Jacobs: *Medical-Surgical Nursing: Clinical Management for Continuity of Care,* 5th ed.)

Confusional States

OVERVIEW

- Confusion is a mental state marked by alterations in thought and attention deficit followed by problems in comprehension. Confusion is accompanied by a loss of short-term memory and often irritability alternating with drowsiness.
- Classification of types of confusion
  (1)delirium
    - reduced ability to focus, sustain, or shift attention
    - change in cognition
    - changes develop over a short period of time and may fluctuate during the course of the day
    - common causes—substance abuse, substance withdrawal

  (2) dementia (chronic form of confusion)
    - memory impairment
    - cognitive disturbances: aphasia, apraxia, agnosia, etc.
    - significant decline in social or occupational functioning
    - gradual onset with progressive decline
- Three mechanisms account for the development of acute confusion: (1) damage to the brain with swelling or loss of oxygen, blood, or both; (2) impairment of the action of the nervous system by chemicals or other substances (metabolic disorder); and (3) the rebound overactivity of a previously depressed center in the brain.
- Chronic confusional states (dementia) are disorders caused by brain tissue destruction, biochemical imbalances, or compression of the brain.
- Common causes of confusion include:
  — trauma
  — alcohol withdrawal

— drug ingestion
— fever
— heart failure
— hypoxia
— hypoglycemia
— severe fluid and electrolyte imbalance
— sepsis
— liver and renal failure
— poisons
— Alzheimer's disease
— neoplasms
— stroke
— viruses (Creutzfeldt-Jakob disease)

CLINICAL MANIFESTATIONS

- attention deficit
- restlessness
- emotional lability
- insomnia and vivid nightmares
- anxiousness
- agitation
- fluctuations in cognition
- difficulty with immediate recall and ability to abstract
- loss of orientation to time
- hallucinations, illusions, and delusions

ACUTE AND SUBACUTE CARE

Medical Management

- determination and correction of the cause
- control of symptoms
  — hypnotics
  — sedatives
- nutritional support

Surgical Management

There are no surgical interventions unless confusion is due to a structural disorder, such as a tumor or hematoma.

Nursing Management

- Assess mental and behavioral status, compare to previous assessments and note trends.

- Maintain consistency in environment and routine.
- Give simple instructions and explanations.
- Reorient as necessary.
- Provide clock and calendar in room.
- Keep room quiet and softly lit without producing shadows.
- Administer hypnotics and sedatives and monitor effectiveness.
- Allow use of familiar objects from home.
- Implement safety measures:
  - — room close to nursing station
  - — bed in low position, side rails up
  - — mechanical and chemical restraints as indicated
- Allow for uninterrupted sleep.
- Keep client active during the daytime hours to promote sleep.
- Encourage balanced diet.

See care of client, "Alzheimer's Disease," p. 29.

COMMUNITY AND SELF-CARE

- Instruct family regarding:
  - — safety measures
  - — measures to decrease confusion:
    - frequent reorientation
    - quiet environment
    - simple instructions
  - — use of hypnotics and sedatives
  - — importance of balanced diet
- Refer to available community resources.

(For more information, see pp. 768–770 of Black and Matassarin-Jacobs: *Medical-Surgical Nursing: Clinical Management for Continuity of Care,* 5th ed.)

Conn's Syndrome

OVERVIEW

- Conn's syndrome is a hypersecretion of aldosterone due to an adrenal tumor.

- Conn's syndrome affects females twice as often as males.
- Aldosterone affects the tubular reabsorption of sodium and water and the excretion of potassium and hydrogen ions. Hypersecretion of aldosterone leads to hypokalemia, hypernatremia, hypervolemia, and metabolic alkalosis.

CLINICAL MANIFESTATIONS

- hypertension
- hypernatremia
- hypokalemia with muscle weakness and cardiac dysrhythmias
- metabolic alkalosis
- overt edema is rare because excess water is excreted with potassium ions

ACUTE AND SUBACUTE CARE

Medical Management

- antihypertensive therapy
- potassium replacement
- renal support

Surgical Management

Surgical management is the treatment of choice.

- unilateral or bilateral adrenalectomy (removal of the adrenal gland(s))

Nursing Management

Medical

- Administer ordered antihypertensives.
- Administer potassium replacement therapy.
- Monitor blood pressure.
- Monitor intake and output.
- Monitor electrolyte levels and renal function studies.

Surgical

- See "Cushing's Syndrome," p. 204.

COMMUNITY AND SELF-CARE

Instruct client regarding:

- importance of medication and treatment regime
- dietary modifications
- importance of follow-up visits

Post Adrenalectomy

- importance of daily hormonal replacement
- medication injection technique should client not tolerate oral medication
- signs of under- and over-dosage
- need to call for dosage adjustment if experiencing physical or emotional stress
- dietary modifications
- need for Medic Alert bracelet and card

(For more information, see pp. 2055–2056 of Black and Matassarin-Jacobs: *Medical-Surgical Nursing: Clinical Management for Continuity of Care,* 5th ed.)

Corneal Dystrophies

OVERVIEW

- Corneal dystrophies are a group of hereditary and acquired disorders of unknown etiology, characterized by deposits in the layers of the cornea and alteration of corneal structure.
- Specific dystrophies characteristically appear at different ages. They may be stationary or slowly progressive. The most common, Fuch's dystrophy, usually begins in the second or third decade, affects women more than men, and is slowly progressive.

CLINICAL MANIFESTATIONS

- cloudy cornea
- visual impairment

ACUTE AND SUBACUTE CARE

Medical Management

None

Surgical Management

- keratoplasty (corneal transplantation) obtained from cadaver donors

Nursing Management

In addition to routine postoperative care:
- Maintain eye patch and shield in place.
- Administer PRN analgesics.
- Monitor for signs/symptoms of increased ocular pressure (pain, nausea).
- Assist with ambulation and activities of daily living (ADL).
- Administer antibiotic/steroid eye drops.

COMMUNITY AND SELF-CARE

Instruct client regarding:
- technique for instilling eye drops
- importance of eye protection (glasses, shields)
- eye care
- importance of not rubbing the eye
- signs/symptoms of graft rejection:
  - — redness
  - — swelling
  - — decreased vision
  - — pain
- the need to evaluate the vision in the operative eye each day and if no improvement is noted or vision is worse, to notify physician. Because graft rejection may occur at any time (even years) after the surgery, advise client to make the vision check a routine part of ADLs for the rest of his/her life.
- signs/symptoms of increased intraocular pressure (pain, nausea, decreased vision)
- signs/symptoms of infection (redness, swelling, drainage, blurred vision, or pain)
- safety measures for the home environment
- importance of follow-up clinic visits

(For more information, see pp. 96
Matassarin-Jacobs: *Medical-Surgic*
Management for Continuity of Care, 5

Corneal Ulcers

OVERVIEW

- Corneal ulcers that severely damage the integrity of the eye are often caused by a corneal infection (keratitis). Sources of infection include *Staphylococcus Aureus, Pseudomonas Aeruginosa, Streptococcus Pneumoniae, Candida,* and herpes zoster. Clients with a systemic collagen disease, such as rheumatoid arthritis, are susceptible to infection and ulceration. Dry eyes or ineffective eyelid closure predispose the eye to keratitis.

CLINICAL MANIFESTATIONS

- tearing
- photophobia
- blurred vision
- pain that worsens with eye movement
- eye appears infected and indurated

ACUTE AND SUBACUTE CARE

Medical Management

- topical antibiotic, antifungal or antiviral therapy (may need to be instilled every 15 minutes around the clock to prevent progression to perforation)
- analgesics

Surgical Management

- tarsorrhaphy (suturing the eyelid shut)
- conjunctival flap to seal defect if ulcer has perforated
- keratoplasty (corneal transplantation)—large perforations
- enucleation (removal of the eyeball)

ical

- Administer eye drops as ordered.
- Administer PRN analgesics.
- Promote effective rest and sleep.
- Cleanse the eyes to remove crustation.

COMMUNITY AND SELF-CARE

Instruct client regarding:
- technique for instilling eye drops
- signs/symptoms of increasing infection (redness, swelling, drainage, blurred vision, or pain)
- eye care
- measures for a safe home environment
- importance of follow-up clinic appointments

(For more information, see pp. 968–970 of Black and Matassarin-Jacobs: *Medical-Surgical Nursing: Clinical Management for Continuity of Care,* 5th ed.)

Coronary Artery Disease

OVERVIEW

- The heart muscle must have an adequate blood supply to contract properly. When a coronary artery is narrowed or blocked, the area of the heart muscle supplied by that artery becomes ischemic and injured, and infarction (tissue death) may result. The major disorders due to insufficient blood supply to the myocardium are: angina pectoris, congestive heart failure (CHF), and myocardial infarction (MI). These disorders are collectively known as coronary artery disease (CAD), also called ischemic heart disease (ISHD).
- CAD results from the development of obliterative atherosclerotic deposits of cholesterol and lipids within the coronary arteries that narrow and obstruct these vessels. As the vessels become lined and eventually occluded with atherosclerotic plaque, the vessels lose their ability to dilate and supply the heart with blood.

- Coronary artery disease is the leading cause of death in Americans today.
- Risk factors can be presented in three categories:
  (1) Nonmodifiable Risk Factors:
    — heredity; hypertension, dyslipidemia, diabetes, and obesity
    — age; appears predominantly in clients over 40
    — gender; affects men more often than women
    — race; CAD is more prevalent in non-Hispanic whites, the death rate from CAD is highest in blacks
  (2) Modifiable Risk Factors
    — environment; urban, less affluent populations have a higher incidence
    — cigarette smoking; smokers have more than twice the risk of heart attack than do nonsmokers. Clients who quit smoking lose their increased risk in 2–3 years.
    — hypertension; hypertensive clients have a 50 per cent higher chance of mortality.
    — elevated serum cholesterol; clients with elevated serum cholesterol (greater than 259 mg/dl) are three times more likely to develop coronary artery disease.
    — diabetes; frequently appears in middle-aged, overweight clients and contributes to increased risk for coronary artery disease.
  (3) Contributing Factors:
    — obesity
    — lack of exercise
    — excessive response to stress
- Coronary artery disease is a progressive disorder; if not prevented or treated in early stages, it will progress to more severe forms of cardiac disorders. Common sequelae include sudden cardiac death, angina pectoris, and MI. In addition, clients may develop heart failure, chronic dysrhythmias, conduction disturbances, and unstable angina.
- Sudden cardiac death is the descriptive term for death from cardiac causes within 24 hours of the onset of symptoms. CAD makes up 75 per cent of all cases of cardiac death. Primary ventricular fibrillation is the major cause of sudden cardiac death. Dyspnea and fatigue are the most com-

monly reported symptoms experienced immediately preceding sudden cardiac death.

CLINICAL MANIFESTATIONS

Atherosclerosis, by itself, does not necessarily produce symptoms. For manifestations to develop, there must be a critical deficit in blood supply to the heart in proportion to the demands of the myocardium for oxygen and nutrients. When atherosclerosis progresses slowly, the collateral circulation that develops generally can meet the heart's demands. Often, manifestations of CAD do not appear until the lumen of the coronary artery is narrowed by 75 per cent.

- See "Angina Pectoris," p. 56.

ACUTE AND SUBACUTE CARE

Medical Management

- reduction of cholesterol and fat intake
- exercise program
- weight reduction
- smoking cessation
- diabetic management
- hypertension management
- cholestyramine (Questran) and colestipol (Colestid) to decrease serum cholesterol levels

Interventional Cardiology

- Percutaneous Transluminal Coronary Angioplasty (PTCA) — arteries that are occluded or stenosed are dilated with a balloon catheter threaded through a femoral artery.
- Directional Coronary Atherectomy—catheter with a balloon and motorized cutter is passed by the femoral approach and when positioned against the blockage, mechanically debrides the plaque and allows fragments to be suctioned back through the catheter.
- Intracoronary Stents—balloon-expandable or self-expandable tubes that, when placed in a coronary artery, act as a mechanical scaffold to reopen the blocked artery. The procedure for placing a stent is similar to PTCA.

- Laser Ablation—used with balloon angioplasty to vaporize atherosclerotic plaque.

Surgical Management

- Coronary Artery Bypass Graft (CABG)—involves the bypass of a blockage in one or more of the coronary arteries using the saphenous veins or mammary artery as replacement vessels. A median sternotomy approach is used. While the client is on cardiopulmonary bypass and the heart is not beating, the distal end of the vein is sutured to the aorta and the proximal end to the coronary vessel distal to the blockage. The veins are reversed so that their valves do not interfere with blood flow.
- Surgical methods only ease the manifestations. Surgery cannot halt the process of atherosclerosis, although it may prolong life in some cases.

Nursing Management

Postinterventional Cardiology Procedure

- Maintain bedrest, do not raise head of bed greater than 30 degrees.
- Keep affected extremity straight and restrict movement.
  — Monitor catheter insertion site for bleeding or hematoma.
  — Check circulation, movement, and sensation distal to insertion site.
  — Assist with repositioning.
- Monitor vital signs and arterial line pressure readings.
- Monitor cardiac rhythm. ST segment monitor may be used to detect ischemia.
- Administer antiplatelet medication as ordered.
- Monitor heparin infusion.
- Monitor coagulation studies.
- See “Angina Pectoris,” p. 56.
- See “Cardiac Surgery,” p. 122.

COMMUNITY AND SELF-CARE

Medical

Instruct client regarding:
- dietary modifications
- establishing an exercise regime
- stress management
- Facilitate referral to smoking cessation program.

Postinterventional Cardiology

Instruct client regarding;
- observation of insertion site for bleeding or hematoma formation
- lifting restrictions
- driving restrictions
- signs/symptoms to report to physician
- anticoagulant and antiplatelet agents

Surgical

See "Cardiac Surgery," p. 122.

(For more information, see pp. 1238–1251 of Black and Matassarin-Jacobs: *Medical-Surgical Nursing: Clinical Management for Continuity of Care,* 5th ed.)

Crohn's Disease (Regional Enteritis)

OVERVIEW

- Crohn's disease is a type of inflammatory bowel disease characterized by periods of exacerbation and remission. The disease usually is slow and unaggressive and involves the entire thickness of the bowel wall (transmural) and particularly the submucosa. Lesions typically develop in several separate segments of the bowel.
- The lesions ulcerate and fissures develop, which can lead to fistulas and abscesses. The small bowel wall becomes congested and thickened and the lumen narrows. In late disease, the intestinal wall becomes permanently fibrosed, thickened, and narrowed.

- Transient arthritis develops in 20 per cent of clients with Crohn's disease.
- The disease is considered autoimmune, and there may be a genetic or hereditary factor.
- It is most common in whites, Jewish people, and people in their twenties. Both sexes are affected equally.

CLINICAL MANIFESTATIONS

- intermittent abdominal pain, weight loss
- steatorrhea
- soft or semi-liquid diarrheal stool
- anorexia, anemia, debility, fatigue
- nutritional deficits
- malnutrition causing:
  - — loss of immunocompetence (decreased resistance to infection)
  - — diminished wound healing
  - — decreased iron-binding capacity
  - — diminished pancreatic enzyme output
- acute inflammatory symptoms:
  - — right lower quadrant pain
  - — cramping, tenderness
  - — flatulence, nausea, diarrhea
  - — borborygmus (stomach rumbling), increased peristalsis

ACUTE AND SUBACUTE CARE

MEDICAL MANAGEMENT

- anti-inflammatory therapy, including steroids
- fluid, electrolyte and blood replacement
- antidiarrheal preparations (Imodium)
- hydrophilic mucilloids (e.g., psyllium or methylcellulose)
- antispasmodics
- antibiotic agents and sulfonamides (e.g., sulfasalazine)
- bowel rest
- total parenteral nutrition (TPN)
- antacids and histamine receptor antagonists
- anticholinergics during acute exacerbations
- diet high in protein and calories

Surgical Management

Surgery is used only to treat complications of Crohn's disease because there is a 50 per cent chance of recurrence, even when the diseased portion is removed.

- ileotransverse colectomy, segmental colectomy, or total colectomy with ileorectal anastomosis for colon disease

Nursing Management

- Administer antidiarrheals as prescribed.
- Monitor the number, color, and consistency of stools—hematest all stools.
- Monitor intake and output; daily weights.
- Provide good perianal skin care—cleanse skin with warm water after each bowel movement and apply protective moisture barrier product.
- Administer TPN as prescribed.
- Monitor nutritional intake.
  - — Monitor intake of fluids and food—encourage small servings of bland and easily digested foods.
  - — Offer nutritional supplements.
- Assess quality of pain and note any changes, as this may signal the onset of complications.
- Administer pain medications as prescribed and assess effectiveness.
- Discuss stress management and relaxation techniques (stress may cause exacerbations).

COMMUNITY AND SELF-CARE

- Instruct client regarding:
  - — diet high in calories and proteins
  - — TPN administration and care of venous access device
  - — perianal skin care
  - — side effects of steroids
  - — importance of follow-up physical examinations and colonoscopy every 1–2 years
  - — signs/symptoms of fluid/electrolyte imbalance
  - — exacerbating factors—dietary indiscretion, emotional upsets, or illness
  - — keeping a record of stools (consistency, color, and the presence of blood)

— reporting significant weight loss to physician
— signs/symptoms of nutritional deficiency
- Make home health referral for TPN administration.
- Refer to Crohn's and Colitis Foundations of America for support groups and information.

(For more information, see pp. 1795–1808 of Black and Matassarin-Jacobs: *Medical-Surgical Nursing: Clinical Management for Continuity of Care,* 5th ed.)

Creutzfeldt-Jakob Disease

- Creutzfeldt-Jakob disease (CJD) is a subacute CNS disorder that produces progressive dementia, myoclonus, and distinctive EEG changes. CJD is a unique disease that can apparently arise from two separate mechanisms; genetic and infectious. Persons with the genetic form have been shown to have a mutated gene present. The infectious form does not develop from a known virus or other pathogen.
- Several reports document human-to-human spread of CJD from cornea transplants, human pituitary growth hormone injections, and reuse of stereotactic EEG electrodes that had previously implanted in a person with CJD. (Apparently, there was a group of infected cadavers that were used for growth hormone replacement).
- The incidence of CJD peaks at 40–70 years of age. It affects both sexes equally.
- Clinical manifestations include vague psychiatric or behavior changes, suggesting a personality change, weight loss, anorexia, insomnia, malaise, and dizziness for a period of weeks to months. In the early stages there is progressive memory loss, visual impairment, and dysphagia. Within a few weeks or months a relentlessly progressive dementia develops; deterioration is noted from week to week.
- No effective treatment is available, and CJD appears to be uniformly fatal.
- Nursing care is directed at supportive care for preventing skin breakdown, nutritional support,

and providing emotional support to the client and family.

(For more information, see pp. 872–873 of Black and Matassarin-Jacobs: *Medical-Surgical Nursing: Clinical Management for Continuity of Care,* 5th ed.)

Cushing's Syndrome

OVERVIEW

- Cushing's syndrome results from overactivity of the adrenal gland, resulting in hypersecretion of glucocorticoids.
- When Cushing's syndrome develops, the normal function of the glucocorticoids becomes exaggerated and the classic picture of the syndrome emerges.
- Cushing's syndrome occurs mainly in women.
- Average age of onset is 20–40 years of age.
- Hypersecretion of cortisol can be caused by:
  — adrenal tumor (85 per cent are benign)
  — adrenal hyperplasia caused by overproduction of ACTH secondary to pituitary hypersecretion and pituitary tumors.
  — administration of exogenous steroids

CLINICAL MANIFESTATIONS

- persistent hyperglycemia
- weakness
- ecchymosis (secondary to capillary fragility)
- osteoporosis (due to bone matrix wasting), compression fractures, stress fractures
- hypokalemia
- hypertension, edema (due to sodium and water retention)
- abnormal fat distribution
  — moon-shaped face
  — dorsocervical fat pad (buffalo hump)
  — truncal obesity with slender limbs
- pink and purple striae appear on the breasts, axillary areas, abdomen, and legs

- increased susceptibility to infection
- decreased resistance to stress
- poor wound healing
- virilism in women, including acne, thinning of scalp hair, and hirsutism
- memory loss, poor concentration, euphoria, and depression

ACUTE AND SUBACUTE CARE

Medical Management

- radiation therapy for pituitary tumors and adenomas
  - — external
  - — internal—transphenoidal implant (approach through the inner aspect of the upper lip to implant radiation seeds)
- cytoxic antihormonal agents—interfere with ACTH production or adrenal hormone synthesis (Lysoderm)
- ACTH-reducing agents—cyproheptadine (Periactin)

Surgical Management

Surgical management is the treatment of choice.

- transphenoidal hypophysectomy (approach through the inner aspect of the upper lip for pituitary tumor removal)
- adrenalectomy (removal of adrenal glands)

Nursing Management

Medical

- Monitor closely for signs/symptoms of infection. (Glucocorticoids suppress immune and inflammatory reactions. Cushing's syndrome clients may experience only mild symptoms even in the presence of severe infection.)
- Protect against falls and accidents.
- Monitor vital signs, assess for hypertension.
- Daily weights.
- Monitor intake and output.
- Monitor electrolytes and blood glucose.
- Initiate a progressive activity schedule and assess client's response.

- Monitor skin for breakdown (extremely prone to breakdown secondary to tissue catabolism).
- Reassure client and significant others that mood swings and changes in appearance should gradually return to normal with treatment.

Surgical

In addition to routine postoperative care:

- Adrenalectomy
  - — Monitor for signs of shock (due to hemorrhage).
  - — Administer corticosteroids as prescribed to protect from acute adrenal insufficiency. Even if only one adrenal gland is removed, temporary corticoid support may be needed until remaining gland begins to secrete sufficient amounts of cortisol.
  - — Monitor for signs of Addisonian crisis
    - sudden profound weakness
    - severe abdominal, back, and leg pain
    - hyperpyrexia followed by hypothermia
    - coma
    - renal shutdown
  - — Monitor for signs of wound or respiratory infection.
- Transphenoidal hypophysectomy
  - — Assess for signs of cerebral edema and rising intracranial pressure (elevated blood pressure, widened pulse pressure, bradycardia, altered respiratory pattern).
  - — Monitor for signs of target gland deficiencies (pituitary no longer produces tropic hormones):
    - adrenal insufficiency
    - hypothyroidism
    - diabetes insipidus (ADH deficiency)
  - — Assess for signs of meningitis (elevated temperature, headache, irritability, nuchal rigidity).
  - — Provide frequent oral hygiene.
  - — Observe client for rhinorrhea after nasal packing removed—can indicate a cerebrospinal fluid leak.

COMMUNITY AND SELF-CARE

Instruct client regarding:

- importance of taking daily replacement hormone
- medication injection technique if client not able to tolerate oral medications
- signs of under- and over-dosage
- need to call for dosage adjustment if experiencing physical or emotional stress
- dietary modifications—low-calorie, low-sodium, low-carbohydrate diet with ample protein and potassium
- post hypophysectomy
  - need to report persistent postnasal drainage
  - need to avoid sneezing, coughing, and bending from the waist for specified period of time
  - need for Medic Alert bracelet or card

(For more information, see pp. 2049–2055 of Black and Matassarin-Jacobs: *Medical-Surgical Nursing: Clinical Management for Continuity of Care,* 5th ed.)

Cystic Fibrosis

OVERVIEW

- Cystic fibrosis (CF) is a hereditary, chronic disease characterized by abnormal secretion of the exocrine glands.
- Pancreatic exocrine function is affected by decreased lipase released into the bowel. This results in malabsorption of lipids and causes blockage of the pancreatic ducts with thick mucous. Pancreatic degeneration, fibrosis, and atrophy of tissues follow, with eventual development of fatty infiltration and loss of function. The lack of pancreatic enzyme causes steatorrhea.
- Pulmonary symptoms are the most obvious complications and develop secondary to increased viscosity of bronchial secretions with subsequent obstruction of glandular ducts. These clients have respiratory compromise with frequent bronchopneumonia and chronic bronchitis.

CLINICAL MANIFESTATIONS

- small stature, appear emaciated
- barrel-chested
- clubbed fingers
- steatorrhea

ACUTE AND SUBACUTE CARE

Medical Management

- dietary modifications
- pancreatic enzyme administration
- fat soluble vitamins
- respiratory complication management
  — pulmonary hygiene
  — IV antibiotics

Nursing Management

- Assess respiratory status and implement pulmonary hygiene measures.
- Monitor arterial blood gas results.
- Administer supplemental oxygen and monitor oxygen saturations.
- Administer antibiotic therapy.
- Suction PRN and instruct on self-suctioning technique.
- Administer pancreatic enzyme replacement.
- Encourage dietary management—high protein, high calorie, high salt, low fat.

COMMUNITY AND SELF-CARE

Instruct client regarding:
- importance of pulmonary hygiene
- pancreatic enzyme replacement therapy
- dietary modifications
- importance of follow-up visits
- Refer to available community resources.

(For more information, see p. 1932 of Black and Matassarin-Jacobs: *Medical-Surgical Nursing: Clinical Management for Continuity of Care,* 5th ed.)

D

Deep Vein Thrombosis

OVERVIEW

- Deep vein thrombosis (DVT) refers to thrombophlebitis of the deep veins. Veins damaged by deep vein thrombosis increase the risk for another DVT, pulmonary embolism, and venous stasis ulcers.
- Thrombus development is a localized process. It begins by platelet adherence to the endothelium. As the thrombi become larger in diameter and length, they obstruct the vein.
- Etiologic factors for thrombus formation include:
  (1) venous stasis
    — causes
      - immobilization without normal calf muscle use
      - obesity
      - pregnancy
      - congestive heart failure
  (2) hypercoagulability
    — causes
      - malignant neoplasms
      - dehydration
      - blood dyscrasias
      - oral contraceptives
  (3) injury to the vein wall
    — causes
      - intravenous injection
      - Buerger's disease
      - fractures and dislocations
      - certain antibiotics
- DVT is more common in women than men. About one-third of clients over 40 years of age who have had major surgery or an acute myocardial infarction develop DVT.
- Risk factors associated with DVT include:
  — surgery
  — age > 40 years

— immobility
— congestive heart failure
— myocardial infarction
— malignancy
— history of DVT
— pregnancy
— trauma
— estrogen therapy or oral contraceptives
— obesity
— varicose veins

- Pulmonary emboli, most of which start as thrombi in the large deep veins of the leg, are an acute and potentially lethal complication of DVT. Usually 24–48 hours after formation, thrombi undergo lysis or become organized and adhere to the vessel wall, diminishing the risk of embolization.
- Measures to prevent DVT include:
  — active and passive range of motion exercises if immobilized
  — early postoperative ambulation
  — postoperative deep-breathing exercises
  — compression stockings
  — avoidance of standing or sitting in one position for prolonged periods
  — intermittent sequential pneumatic compression (IPC) devices
  — pharmacologic prevention with warfarin, platelet antiaggregation agents, heparin, and dextran

CLINICAL MANIFESTATIONS

- may be asymptomatic
- pain in the region of the thrombus
- unilateral swelling distal to the site
- redness and warmth of the leg
- dilated veins
- low-grade fever
- the first manifestation may be signs/symptoms of a pulmonary embolism
- positive Homan's sign—pain in upper calf during forced dorsiflexion of the foot

ACUTE AND SUBACUTE CARE

Medical Management

- bedrest with leg elevation—5–7 days of bedrest allows the thrombus to adhere to the vein wall and decreases embolization
- anticoagulation therapy to prevent clot extension (does not induce thrombolysis)—IV heparin course followed by oral warfarin sodium (Coumadin)
- fibrinolytic agents—dissolve thrombi (streptokinase, urokinase)

Surgical Management

- venous thrombectomy—direct removal of venous thrombi, now rarely performed
- umbrella procedure—under local anesthesia, a filter or an umbrella is inserted into the vena cava to trap emboli

Nursing Management

- Maintain bedrest and provide good skin care.
- Administer anticoagulant therapy and titrate as ordered according to partial thromboplastin (PTT) levels (therapeutic PTT values are usually 1.5–2.0 times normal control levels).
- Administer thrombolytic therapy as ordered. See "Peripheral Vascular Disease: Chronic Arterial," p. 556.
- Encourage in-bed exercises for all but affected limb.
- Administer analgesics.
- Elevate legs above the level of the heart to facilitate blood flow and decrease venous pressure.
- Apply elastic wraps/stockings as ordered.
- Administer warm packs around involved area.
- Initiate Coumadin as ordered (Coumadin takes 24–48 hours to take effect; therefore, heparin is continued until therapeutic level is reached).
- Monitor prothrombin time (PT) to determine Coumadin dose.
  - PT must be measured every day before Coumadin is administered.
  - A PT of 1.3 to 1.5 times the normal control is desired.

— If International normalized ratio (INR) is used to monitor coagulation, the therapeutic level is 2.0–3.0.

- Monitor for manifestations of excess anticoagulation
  - — blood in urine, stool, nasogastric contents
  - — bleeding gums
  - — subcutaneous bruising
  - — flank pain
  - — epistaxis
- Apply pressure to puncture sites.
- Initiate appropriate bleeding precautions.
- Monitor for signs/symptoms of a pulmonary embolus
  - — pleuritic-type chest pain with sudden onset and aggravated by breathing
  - — hemoptysis
  - — cough
  - — diaphoresis
  - — dyspnea
  - — apprehension
- Advance activity as ordered.

COMMUNITY AND SELF-CARE

Instruct client regarding:

- disease process and treatment regime
- the importance of long-term anticoagulation therapy (3–6 months)
- signs of hypocoagulation and need to report to physician
  - — bleeding gums
  - — blood in urine or stool
  - — nosebleed
  - — inability to stop bleeding from a minor cut
- safety measures to prevent bleeding
  - — soft toothbrush
  - — electric razor
  - — fall prevention
  - — gloves when doing yard work
- measures to prevent recurrence of DVT
  - — avoid standing or sitting for long periods of time
  - — no crossing legs
  - — no constrictive clothing
  - — elevate legs when sitting

— elastic stockings
- importance of wearing Medic-Alert identification
- need to alert dentist and physician of anticoagulation status

(For more information, see pp. 1432–1436 of Black and Matassarin-Jacobs: *Medical-Surgical Nursing: Clinical Management for Continuity of Care,* 5th ed.)

Dermatitis, Atopic

OVERVIEW

- Atopic dermatitis is a common, chronic, relapsing, pruritic type of eczema. The word "atopic" refers to a group of three associated allergic disorders: asthma, allergic rhinitis (hay fever), and atopic dermatitis.
- The exact cause of atopic dermatitis is unknown. However, 75–80 per cent of clients with this disorder have a personal or family history of allergic disorders.
- Atopic dermatitis affects 0.5–1 per cent of people around the world.
- Complications may include development of viral, bacterial, and fungal skin infections.

CLINICAL MANIFESTATIONS

Acute form (may begin in infancy)
- red, oozing, crusting rash

Chronic form
- thickened, dry texture of the skin
- brownish-gray color and scales on the skin
- localized areas of rash as client ages; found on elbow bends, back of knees, neck, sides of face, eyelids and the back of hands and feet
- pruritus, which can lead to excoriated lesions, infection, and scarring

ACUTE AND SUBACUTE CARE

Medical Management

- daily skin care to hydrate and lubricate the skin (may be accomplished by soaks and wet wraps)

- identification and elimination of factors causing flare-ups
- topical corticosteroids, occlusives, moisturizers, or tar preparations
- systemic antibiotics and antihistamines
- a short course of oral steroids may be used, though rarely
- dietary restriction of known allergens (common allergens are eggs, cow's milk, soy, wheat, nuts, and fish)

Nursing Management

- Instruct client to bathe at least once daily for 15–20 minutes. Apply prescribed emollient or topical preparations within 2–4 minutes after the bath before drying. Elderly clients do not need to bathe daily but should use moisturizers.
- Use only warm water—never hot.
- Apply prescribed topical preparations 2 to 3 times per day.
- Instruct client not to scratch and to keep fingernails short, smooth, and clean.
- Encourage client and significant others to share feelings with each other regarding the client's appearance and the chronic nature of eczema.
- Reinforce client's sense of identity and self esteem.
- Encourage client to teach others that eczema is not contagious unless severely infected.

COMMUNITY AND SELF-CARE

Instruct client regarding:
- use of superfatted soaps
- avoidance of bubble bath
- washing all clothes before wearing to remove formaldehyde and other chemicals
- avoidance of fabric softeners
- use of mild detergent and adding second rinse cycle
- wearing light cotton-blend clothing
- maintaining surroundings at 68–75 degrees and humidity at 45–55 per cent
- use of sunscreen
- signs of infection and to report these to physician

- how to determine need for treatment modalities, e.g., when to initiate wet wraps
- avoidance of known allergens
- medications—use and side effects
- techniques for self care (e.g., use of topicals, wet wraps)

(For more information, see pp. 2209–2210 of Black and Matassarin-Jacobs: *Medical-Surgical Nursing: Clinical Management for Continuity of Care,* 5th ed.)

Dermatitis, Contact

- Contact dermatitis is an inflammatory response of the skin to chemical or physical allergens.
- Clinical manifestations range from mild erythema or vesicles to ulceration.
- Management includes determination of the causative agent and use of topical medications, wet dressings, antihistamines, or steroids.

(For more information, see pp. 2209–2210 of Black and Matassarin-Jacobs: *Medical-Surgical Nursing: Clinical Management for Continuity of Care,* 5th ed.)

Dermatitis, Stasis

- Stasis dermatitis is the development of areas of very dry skin and sometimes shallow ulcers (stasis ulcers) on the lower legs primarily due to venous insufficiency.
- The process of dermatitis begins with edema of the leg due to slowed venous return (clients usually have a history of varicose veins or deep vein thrombosis). As venous stasis continues, the tissue becomes hypoxic from inadequate blood supply. As the blood pools, hemoglobin is released from the red blood cells and deposited in the tissues. The tissues begin to necrose and are very slow to heal because of the lack of oxygenated blood.

- Clinical manifestations are itching, brown-stained skin, a feeling of heaviness in the legs, and open shallow lesions.
- Treatment includes wet to dry dressings for debridement of the area, Unna's boot, and skin grafts.
- Nursing management includes instructing the client on ways to promote venous return: leg elevation, support hose, and avoidance of standing or sitting in one position for long periods of time.

(For more information, see pp. 2207–2208 of Black and Matassarin-Jacobs: *Medical-Surgical Nursing: Clinical Management for Continuity of Care, 5th ed.)*

Diabetes Insipidus

OVERVIEW

- Diabetes insipidus (DI) is a deficiency of antidiuretic hormone (ADH) resulting in the inability to conserve water.
- The major functions of ADH are to: (1) promote water reabsorption by the kidneys, and (2) control the osmotic pressure of the extracellular fluid. When ADH production decreases excessively, the kidney tubules fail to reabsorb water and, consequently, the client excretes large amounts of dilute urine.
- Causes of DI are categorized as:
  - — central or neurogenic—CNS interruption of the anatomic integrity of the posterior pituitary; localized or generalized edema from trauma; vascular lesions
  - —complete—disruption to the hypophyseal tract and complete absence of ADH
  - —nephrogenic—an inherited defect, the kidneys cannot respond to ADH
  - —idiopathic—unknown cause
- Risk factors for diabetes insipidus include:
  - — head injury
  - — neurosurgery
  - — hypothalamic tumors
  - — pituitary tumors

- certain medications—Dilantin, lithium, and narcotic antagonists
- CNS infection

CLINICAL MANIFESTATIONS

- polyuria
- polydypsia—client must drink fluid almost continuously to avoid severe dehydration and hypovolemic shock
- dry cool skin, dry mucous membranes
- tachycardia
- weight loss
- excretion of urine with abnormally low specific gravity

ACUTE AND SUBACUTE CARE

Medical Management

- vasopressin or synthetic ADH to control polydypsia and polyuria
- fluid therapy

Surgical Management

- If diabetes insipidus is secondary to a tumor, excision of the tumor may be curative.

Nursing Management

Medical

- Strict intake and output.
- Monitor electrolyte levels.
- Maintain adequate hydration.

Surgical

- If client undergoes surgical resection of a pituitary tumor, see nursing care for the hypophysectomy patient, "Pituitary Tumors," p. 567.

COMMUNITY AND SELF-CARE

Instruct client regarding:

- importance of vasopressin therapy
- signs of under- or over-dosage
- when to seek medical attention

(For more information, see pp. 2067–2068 of Black and Matassarin-Jacobs: *Medical-Surgical Nursing: Clinical Management for Continuity of Care,* 5th ed.)

Diabetes Mellitus

OVERVIEW

- Diabetes mellitus is a metabolic disorder characterized by glucose intolerance. It is a systemic disease caused by an imbalance between insulin supply and insulin demand.
- Insulin is produced by the pancreas and normally maintains the balance between high and low blood glucose levels. In diabetes mellitus, either there is not enough insulin or the insulin that is produced is ineffective, resulting in high blood glucose levels.
- Diabetes mellitus also causes disturbances of protein and fat metabolism, which are associated with microvascular, macrovascular, and neuropathic changes.
- There are two main types of diabetes mellitus:
  (1) Insulin dependent diabetes mellitus (IDDM) Type I—also called juvenile diabetes, labile or brittle diabetes. It usually occurs before 30 years of age, but may occur at any age. There is little or no endogenous insulin production and insulin injections are required. It is believed to be caused from:
    — genetic predisposition
    — autoimmune response causing the body to develop islet cell antibodies and anti-insulin antibodies. The antibodies attack the beta cells of the pancreas where insulin is produced and the insulin molecules themselves.
    — certain viral diseases common in the spring and fall are etiologic factors in clients who are predisposed.
  (2) Non-insulin dependent diabetes mellitus (NIDDM) Type II—also called adult onset or mild diabetes. Usually occurs in clients over 30 years of age but can occur in children. There is

below normal, normal, or above normal insulin production with insulin injections being required in only 20–30 per cent of clients. Hyperglycemia develops when the pancreas cannot secrete enough insulin to match the body's needs or when the number of insulin receptor sites is decreased or altered (as in obesity). It is believed to be caused from:
— genetic predisposition
— obesity
— increasing age (the pancreas becomes more sluggish)

- Metabolic effects of diabetes include:
  — decreased utilization of glucose—since insulin is needed as a carrier for glucose to go into the cells, glucose remains in the blood, and glucose levels rise
  — increased fat metabolism—the body breaks down fat for energy since glucose is not available. Fat metabolism produces ketones, which can lead to metabolic acidosis
  — increased protein utilization—without insulin to stimulate protein synthesis, there is increased catabolism and, therefore, protein wasting
- Complications of diabetes include:
  — neuropathy—nerve fibers do not receive adequate nutrients and oxygen across the membrane, so transmission of nerve impulses slows. Also, sorbitol accumulates in the nerve tissue affecting sensory and motor function. Clients may experience pain or tingling in the extremities; inability to perceive pain (especially in the lower extremities); paresthesias; sensory loss; and decreased or absent reflexes. Autonomic neuropathy also can develop which may manifest itself as: gastroparesis (slowed digestion); inability to recognize hypoglycemic symptoms; urinary incontinence or retention; orthostatic hypotension; and impotence in males.
  — retinopathy—microangiopathy or vascular degeneration of the small vessels supplying the eyes eventually can lead to partial or total permanent blindness
  — nephropathy—damage and eventual obliteration of the capillaries supplying the glomerulus

leads to pathologic changes that cause renal disease and possibly chronic renal failure
  - cataracts, glaucoma, pyelonephritis and infections—these are more common in diabetic clients
  - peripheral vascular lesions, coronary artery disease, stroke, and hypertension—may result from disorders of the macrocirculation
- There are approximately 14 million Americans with diabetes and 7 million of these are undiagnosed. Eighty-five to 90 per cent of clients are non-insulin dependent (NIDDM).
- Diabetes with its complications is the third leading cause of death by disease in the United States.
- Risk factors for Type II DM include a family history of diabetes, age, ethnicity, android (upper body or apple-type) fat distribution, dietary habits, lack of exercise, gestational diabetes, female with hirsuitism, and/or polycystic ovarian disease, and obesity.
- The prevalence of Type II DM has increased in American Indians, Blacks, Hispanics, and the elderly.

CLINICAL MANIFESTATIONS

- polyuria—frequent urination (glucose acts as an osmotic diuretic and pulls fluid with it when excreted through the kidneys)
- polydipsia—excessive thirst due to fluid loss
- polyphagia—hunger due to unavailability of glucose for energy
- weight loss—due to protein wasting
- recurrent blurred vision
- pruritus, skin infections, vaginitis
- ketonuria
- weakness, fatigue, dizziness

ACUTE AND SUBACUTE CARE

Medical Management

Diabetes management must be individualized and take into account the client's age, maturity, lifestyle, nutritional needs, activity level, occupation and ability to independently perform the skills required by the treatment plan.

- dietary regulation, discouraging foods with high sugar and fat content and correction of or avoidance of obesity
- oral hypoglycemic agents (sulfonylurea) for some NIDDM clients
- insulin therapy—required for IDDM clients and may be required for some NIDDM clients if diet, exercise and oral hypoglycemic agents are ineffective
- exercise regime

Surgical Management

- pancreas transplant—usually performed for clients who have IDDM and who have had a kidney transplant

Nursing Management

- Discuss the basic pathophysiologic mechanism of diabetes mellitus—monitor for responses of denial or anger in the newly diagnosed client.
- Consult physician before starting an exercise program.
- Monitor blood glucose levels by meter or laboratory as ordered. Ensure accuracy of meter results by performing controls and quality control measures as outlined by your health care institution.
- Monitor for signs/symptoms of hypoglycemia (especially at times of peak insulin action) or hyperglycemia and treat accordingly (see "Hypoglycemia," p. 395, and "Hyperglycemia and Diabetic Ketoacidosis," p. 368).
- Be aware that "feeding" a client for hypoglycemia may be ineffective in a client with gastroparesis and subcutaneous or intravenous treatment may be necessary (instruct client and significant other also).
- Ensure that the client receives meals as ordered. If meals are missed due to NPO status, replace meals with IV $D_{10}W$ or adjust insulin doses as ordered.
- Administer insulin injections and supplemental doses as needed for high blood sugars, according to physician orders.
- Be aware that a client with autonomic nervous system neuropathy may not demonstrate any signs/

symptoms of hypoglycemia during a hypoglycemic reaction (instruct client and significant other on this).

- Develop an individualized teaching plan, including client and significant others, that addresses the following (as appropriate to client's needs):
  - — blood glucose monitoring—visually or with meter
  - — include when to test, technique, goals for good control, how to read test results, what to do for abnormal results and quality control measures
  - — urine ketone testing and dangers of ketones
  - — normal blood sugar range
  - — dietary management (obtain Dietician consult)
- If on oral hypoglycemic agents or insulin, discuss:
  - — eating meals and snacks at regular times and in amounts prescribed
  - — caloric intake:
    - 50–60 per cent from carbohydrates
    - less than 30 per cent from fat
    - 20–35 grams of fiber per day
    - 10–20 per cent from protein
    - 15–30 grams of carbohydrate prior to exercise
  - — sick day rules
  - — insulin administration
    - times of peak action
    - insulin storage
    - preparation and injection
    - site selection and rotation
    - techniques for self-injection
  - — use of oral hypoglycemic agents and side effects
  - — foot care is very important in diabetes to decrease the risk of infection. Foot care includes:
    - daily inspection of feet for trauma, injury
    - wearing properly fitting shoes and avoiding tight hoisery
    - washing feet and drying especially between the toes
    - nail care by trained professionals.
  - — regular planned exercise program, effects of exercise and ways to compensate
  - — signs/symptoms of hypoglycemia/hyperglycemia and management (see "Hypoglycemia," p.

395, and "Hyperglycemia and Diabetic Ketoacidosis," p. 368)
- — glucagon administration by significant other
- — need to always carry fast-acting sugar for treatment of hypoglycemia
- — complications of diabetes and when to call physician

COMMUNITY AND SELF-CARE

- Instruct client regarding information included under "Nursing Management." Be sure the regimen has been individualized to client's typical daily routine.
- Discuss need for follow-up care and to maintain log of daily glucose levels and insulin.
- Instruct to obtain a Medic-Alert bracelet, necklace or to carry an identification card.
- Assess need for follow-up with home health care agency.
- Refer to American Diabetes Association as appropriate.

See also "Hypoglycemia," p. 395; "Hyperglycemia and Diabetic Ketoacidosis," p. 368; and "Hyperglycemic, Hyperosmolar, Nonketotic Coma," p. 371.

(For more information, see pp. 1955–1981 of Black and Matassarin-Jacobs: *Medical-Surgical Nursing: Clinical Management for Continuity of Care,* 5th ed.)

Diabetic Retinopathy

OVERVIEW

- Diabetic retinopathy is a progressive disorder of the retina characterized by microscopic damage to the retinal vessels, resulting in occlusion of the vessels. As a result of inadequate blood supply, sections of the retina deteriorate, and vision is permanently lost.
- Diabetic retinopathy is one of the leading causes of blindness worldwide.

- All diabetics are prone to develop retinopathy, and studies indicate a strong correlation between the incidence and severity of retinopathy with both the duration of the disease and erratic blood glucose control.

CLINICAL MANIFESTATIONS

- wide range of visual disturbances
- experience black spots or floaters (areas of ischemia become blind spots)
- decreased central vision

ACUTE AND SUBACUTE CARE

Medical Management

None

Surgical Management

- argon laser treatment to photocoagulate blood vessels
- vitrectomy (removal of a portion of the vitreous)

Nursing Management

Postoperative Care

In addition to routine postoperative care:
- Monitor for signs of increased intraocular pressure (nausea, pain).
- Monitor blood glucose levels.
- Assist with ambulation and activities of daily living.
- Discuss measures to prevent increased intraocular pressure—see below.

COMMUNITY AND SELF-CARE

- Instruct client regarding:
  — progressive nature of disease
  — importance of maintaining stable blood glucose levels
  — measures to prevent increased intraocular pressure:
    - no lifting heavy objects
    - no straining with stool
    - no bending from the waist

- avoidance of coughing and vomiting
- importance of follow-up clinic appointments
- safety measures for the home environment
- Refer to available community resources.

(For more information, see pp. 964–965 of Black and Matassarin-Jacobs: *Medical-Surgical Nursing: Clinical Management for Continuity of Care,* 5th ed.)

Dialysis

OVERVIEW

- Dialysis is used to relieve symptoms of renal failure temporarily until the client regains kidney function, or to sustain life in the client with irreversible kidney disease.
- Goals of dialysis therapy are to:
  - remove the end products of protein metabolism from the blood
  - maintain a safe concentration of serum electrolytes
  - correct acidosis and replenish the blood's bicarbonate buffer system
  - remove excess fluid from the blood.
- There are two types of dialysis:

  (1) Peritoneal dialysis involves repeated cycles of instilling dialysate into the peritoneal cavity through a catheter, allowing time for substance exchange and then removing the dialysate.
  - There are two types of peritoneal dialysis:

    (a) Continuous Ambulatory Peritoneal Dialysis (CAPD)—the dialysate is instilled into the abdomen and left in place for 4–10 hours. The empty bag is disconnected and carried with the client until it is time to drain the dialysate. The dialysate is drained into the bag, and the process usually is repeated four times in 24 hours.

    (b) Automated Peritoneal Dialysis (APD)—similar to CAPD but requires a peritoneal cycling machine.

- Continuous Cycle Peritoneal Dialysis (CCPD)—three cycles at night and one in the morning.
- Intermittent Peritoneal Dialysis—dialysis is performed for 10–14 hours, 3–4 times weekly, with use of a peritoneal cycling machine.

— Complications of peritoneal dialysis include peritonitis, catheter displacement or plugging.

— Pain during peritoneal dialysis may result from rapid instillation, incorrect dialysate temperature or pH, dialysate accumulation under the diaphragm, or excessive suction during outflow.

(2) Hemodialysis involves diverting toxic-laden blood from the client into a dialyzer and then returning clean blood to the client. Hemodialysis clears waste products from the body; restores fluid, electrolyte and acid base balance; and reverses some of the untoward manifestations of irreversible renal failure.

— The major routes of access are external arteriovenous shunts for acute dialysis and internal arteriovenous fistulas and grafts for chronic dialysis.

— Hemodialysis for irreversible renal failure must be done for the client's lifetime unless a transplant is performed.

— A typical schedule is 3–4 hours of treatment, 3 days per week.

— Complications include hypotension, hypertension, cardiac dysrhythmias from potassium imbalance, air embolus, hemorrhage from heparinization, muscle cramps, infection, hepatitis B, dialysis disequilibrium syndrome (develops as a result of rapid changes in the composition of extracellular fluid and involves nausea, vomiting, mental confusion, deterioration of the level of consciousness, twitching, headache, and seizures), and restless legs syndrome (an irresistible urge to move the legs when awake and inactive, especially just prior to falling asleep; clients report a creeping, crawling sensation in their calves that is only relieved by movement, particularly walking). Aluminum intoxication—accumulation from phosphate binding.

ACUTE AND SUBACUTE CARE

NURSING MANAGEMENT

- Monitor for fluid volume excess or deficit:
  - — intake and output
  - — vital signs, including postural blood pressure
  - — obtain weights pre- and post-dialysis.
- Encourage client/family to discuss feelings regarding chronic illness, chronic dialysis, and changes in lifestyle and body image.
- Peritoneal Dialysis:
  - — Assess for signs/symptoms of infection or peritonitis.
  - — Maintain aseptic technique when accessing peritoneal catheter.
  - — Keep dressing dry at all times.
  - — Relieve discomfort by slowing the rate of flow, lowering the head of the bed, massaging the abdomen, or repositioning the client.
  - — Provide small frequent meals if abdominal distention is present.
  - — Encourage turning, coughing, and deep breathing (the client is at increased risk for respiratory problems due to increased pressure and reduced excursion of the diaphragm).
- Hemodialysis:
  - — Maintain a sterile dressing over the access site.
  - — Protect the access site from trauma that may cause clotting, bleeding, or physical disruption of the device.
  - — No blood pressures or laboratory draws on affected side.
  - — Wash fistula or graft site with warm soap and water between dialysis treatments.
- See also "Renal Failure, Chronic," p. 618, and "Renal Failure, Acute," p. 615.

COMMUNITY AND SELF-CARE

- Instruct client regarding:

— set-up and maintenance of dialysis and signs/symptoms to report to physician
— hemodialysis regimen and signs/symptoms to report to physician
— care of catheters, fistula, or graft as appropriate
— possible changes in lifestyle and activities

- Make referrals to support groups as needed.
- Make referral to home health care agency as needed.

See also "Renal Failure, Chronic," p. 618 and "Renal Failure, Acute," p. 615 for related information.

(For more information, see pp. 1647–1660 of Black and Matassarin-Jacobs: *Medical-Surgical Nursing: Clinical Management for Continuity of Care,* 5th ed.)

Dislocation and Subluxation

OVERVIEW

- Dislocation and subluxation are both displacements of a joint from its normal position. Dislocation is the separation of both articulating surfaces. Subluxation occurs when the articulating surfaces lose partial contact. These injuries usually occur from direct or indirect pressure to the joint.
- The displaced bone may impede blood supply, tear ligaments, rupture blood vessels, damage nerves, or rupture muscle attachments.

CLINICAL MANIFESTATIONS

- deformity of affected extremity
- altered length of extremity
- joint pain and loss of function

ACUTE AND SUBACUTE CARE

Medical Management

- closed reduction followed by immobilization with a splint or cast—see "Fracture, General Information," p. 279

Surgical Management

- open reduction — see "Fracture, General Information," p. 279

Nursing Management

- Administer analgesics.
- Monitor for signs/symptoms of nerve damage — paresthesias, numbness, paralysis.
- Monitor for signs of impeded blood supply — coolness, pain, pallor.
- Collaborate with Physical Therapy for prescribed exercises and adaptive devices.
- See "Casts," p. 131, for cast care.

COMMUNITY AND SELF-CARE

- Instruct client regarding:
  - — prescribed exercises
  - — signs/symptoms of complications
- See "Casts," p. 131.

(For more information, see pp. 2161–2164 of Black and Matassarin-Jacobs: *Medical-Surgical Nursing: Clinical Management for Continuity of Care,* 5th ed.)

Disseminated Intravascular Coagulation (DIC)

OVERVIEW

- Disseminated intravascular coagulation (DIC) is a complex coagulation disorder characterized by two apparently conflicting manifestations: (1) diffuse fibrin disposition within arterioles and capillaries, with resultant widespread clotting, and (2) hemorrhage from the kidneys, brain, adrenals, heart, and other organs.
- DIC is characterized by the following chain of events:

  (1) Certain disease states cause the release of thromboplastic substances that activate thrombin, which activates fibrinogen and results in

deposition of fibrin throughout the microcirculation.

(2) Platelet aggregation is increased; this enables fibrin clots and microthrombi to form in the brain, kidneys, heart, etc.

(3) Red blood cells become trapped in the fibrin strands and are destroyed (hemolysis).

(4) Platelets, prothrombin, and clotting factors are consumed in the process, which compromises coagulation and predisposes to bleeding.

(5) Excessive clotting activates the fibrinolytic mechanism, which causes the production of fibrin degradation products that inhibit platelet clotting functions and cause further bleeding.

(6) With clots being lysed and clotting factors depleted, the blood loses its ability to clot.

- Conditions that precipitate DIC include:
  — shock
  — cirrhosis
  — transfusion reaction
  — glomerulonephritis
  — hepatitis (acute fulminant)
  — acute bacterial and viral infections
  — tissue damage due to trauma, burns, transplant rejection, or surgery
  — neoplasms
- The prognosis for DIC varies from self-limiting to death within days.

CLINICAL MANIFESTATIONS

Onset is usually acute and develops within hours to days after the initial assault to the body system.

- purpura
- petechiae
- ecchymosis
- prolonged bleeding from venipuncture sites
- uncontrolled hemorrhage during surgery or childbirth
- oliguria and renal failure
- convulsions, coma
- prolonged prothrombin time, low platelet count

ACUTE AND SUBACUTE CARE

Medical Management

- identification/treatment of underlying cause
- heparin therapy (use is controversial)
- fresh frozen plasma and platelet infusions
- packed red blood cell administration
- cryoprecipitate infusion for depletion of factors V and VIII
- aminocaproic acid (Amicar)

Nursing Management

- Administer ordered therapies.
- Assess all body systems for signs/symptoms of bleeding.
- Monitor laboratory results—prothrombin time, partial thromboplastin time, platelet count, CBC.
- Institute bleeding precautions:
  — no intramuscular or subcutaneous injections
  — apply pressure to venipuncture sites
  — reposition frequently and gently
  — no aspirin or nonsteroidal anti-inflammatory drugs.

COMMUNITY AND SELF-CARE

The condition will be resolved prior to discharge, and care will be based on underlying etiologic factor(s).

(For more information, see pp. 151—1512 of Black and Matassarin-Jacobs: *Medical-Surgical Nursing: Clinical Management for Continuity of Care,* 5th ed.)

Diverticular Disease

OVERVIEW

- A diverticulum is a blind outpouching or herniation of intestinal mucosa through the muscular coat of the large intestine. Diverticular disease is a term used to describe diverticulosis and diverticulitis.

- Diverticulosis is the presence of non-inflamed outpouchings (diverticulum) in the intestine. It is caused by atrophy or weakness of the bowel muscle, increased intraluminal pressure, obesity or chronic constipation.
- Diverticulitis is inflammation of a diverticulum. It occurs when undigested food blocks the diverticulum, leading to a decrease in blood supply to the area, predisposing the bowel to invasion of bacteria into the diverticulum.
- Risk factors include:
  — chronic constipation (usually due to a low fiber diet) for diverticulosis
  — ingestion of indigestible roughage (e.g., corn, popcorn, vegetables with seeds) for diverticulitis.

CLINICAL MANIFESTATIONS

- episodic, dull or steady left quadrant or mid-abdominal pain
- constipation, diarrhea or both
- increased flatus
- mucous in the stools
- rectal bleeding in 15 per cent of clients
- anorexia
- low grade fever

ACUTE AND SUBACUTE CARE

Medical Management

- Asymptomatic disease
  — high fiber diet
  — prevention of constipation
- Diverticulitis
  — NPO, nasogastric suctioning, antibiotics and parenteral fluids until inflammation decreases

Nursing Management

- Acute management
  — Keep client NPO.
  — Maintain nasogastric tube to suction
  — Administer IV antibiotics.
  — Slowly progress diet as symptoms subside.

COMMUNITY AND SELF-CARE

Instruct client regarding:

- prescribed antibiotics
- high fiber diet and avoidance of popcorn, seeds, or corn
- prevention of constipation with bran and bulk laxatives (hydrophilic colloids)
- drinking at least 8 glasses of water daily
- weight reduction (if obese)
- avoidance of activities that increase intra-abdominal pressure, such as bending, lifting, stooping, coughing, or vomiting
- notification of physician of any changes in bowel patterns (constipation or diarrhea) or stools (presence of mucous or blood), or if fever, abdominal pain, or urinary symptoms develop

(For more information, see pp. 1818–1819 of Black and Matassarin-Jacobs: *Medical-Surgical Nursing: Clinical Management for Continuity of Care,* 5th ed.)

Dysmenorrhea

OVERVIEW

- Dysmenorrhea is painful menstrual flow.
- Primary—caused by prostaglandin excess or increased sensitivity to prostaglandins with no pathologic pelvic disorder.
- Secondary—begins with an underlying disease condition.
- Risk factors for primary dysmenorrhea include:
  - — elevated uterine prostaglandins
  - — endocrine factors
  - — myometrial factors
  - — biochemical factors
  - — psychosocial factors
  - — obese, sedentary women
- Risk factors for secondary dysmenorrhea include:
  - — pelvic inflammatory disease (PID)
  - — endometriosis
  - — adenomyosis
  - — uterine prolapse

— uterine myomas
— polyps

CLINICAL MANIFESTATIONS

PRIMARY

- dysmenorrhea begins 1–2 months after menarche
- usually decreases after childbirth
- prolonged menstrual flow
- discomfort usually begins 1–2 days before onset of menstrual flow
- fifty per cent experience nausea, vomiting, diarrhea, syncope, headache, and leg pain

ACUTE AND SUBACUTE CARE

MEDICAL MANAGEMENT

Primary

- biofeedback, therapeutic touch
- acupuncture
- oral contraceptives
- exercise
- prostaglandin synthesis inhibitors (ibuprofen [Motrin], indomethacin [Indocin])

Secondary

- correct underlying cause

NURSING MANAGEMENT

- Monitor for side effects of medications.
- Supportive care.

COMMUNITY AND SELF-CARE

Instruct client regarding:
- medications and contraceptive therapy
- adequate nutrition, rest, sleep, and exercise
- stress management

(For more information, see pp. 2386–2387 of Black and Matassarin-Jacobs: *Medical-Surgical Nursing: Clinical Management for Continuity of Care,* 5th ed.)

Dysphagia

- Dysphagia is defined as difficulty swallowing and is the most common manifestation of esophageal disease.
- The causes of dysphagia include: neuromotor malfunction; mechanical obstruction; cardiovascular abnormalities; neurologic diseases.
- Cerebrovascular accident (CVA) is the most frequent cause of dysphagia.
- Endoscopy may be performed when food is lodged in the esophagus.
- Other treatment options include swallowing and speech therapy.

(For more information, see p. 1732 of Black and Matassarin-Jacobs: *Medical-Surgical Nursing: Clinical Management for Continuity of Care,* 5th ed.)

Dysrhythmias

OVERVIEW

- Dysrhythmias are common in persons with cardiac disorders, but also occur in persons with normal hearts. The most serious complication of dysrhythmia is sudden death.
- Dysrhythmias result from disturbances in three major mechanisms;
  (1) Automaticity—the sinoatrial (SA) node is the normal pacemaker of the heart. If the SA node fails to initiate an impulse, every other muscle cell in the myocardium can start the impulse. Abnormal automaticity is an unusual condition of latent pacemaker cells in which their firing rate is increased beyond their inherent rate. Enhanced automaticity can cause atrial, junctional, and ventricular ectopic beats and rhythm.
    — Abnormal automaticity is commonly caused by ischemia, hyperkalemia, hypocalcemia, hypoxia, digitalis toxicity, or increase in catecholamines.

(2) Conduction—the speed the impulse travels through the SA node, AV node, and Purkinje fibers. Blocks that slow or stop an impulse can occur anywhere along the pathway. Conduction disturbances can lead to decreased cardiac output and life-threatening dysrhythmias.
— Blocks develop as a result of ischemia of the tissues, scarring of conduction pathways, compression of the AV bundle, electrolyte imbalances, digitalis toxicity, or MI.

(3) Reentry—activation of muscle for a second time by the same impulse. The waves of electrical impulse keep going due to a combination of slow conduction and blocks. The conduction system is delayed or blocked in one or more segments while being conducted normally through the rest.
—Hyperkalemia and myocardial ischemia are the two most common causes of reentry mechanism.

- Disorders arising in the atrium:

(1) Sinus Tachycardia—rapid, regular rhythm at a rate of 100-180 beats per minute with normal P wave and QRS complex. It often occurs in response to an increase in sympathetic stimulation or a decrease in vagal stimulation.
— Causes
  - fever
  - fluid volume loss
  - emotional/physical stress
  - caffeine or nicotine
  - heart failure
  - hypercalcemia
  - hyperthyroidism
  - medications—nitrates, atropine, epinephrine, and isoproterenol

— Clinical manifestations
  - occasional palpitations
  - decreased activity tolerance
  - hypotension
  - angina pectoris

— Medical management
  - correct the underlying cause
  - antidysrhythmic therapy:
    - digitalis

- beta-adrenergic blocking agents (e.g., propranolol)
- calcium channel blockers—diltiazem, nifedipine

– bedrest to decrease metabolic demand
– supplemental oxygen

(2) Sinus Bradycardia—SA node fires at a rate less than 60 beats per minute with normal P wave and QRS complex. Sinus bradycardia may result from increased vagal stimulation.

— Causes:
 - Valsalva's maneuver (increased vagal tone)
 - medications—digitalis, quinidine, verapamil
 - myocardial infarction
 - hyperkalemia
 - hypothyroidism

— Clinical manifestations
 - may be asymptomatic
 - fatigue
 - hypotension
 - lightheadedness or syncope
 - shortness of breath
 - ectopic beats
 - decreased level of consciousness

— Medical management
 - correct the underlying cause
 - antidysrhythmic therapy:
   - beta-adrenergic agonists (isoproterenol)
   - vagolytics (atropine)
 - transcutaneous pacing
 - temporary/permanent pacemaker placement

(3) Sinus Dysrhythmia—changes in the automaticity of the SA node that cause it to fire at varying speeds. The heart rate ranges between 60 and 100 BPM. ECG has normal P wave, PR interval, and QRS complex; the only abnormality is an irregular P-P interval.

— Causes
 - alteration in vagal tone—speeds up with inhalation and slows down during exhalation

— Clinical manifestations—usually asymptomatic
— Medical management—intervention usually not required.

(4) Premature Atrial Contractions (PACs)—most often result from enhanced automaticity of the atrial muscle. PACs are early beats arising from ectopic atrial foci interrupting the normal rhythm. ECG shows P waves that occur early and differ from normal sinus P waves in direction, size, and/or shape.
— Causes
  - stress
  - fatigue
  - alcohol
  - smoking
  - valvular disease
  - coronary artery disease
  - heart failure
  - medications—digitalis, quinidine, and procainamide
— Clinical manifestations
  - palpitations or "missed beats"
— Medical management
  - correct the underlying cause
  - antidysrhythmic therapy:
    - quinidine
    - procainamide

(5) SA Conduction Defects—the impulse from the SA node is either (a) not generated in the SA node (sinus arrest) or (b) not conducted from the SA node (sinus exit block). During SA arrest neither the atria nor the ventricles are stimulated, which produces a pause in the rhythm. In sinus exit block, there is a conduction delay between the SA node and the atrial muscle, but the rhythm of SA node discharge remains constant and uninterrupted. During SA arrest, neither the atria nor the ventricles are stimulated. An entire PQRST will be missing for one or more cycles. In sinus exit block, the ECG characteristically displays a normal sinus rhythm that has intermittent pauses.
— Causes
  - coronary artery disease

- myocardial infarction
- hypertensive disease
- medications—digitalis and calcium channel blockers

— Clinical manifestations
- may be asymptomatic
- lightheadedness or syncope

— Medical management—intervention usually not necessary.
- correct the underlying cause
- antidysrhythmic therapy:
  - vagolytics (atropine)
  - sympathomimetics (isoproterenol)

— Surgical management
- pacemaker insertion—see "Pacemakers," p. 513

(6)Paroxysmal Atrial Tachycardia (PAT)—is the sudden onset and sudden termination of a rapid firing from an ectopic atrial pacemaker. PAT is identified as three or more consecutive atrial beats at a rate greater than 150 BPM, alternating with normal sinus rhythm. PAT is caused by the reentry phenomenon. The P waves are upright in Lead II, narrow and peaked. At faster rates, the P waves may become lost in the preceding T wave.

— Causes
- digitalis toxicity
- myocardial infarction
- cardiomyopathy
- caffeine, smoking, alcohol
- valvular disease

— Clinical manifestations
- palpitations
- lightheadedness
- syncope

— Medical management
- vagotonic maneuvers (stimulating the vagus nerve to slow the heart) — carotid sinus massage, Valsalva's maneuver (bearing down as with a bowel movement)
- antidysrhythmic therapy:
  - propranolol
  - adenosine
  - verapamil

—synchronized cardioversion—the use of electricity to convert a dysrhythmia to normal sinus rhythm. The electrical discharge is synchronized with the client's QRS complex to avoid discharge during the repolarization phase when the ventricles are most vulnerable to develop ventricular fibrillation (VF).

(7) Atrial Flutter—rapid firing of an ectopic atrial focus. Atrial rate is 220-350 beats per minute. P waves are bidirectional, producing a "saw-toothed" pattern. The AV node cannot conduct all the atrial impulses that bombard it; therefore, the ventricular rate is always slower than the atrial rate.

— Causes
  - coronary artery disease
  - mitral valve disease
  - pulmonary embolism
  - hyperthyroidism
  - post cardiac surgery
— Clinical manifestations
  - palpitations
  - chest pain
— Medical management
  - synchronized cardioversion
  - antidysrhythmic therapy:
    - digitalis
    - quinidine
    - verapamil
    - propranolol
    - procainamide

(8) Atrial Fibrillation—rapid, chaotic atrial depolarization. Ectopic atrial foci produce impulses between 400 and 700 BPM. ECG reveals erratic or no P waves and a baseline that appears to be irregular and undulating. The ventricular rhythm is irregular with rates ranging from 160 to 180 beats per minute.

— Causes
  - increased atrial pressure
  - sick sinus syndrome
  - pericarditis
  - hypoxia
—Clinical manifestations
  - may be asymptomatic

- irregular pulse
- palpitations
- pulse deficit between apical and radial pulses

— Medical management
- synchronized cardioversion
- antidysrhythmic therapy:
  - digoxin
  - calcium channel blockers—diltiazem, verapamil
  - beta-blockers
- anticoagulant therapy to decrease the risk of thrombi formation from blood that pools in the atria because of inadequate contraction of the atrial muscle

- Disorders arising within the atrioventricular (AV) junction

(1) Junctional Rhythms—upward spread of an impulse from the AV junction to the atria rather than the normal downward transmission of impulses from SA node to the AV junction. ECG shows P wave inversion in Lead II and PR interval less than 0.12 second. The major junctional dysrhythmias are (a) premature junctional contractions—single, early firing of a junctional ectopic focus, (b) junctional escape rhythm—if the SA node experiences decreased automaticity, a junctional escape rhythm at a rate of 40–60 beats per minute will take over, and (c) junctional tachycardia—a junctional rate that exceeds 60 beats per minute.

— Causes
- ischemia
- myocardial infarction
- post cardiac surgery
- digitalis toxicity
- quinidine toxicity
- hyperkalemia

— Clinical manifestations
- activity intolerance
- lightheadedness

— Medical management
- carotid massage (rapid junctional rhythm)
- synchronized cardioversion
- antidysrhythmic therapy:

- propranolol
- quinidine
- digitalis

- pacemaker insertion—see "Pacemakers," p. 513

(2) First-Degree Atrioventricular Block—conduction in atrioventricular node is slowed. ECG shows a regular rhythm, each P wave is followed by a QRS complex, and the PR interval is greater than 0.20 second.

— Causes
- coronary artery disease
- increased vagal tone
- congenital anomalies
- digitalis

— Clinical manifestations
- none

— Medical management—usually requires no intervention.
- discontinuation of digitalis if due to toxicity

(3) Second-Degree Atrioventricular (AV) Block

(a) Mobitz Type I (Wenckebach Phenomenon)—recurrent cycles in which the PR interval becomes progressively prolonged until eventually a QRS complex is dropped.

— Causes
- coronary artery disease
- digitalis toxicity
- myocardial infarction

— Clinical manifestations
- usually asymptomatic
- irregular pulse
- vertigo
- weakness

(b) Mobitz Type II—PR intervals remain constant; P waves are normal and are followed by normal QRS complexes until suddenly a ventricular beat is dropped.

— Causes:
- ischemia
- digitalis or quinidine toxicity
- myocardial infarction

— Clinical manifestations
- irregular pulse

- weakness
- syncope
- Medical management
  - Type I—intervention not required as long as the ventricular rate remains adequate for perfusion.
    - correct underlying cause
    - assessment for progression to a higher degree of block
  - Type II
    - assessment for progression to a higher degree of block
    - antidysrhythmic therapy:
      - atropine
      - isoproterenol
    - temporary or permanent pacemaker placement—see "Pacemakers," p. 513
    - withholding of cardiac depressant drugs (digitalis)

(4) Third-Degree AV Block (complete heart block)—all impulses from the atria are blocked, and the action of the atria and ventricles becomes completely disassociated; that is, the atria and the ventricles each have their own pacemaker and beat independently of each other. ECG shows regular P to P intervals, regular R to R intervals, and no consistent PR intervals. The atrial rate is always faster than the ventricular rate.

- Causes
  - fibrotic or degenerative changes in the conduction system
  - myocardial infarction
  - myocarditis
  - congenital anomalies
  - drug toxicities (digitalis, procainamide, quinidine, verapamil)
  - post cardiac surgery
- Clinical manifestations
  - angina
  - hypotension
  - heart failure
  - signs/symptoms of decreased cardiac output

— Medical management
  - transcutaneous pacing
  - pacemaker insertion—see "Pacemakers," p. 513
  - antidysrhythmic therapy:
    - atropine
    - catecholamine infusions (dopamine, epinephrine)

- Disorders arising in the ventricles

Ventricular dysrhythmias arise below the level of the AV junction. Ventricular dysrhythmias are generally more serious and life-threatening than are atrial or junctional dysrhythmias because they develop more often in association with intrinsic heart disease. Also, ventricular dysrhythmias usually cause greater hemodynamic compromise (e.g., hypotension, heart failure, and shock). The independent contraction of the ventricles results in reduced stroke volume and, therefore, reduced cardiac output.

(1) Premature Ventricular Contractions (PVCs)—are caused by the firing of an irritable focus in the ventricle. On the ECG, a wide and bizarre QRS complex appears early, interrupting the underlying rhythm.

— Causes
  - hypoxia
  - hypokalemia
  - hypocalcemia
  - coronary artery disease
  - acidosis
  - heart failure
  - medications — digitalis, tricyclic antidepressants
  - alcohol, caffeine, nicotine
  - myocardial infarction

— Clinical manifestations
  - isolated PVCs; asymptomatic
  - signs/symptoms of decreased cardiac output

— Medical Management

PVCs are innocuous as long as they remain infrequent or isolated. They require intervention when they are: (1) frequent (more than 6 per minute), (2) coupled with normal beats (bigeminy), (3) multiform, (4) occurring in pairs, (5) occurring as a result of acute myocardial infarction, or (6) falling on the T wave (vulnerable period).

- Type I and Type II antidysrhythmics (quinidine, lidocaine, Tambocor, propranolol)

(2) Ventricular Tachycardia (VT)—occurs when an irritable ectopic focus in the ventricles takes over the role of the pacemaker. It is characterized by a rapidly occurring series of PVCs (three or more) with no normal beats between. P waves are absent; QRS complex is wide and bizarre. The ventricular rate ranges between 130 and 170 BPM.

— Causes
- coronary artery disease
- cardiomyopathy
- myocardial infarction
- mitral valve prolapse
- digitalis toxicity

— Clinical manifestations

VT, an extremely dangerous dysrhythmia, produces a very low cardiac output that can quickly lead to cerebral and myocardial ischemia.
- may be asymptomatic
- hypotension
- nonpalpable peripheral pulse
- change in level of consciousness
- at any time, ventricular tachycardia can deteriorate into ventricular fibrillation

— Medical management
- defibrillation if client loses consciousness
- synchronized cardioversion
- antidysrhythmic therapy:
  - lidocaine
  - procainamide
  - bretylium
  - magnesium sulfate

(3) Torsades de Pointes—a form of ventricular tachycardia in which the QRS complexes appear to be constantly changing. Delayed repolarization is revealed as a prolonged QT interval and a broad flat T wave in the preceding sinus rhythm. The ventricular rate is 150-300 BPM with a wide and bizarre QRS.

- Causes
  - drug toxicity (procainamide, quinidine, disopyramide)
  - electrolyte imbalance (hypokalemia, hypomagnesemia)
- Clinical manifestations
  - palpitations
  - syncope
  - rhythm often precedes ventricular fibrillation and sudden death
- Medical management
  - temporary overdrive ventricular or atrial pacing (only if QT interval is prolonged)
  - discontinuation of offending agents
  - magnesium sulfate infusion

(4) Ventricular Fibrillation (VF)—characterized by an extremely rapid, erratic impulse formation and conduction. ECG tracing displays bizarre fibrillatory wave patterns, and it is impossible to identify P waves, QRS complexes, and T waves. Ventricular fibrillation causes abrupt cessation of effective blood flow and death results within minutes without immediate intervention.

- Causes
  - severe myocardial damage
  - hypothermia
  - R-on-T phenomenon—the downward slope of the T wave is the most vulnerable period. If the heart is stimulated at this time, it often cannot respond in an organized fashion and VT or VF may be precipitated.
  - hypoxia
  - electrocution
  - electrolyte imbalance
  - drug toxicity (quinidine, procainamide, digitalis)
- Clinical manifestations
  - unresponsiveness
  - no palpable pulse
- Medical management
  - CPR and defibrillation
  - epinephrine in order to increase myocardial responsiveness to defibrillation

- lidocaine, bretylium, magnesium sulfate, sodium bicarbonate

(5) Bundle Branch Block (BBB)—impaired conduction in one of the bundle branches (distal to the bundle of His), and thus the ventricles do not depolarize simultaneously. The ECG tracing shows a wide or notched QRS complex. These disturbances in conduction result in either a right bundle branch block (RBBB) or a left bundle branch block (LBBB). Because of its association with left ventricular disease, LBBB has a worse prognosis. The left bundle branch is composed of anterior and posterior fascicles of which one or both may be involved.

— Causes
- myocardial fibrosis
- coronary artery disease
- myocardial infarction
- cardiomyopathies
- pulmonary embolism
- congenital anomalies

— Clinical manifestations
- asymptomatic

— Medical management

No specific intervention, however, if RBBB exists along with block in one of the fascicles of the left bundle, the one remaining fascicle represents the only conduction pathway; therefore, a pacemaker may be inserted.

(6) Wolff-Parkinson-White syndrome (WPW)—a pre-excitation syndrome that occurs when part or all of the ventricle is re-entered by a depolarization wave traveling down a congenital or acquired conducting pathway between the atrium and ventricle. Clients with WPW develop sudden attacks of very rapid supraventricular dysrhythmias.

— Clinical manifestations
- may be asymptomatic
- shortness of breath
- palpitations
- syncope

— Medical management
- vagotonic maneuvers

- cardioversion
- adenosine, amiodarone, esmolol
- chemical ablation—alcohol or phenol is injected into involved areas of the myocardium through an angioplasty catheter
- radiofrequency ablation (RFA)—a steerable pacing catheter directs low-power, high frequency current to a localized accessory pathway
- mechanical ablation—abnormal pathway is surgically dissected or treated with a cryoprobe. Prior to surgery, the myocardium is mapped to isolate the area to be treated.

(7) Ventricular Asystole (Cardiac Standstill)—represents the total absence of ventricular electrical activity. ECG shows an absence of any rhythm.

— Causes
- can occur as a primary event
- may follow VF or pulseless electrical activity
- complete heart block with no escape pacemaker

— Clinical manifestations
- faintness followed within seconds by loss of consciousness
- seizures
- apnea
- if untreated, death

— Medical management
- CPR
- epinephrine, atropine
- transcutaneous pacing
- correction of underlying cause

ACUTE AND SUBACUTE CARE

Surgical Management

Surgery can be used to treat dysrhythmias when medications or cardioversion fail. Surgical methods include:

- pacemaker placement—see "Pacemakers," p. 513
- automatic implantable cardioverter defibrillator (AICD)—placement of a system that consists of a pulse generator and sensor that continuously monitors the heart's rhythm and delivers a counter-

shock when it detects a dysrhythmia. It can also detect and treat VT with cardioversion. This implanted system does not require as much energy as external defibrillation because less energy is lost when the impulse is directly applied to the heart. The AICD is implanted surgically into a pouch in the abdominal wall through a thoracotomy incision or transvenously. The two conditions the Food and Drug Administration has approved for AICD placement are (1) survival of one or more episodes of sudden death resulting from ventricular tachycardia or ventricular fibrillation, and (2) recurrent refractory, life-threatening ventricular dysrhythmias that can develop into ventricular tachycardia or ventricular fibrillation despite antidysrhythmic therapy. See "Cardiac Surgery," p. 122.

Nursing Management

Medical

- Monitor heart rhythm continuously.
- Assess skin temperature, lung sounds, heart sounds, and peripheral pulses.
- Monitor laboratory values—drug levels, enzyme levels, electrolyte levels.
- Administer antidysrhythmics as ordered.
- Administer supplemental oxygen therapy as ordered.
- Maintain a quiet, restful environment.

Surgical

- See "Pacemakers," p. 513.
- See "Cardiac Surgery," p. 122.

COMMUNITY AND SELF-CARE

- Instruct the client regarding:
  — importance of taking antidysrhythmic agents as prescribed
  — signs/symptoms to report
  — activity guidelines
  — importance of household member(s) to be trained in CPR
  — how to obtain emergency medical attention

— importance of follow-up laboratory/clinic visits
- See "Pacemakers," p. 513.
- See "Cardiac Surgery," p. 122.
- Additional instructions for AICD clients:
  — AICD follow-up testing (every 2 months)
  — need to wear medical alert identification and to carry a cardioverter defibrillator identification card
  — avoidance of contact sports
  — avoidance of strong magnetic fields
  — need to inform doctors/dentists of the device
  — procedure to follow if shock occurs
  — need to report audible beeping tones coming from the pulse generator in the abdomen

(For more information, see pp. 1295–1314 of Black and Matassarin-Jacobs: *Medical-Surgical Nursing: Clinical Management for Continuity of Care,* 5th ed.)

Encephalitis (Viral)

- Encephalitis is inflammation of the brain parenchyma.
- The two most common causes of encephalitis are arbovirus and herpes simplex Type I virus.
  (1) Arbovirus encephalitis is transmitted via a mosquito or tick bite. It commonly occurs in late summer and early fall. Clinical manifestations are gradual in onset: headache, nausea, vomiting, listlessness, and fever. After a few days, seizures, stiff neck, and coma develop. Fever and neurologic signs subside within 2 weeks unless the client develops irreversible central nervous system changes or dies.
  (2) Herpes simplex virus encephalitis occurs at any time of the year and particularly in middle-aged adults. Clinical manifestations are acute with headache, fever, vomiting, visual field deficits, and seizures. Temporal lobe swelling can lead to herniation, coma, and brain death. The prognosis is grave with a mortality rate above 30 per cent. The client may die within 2 weeks and of those who survive, many are left with severe neurologic and mental disabilities. Medical intervention is a 10-day course of intravenous acyclovir. Nursing management includes protection from injury due to combative, restless, or confused behavior and support to the client's family.

(For more information, see p. 859 of Black and Matassarin-Jacobs: *Medical-Surgical Nursing: Clinical Management for Continuity of Care,* 5th ed.)

Endometrial (Uterine) Cancer

OVERVIEW

- Endometrial cancer is cancer of the uterus. It is the second most common genital malignancy. One in 100 women in the United States will develop uterine cancer.
- The exact mechanism of malignant change is unknown but believed to be related to the hormone estrogen.
- Risk factors include:
  — exogenous estrogen replacement therapy for long periods without concomitant progesterone therapy
  — obesity (increased estrogen production and storage)
  — history of pelvic irradiation
  — hyperestrogenism (early menarche, late menopause, dysfunctional uterine bleeding, delayed onset of ovulation)
  — old age
  — history of other reproductive cancer
  — family history
  — history of infertility or habitual abortion
  — history of diabetes or hypertension
  — white race
  — postmenopausal bleeding
- Primary prevention includes weight loss and proper use of estrogen.
- Early detection is important. Women at menopause and older should have a yearly pelvic examination and Pap smear. Women at high risk should have periodic endometrial tissue sample biopsies.

CLINICAL MANIFESTATIONS

- abnormal uterine bleeding, especially postmenopausal

ACUTE AND SUBACUTE CARE

Medical Management

- progesterone

- chemotherapy and hormonal therapy with estrogen and tamoxifen is used to treat late stages
- irradiation

Surgical Management

- total abdominal hysterectomy and bilateral salpingo-oophorectomy (TAH-BSO) alone or in combination with radiation therapy

Nursing Management

See "Uterine Tumors, Benign," p. 743, for care following a TAH-BSO; "Radiation Therapy," p. 605; and "Chemotherapy," p. 149.

(For more information, see pp. 2404–2406 of Black and Matassarin-Jacobs: *Medical-Surgical Nursing: Clinical Management for Continuity of Care,* 5th ed.)

Endometriosis

OVERVIEW

- Endometriosis is an abnormal condition in which endometrial tissue, which normally lies in the uterine cavity, is located in other sites.
- The abnormally located tissue usually is confined to the pelvic cavity, typically the ovary or dependent portion of the pelvic peritoneum. Tissue also may be found outside the pelvis, although rarely.
- The misplaced tissue responds to hormonal stimulation and bleeds, leading to scarring, inflammation, and adhesions.
- This disorder most commonly is found in premenopausal women aged 30–40 years. It appears to be a hereditary disorder, although the cause is unknown.

CLINICAL MANIFESTATIONS

- one fourth of women are asymptomatic
- pain, beginning before the menstrual period and lasting until several days after the period ends

- dyspareunia (pain during vaginal intercourse)
- menstrual irregularities
- infertility in the absence of tubal obstruction

ACUTE AND SUBACUTE CARE

Medical Management

- analgesics
- oral contraceptives, progesterone or both to induce a pseudopregnancy (symptoms subside during pregnancy)
- Danazol (an antigonadotropin testosterone derivative) to induce ovarian suppression or pseudo–menopause

Surgical Management

- carbon dioxide laser treatment to vaporize adhesions and endometrial implants
- removal of the uterus, as many implants as possible, and some ovarian tissue if the client does not wish to have any more children
- radical surgery involving removal of the uterus, ovaries, tubes, and as many implants as possible—although this procedure is almost completely effective, it does cause surgically induced menopause and sterility

Nursing Management

- Provide information about the disease, its treatment, and ways to cope with the symptoms.
- Provide information and support in regard to infertility.
- Other teaching and interventions depend upon the specific treatment for the client.

(For more information, see pp. 2398–2400 of Black and Matassarin-Jacobs: *Medical-Surgical Nursing: Clinical Management for Continuity of Care,* 5th ed.)

Endotracheal Tubes

OVERVIEW

- An endotracheal tube is a long, slender, hollow tube inserted into the trachea via the nose or mouth. It passes through the vocal cords and the distal tip is positioned just above the bifurcation of the main stem of the bronchus. For short-term management, oral intubation may be used due to the risk of sinusitis with nasal intubation. A tracheostomy may be performed for prolonged intubation.
- Indications for endotracheal intubation include:
  — relief of airway obstruction
  — prevention of aspiration
  — facilitation of tracheal suctioning
  — facilitation of artificial ventilation
- After placement of an endotracheal tube, tube placement can be verified by bilateral auscultation and chest x-ray examination to ensure aeration of both sides of the chest. The point at which the tube meets the lips or nostrils is recorded in the nurse's notes, using the numbers listed on the side of the tube. The tube is secured with adhesive tape or specially designed endotracheal tube holders.
- Endotracheal tubes have soft plastic cuffs designed to inflate with a high enough volume of air to seal the trachea while exerting the lowest possible pressure on the tracheal wall. Low cuff pressure is necessary to prevent impeded circulation to the tracheal mucosa, which may lead to stenosis and necrosis of the trachea.
- Extubation is the removal of the endotracheal tube. This is done when the client demonstrates adequate arterial oxygen levels, tidal volume, vital capacity, and negative inspiratory force, as well as a level of consciousness to sustain spontaneous respiration. If the client has been on mechanical ventilation, the client will need to be weaned from the ventilator prior to extubation (see "Mechanical Ventilation," p. 467). Only health team members qualified to reintubate can extubate a client. Extubation requires a physician order.

- To extubate, the endotracheal tube is suctioned, the cuff deflated, and the tube removed.
- After extubation, the client is placed on oxygen and assessed for signs of respiratory distress, hypoxia (restlessness, irritability, tachycardia, tachypnea), and decreased PaO_2 or increased $PaCO_2$.
- Possible complications due to endotracheal intubation are tracheal necrosis, tracheal trauma from self-extubation, and aspiration from inability to seal the airway.

ACUTE AND SUBACUTE CARE

Nursing Management

- Discuss the purpose of the tube.
- Discuss that suctioning will last about 15 seconds at most.
- Provide reassurance.
- Use a suction catheter that does not exceed one-half the diameter of the airway being suctioned.
- Suction PRN. Provide oxygen and hyperinflate the client's lungs by delivering breaths with a manual resuscitation bag before and after suctioning.
- Limit suctioning to 15 seconds.
- Keep the suction level below 120 mm Hg.
- During suctioning, monitor for cardiac dysrhythmias.
- Assess for clinical manifestations of airway obstruction requiring suctioning: noisy, wet respirations; visible mucous bubbling into the artificial airway; rhonchi identified by auscultation; restlessness; increased pulse and respirations; and an increase in peak inspiratory pressures, if client is on continuous mechanical ventilation.
- Provide adequate hydration and humidification to thin secretions.
- Instill normal saline via the endotracheal tube just before suctioning to loosen secretions.
- Monitor color, odor, and amount of sputum.
- Provide a means of communication for the client—pen and pad of paper or a picture board.
- Perform frequent oral hygiene.
- Perform oral suctioning above the cuff frequently.

- Monitor the cuff pressure (should be below 20 cm H_2O).
- Use the minimal leak technique to inflate the cuff.
- To deflate the cuff:
  — suction the trachea
  — suction deep into the oropharynx to remove secretions above the cuff
  — advance the suction catheter to the end of the endotracheal tube. Deflate the cuff while applying suction to the suction catheter, so that any secretions lying above the cuff will be removed.
  — repeat pharyngeal suctioning.
- Monitor for cuff leaks:
  — pilot balloon is not filling when air is injected
  — client is able to talk when cuff is inflated
  — air is heard leaking during positive-pressure breathing

  Anticipate possible reintubation since the client is at risk for aspiration.
- Monitor the point at which the tube meets the lip or nostrils (should match number documented when placed).
- Retape if necessary.
- Assess for nasal or oral breakdown or necrosis, depending upon site of the tube.

See also "Mechanical Ventilation," p. 467.

(For more information, see pp. 1173–1176 of Black and Matassarin-Jacobs: *Medical-Surgical Nursing: Clinical Management for Continuity of Care,* 5th ed.)

Enteral Feedings

OVERVIEW

- Enteral feeding is the instillation of essential nutrients and calories directly into the stomach or intestine via a gastrointestinal tube.
- Major advantages of gastrointestinal feedings over parenteral nutrition are that they help maintain gastrointestinal structure, gastrointestinal motility, and the mucosal barrier.

- Feedings may be given via nasoenteric or nasogastric tubes. The physician may also perform surgery to place a gastrostomy, percutaneous gastrostomy (PEG), jejunostomy, needle catheter jejunostomy tube, or an esophagostomy tube.
- The physician or dietician prescribes the amount, frequency, and type of tube feeding, based on the client's special needs. There are many commercially prepared enteral feedings available. They differ in osmolality, digestibility, caloric density, lactose content, viscosity, fat content, and expense.
- Tube feedings may be administered continuously, intermittently (given amount is administered over set intervals several times daily), or by bolus (a specified volume of formula is poured through an Asepto syringe or funnel attached to the gastrointestinal tube and allowed to drip in by gravity).

ACUTE AND SUBACUTE CARE

Nursing Management

- Initiate tube feeding at a low rate and gradually increase as prescribed until client is receiving the desired amount of formula.
- Keep head of bed elevated 30 degrees for continuous feedings.
- Check the placement of the tube by aspirating for gastric contents and measuring the pH of gastric contents (injecting air into small bore tubes is not always an accurate way to check placement). For bolus feedings, check prior to each feeding. For continuous feedings, check several times per shift.
- Check gastric residuals before each feeding (for bolus feedings) or every 4–8 hours. Notify physician of high residuals (a residual greater than 50 per cent of the previous hour's intake indicates delayed gastric emptying). Reinstill the feeding residual to prevent excessive fluid and electrolyte loss.
- Monitor for signs of intolerance, such as cramping, diarrhea, nausea, vomiting, aspiration, glycosuria and diaphoresis.

- The feeding tube should be flushed with 50–100 mls of water before and after intermittent feedings, every 4 hours during continuous feedings, and before and after any medications are administered through the tube.
- If an obstruction occurs, try flushing the tube with water, cola, or cranberry juice.
- Monitor for diarrhea and report to physician.
- Monitor for constipation. If this occurs, increase water intake or suggest switching to a fiber-enriched formula.
- Monitor for signs/symptoms of dehydration.
- Monitor for possible complications:
  — nausea, vomiting
  — plugging of the tube
  — dislocation of the tube into the trachea or lungs
  — development of ulcerations and dried secretions in the nares
  — tracheoesophageal fistula (may be demonstrated by adding blue food coloring to the formula. If blue fluid is obtained when the lungs are suctioned, a fistula is present.)
- Provide instructions to the client/significant other on home enteral feedings.
- Refer to a home health care agency as appropriate.

(For more information, see pp. 1752–1754 of Black and Matassarin-Jacobs: *Medical-Surgical Nursing: Clinical Management for Continuity of Care,* 5th ed.)

Epilepsy

OVERVIEW

- Epilepsy is a paroxysmal neurologic disorder causing recurrent episodes of (1) loss of consciousness, (2) convulsive movements or other motor activity, (3) sensory phenomena, and (4) behavioral abnormalities.
- A tendency to have a lower threshold for seizures is inherited, but the actual seizure disorder itself is not. This form of epilepsy is called idiopathic

epilepsy. When the cause of seizure is known, the disorder is called secondary epilepsy. These causes include traumatic brain injury, brain tumor, and infection. Approximately two-thirds of epilepsy cases are idiopathic and one-third are secondary.

- The following are important terms that may be used when discussing epilepsy:
  (1) prodromal phase—a vague change that occurs in emotional reactivity or affective responses (e.g., depression or anxiety) that may precede the seizure by minutes or hours
  (2) aura—a brief, sensory experience that occurs a few seconds before the seizure. It may be an odor or a feeling of weakness or dizziness
  (3) ictus —seizure phase
  (4) "epileptic cry"—a cry occurring with some seizures; caused by a thoracic and abdominal spasm, which expels air through the glottis
  (5) seizure—a paroxysmal, uncontrolled, abnormal discharge of electrical activity in the brain's gray matter; causes events that interfere with normal function
  (6) postictal—the postseizure phase during which the client experiences some change in consciousness, behavior or activity
  (7) status epilepticus—the state in which a client has continuous seizures or seizures in rapid succession lasting at least 30 minutes. This is a medical emergency and may result in permanent damage to the brain.
- Approximately 0.5–1.0 per cent of people in the United States have epileptic seizures.

CLINICAL MANIFESTATIONS

Generalized Seizures

One-third of seizures are generalized. There are four types of generalized seizures:

- Tonic clonic (grand mal)
  — aura
  — sudden loss of consciousness
  — tonic phase—entire body stiffens in rigid contraction
    - respirations may be interrupted temporarily and cyanosis may be present

- jaws are fixed and the hands clenched
- eyes open wide, pupils are fixed and dilated
- lasts 30–60 seconds

— clonic phase
- rhythmic, jerky contraction and relaxation of all body muscles, especially the extremities
- incontinence of urine or feces
- saliva blown from the mouth (creates a froth at the lips)
- biting of lips, tongue, and inside of the mouth

This entire episode may last 2–5 minutes, after which the client may go into a postictal sleep lasting 30 minutes to several hours. This may be followed by depression, confusion or headache pain. The client has complete amnesia for the seizure episode.

- Petit mal (absence) seizures
  — brief periods of altered consciousness (periods of "absence") lasting 5–30 seconds
  — usually begin during childhood and diminish or disappear after puberty
- Myoclonic seizures
  — involuntary jerking contractions of a single muscle group or multiple muscle groups
  — client usually loses consciousness for a moment and is confused postictally
- Atonic seizures
  — total loss of muscle tone
  — may be mild with the client briefly nodding the head or may fall to the floor

PARTIAL (FOCAL) SEIZURES

Most common type of epilepsy. There are four types of partial seizures:

- Partial motor seizures
  — begin with convulsive twitching in an upper extremity
  — involuntary movements of an area may spread centrally and involve the entire limb, that side of the face and the lower extremity. This progression or "spread" is known as the Jacksonian march.
- Partial sensory seizures

- experiences sensory phenomena from a focus in a specific area
  - may see flashing lights, or experience numbness or tingling
- Autonomic seizures
  - stimulation of the autonomic system
  - produces epigastric sensations, pallor, sweating, flushing, and pupillary dilation
- Subjective (psychic) seizures—two types:
  - complex partial
    - automatism (such as purposeless repetitive activities, e.g., lip smacking, chewing, patting a part of the body) while in a dreamy state
    - inappropriate or antisocial behavior may occur
  - partial seizures that generalize
    - seizures start from a particular focus, eventually involving the whole body

ACUTE AND SUBACUTE CARE

Medical Management

- antiepileptic drugs—usually single drug therapy is used, e.g., phenytoin (Dilantin), carbamazepine (Tegretol), primidone (Mysoline), valproate (Depakene)

Surgical Management

May be used when seizures do not respond to medication.

- cortical resection of the anterior temporal lobe for complex partial seizures
- corpus callosal resection—palliative surgery to make seizures more tolerable
- temporal lobectomy—curative surgery removes the area where the seizures begin without causing neurologic or cognitive deficit
- surgery to remove operable brain tumor, cyst or abcess

Nursing Management

Medical

- Initiate seizure precautions.

- Monitor for seizure activity.
- Administer anticonvulsants.

During a seizure

- If possible, move to a place of safety.
  - If in bed, raise padded side-rails
  - If sitting or standing, lower to floor
  - Move objects out of the way
- Turn client to one side to maintain patent airway and prevent aspiration.
- Document when seizure started and describe it (presence of aura, tonic clonic movements, area where seizure began, eye deviation, generalized or unilateral activity, labored or frothy respirations, incontinence, and client's behavior during post-ictal period).

  During status epilepticus—an emergency situation in which the client has continuous seizures or seizures in rapid succession without regaining consciousness, lasting at least 30 minutes.
- Be aware that this is a medical emergency and will result in permanent brain damage or death if not treated rapidly.
- Maintain a patent airway and prevent aspiration. (Position on side, suction and provide oxygenation. Endotracheal intubation may be needed.)
- Assess client continuously.
- Protect client from injury.
- Anticipate laboratory studies for blood chemistries, liver function tests, and toxicology.
- Administer IV phenytoin (first line of treatment) and then loading dose of phenytoin. Other medications, such as valium or lorazepam, may be ordered. Because all of these medications can depress respirations, emergency ventilatory equipment should be available.
- Anticipate general anesthesia or a barbiturate coma (induced by pentobarbital), if unable to control with medications.
- Provide emotional support to significant others.

Surgical

Postoperative nursing care is the same as for any client undergoing a craniotomy.

COMMUNITY AND SELF-CARE

- Instruct client/significant other regarding:
  - — medication
    - – importance of taking daily even if no seizures occur
    - – method of action and possible side effects. Gingival hyperplasia (excessive gum tissue growth) may occur with phenytoin. Instruct client to brush teeth two to three times daily. Discuss possible need to have gingival tissues excised every 6–12 months.
    - – diplopia, sedation, bone marrow depression, and ataxia are other possible side effects
  - — avoidance of factors that may trigger seizures (flickering lights, stress, lack of sleep, emotional upset, alcohol use)
  - — using safety measures for certain activities (e.g., swimming or horseback riding) and avoidance of dangerous activities
  - — avoidance of overprotecting the client
  - — local laws on driving motor vehicles
  - — what to do if seizure occurs:
    - – lie on ground (when aura occurs, if client has aura)
    - – loosen clothing
    - – protect head (place something under it)
    - – remove sharp objects from environment
    - – do not restrain the client
    - – do not insert anything into mouth (clients do not swallow their tongues)
    - – position on side to displace the tongue and allow oral secretions to drain from the airway
    - – stay with client until consciousness returns
    - – call ambulance, if: seizure lasts over 10 minutes, respiratory difficulty occurs, injury occurs, another seizure occurs or the client is pregnant
  - — importance of wearing identification stating client has epilepsy and name of physician
- Provide emotional support for possible feelings of anger, poor self image, self consciousness, guilt, or depression.
- Importance of follow-up visits.

- Refer to National Epilepsy League, National Association to Control Epilepsy or local support groups.

(For more information, see pp. 834–842 of Black and Matassarin-Jacobs: *Medical-Surgical Nursing: Clinical Management for Continuity of Care,* 5th ed.)

Epistaxis

OVERVIEW

- Epistaxis (nosebleed) may result from irritation, trauma, infection or tumors. It also may result from systemic disease (hypertension, atherosclerosis, or blood dyscrasias) or systemic treatment (chemotherapy or anticoagulants).

ACUTE AND SUBACUTE CARE

Medical Management

- Application of pressure by pinching the anterior portion of the nose for 5-10 minutes and application of ice compresses.
- Cauterization of the bleeding vessel with silver nitrate.
- Nasal packing is most effective for anterior nasal bleeding. Antibacterial ointment is applied to one-half inch gauze and inserted into the anterior nasal cavities and left in place for 48-72 hours.
- For posterior nasal bleeding, a posterior plug may be needed in addition to nasal packing. A small red rubber catheter is passed through the nose into the oropharynx and mouth. A gauze pack is tied to the catheter, and the catheter is withdrawn, moving the pack into the nasopharynx and posterior nose. Strings from the pack are tied around a rolled gauze. Strings from the oral cavity are taped to the client's face to prevent dislodgement of the plug. Posterior plugs are left in for 5 days.

Surgical Management

- internal maxillary or ethmoid artery ligations, if the above interventions fail

Nursing Management

- Monitor for changes in vital signs.
- Monitor for bleeding from the anterior nares.
- Monitor for posterior bleeding manifested by increased swallowing or presence of blood in the throat.
- Change nasal drip pad PRN.
- Encourage use of humidification, adequate fluids, and frequent mouth care to prevent dryness and crusting of secretions.
- If nasal packing or posterior plugs are present, monitor for hypoxia. Ensure intactness of the packing or plug. Assess the oral cavity for proper placement of the plug. If the plug is visible, notify the physician for repositioning.

COMMUNITY AND SELF-CARE

Instruct client regarding:
- minimal activity for 10 days—avoidance of strenuous exercise
- no blowing of the nose
- sneezing only with the mouth open
- no lifting, stooping, or straining
- use of water soluble lubricant at the entrance of the nose and around the nares for comfort

(For more information, see pp. 1076–1077 of Black and Matassarin-Jacobs: *Medical-Surgical Nursing: Clinical Management for Continuity of Care,* 5th ed.)

Esophageal Neoplasms

OVERVIEW

- Cancer of the esophagus may be manifest as either squamous cell carcinoma or adenocarcinoma of the esophageal mucosa. Adenocarcinoma occurs less often than squamous cell carcinoma.

- The incidence of esophageal cancer is twice as high in men as in women. The incidence of squamous cell cancer of the esophagus in the United States is 4 per 100,000 males.
- Risk factors include long-term use of alcohol and tobacco combined with poor nutrition. The presence of achalasia, hiatal hernia, reflux, and stricture.

CLINICAL MANIFESTATIONS

- dysphagia, odynophagia (pain upon swallowing)—usually not apparent until the tumor involves the circumference of the esophagus

ACUTE AND SUBACUTE CARE

Medical Management

Treatment depends upon the location of the tumor, size of the tumor, metastases, and the condition of the client.

- radiation therapy, used alone or in conjunction with surgery (radiation therapy reduces tumor size and slows tumor growth)
- chemotherapy

Surgical Management

- esophageal dilatation to treat strictures and tumor obstruction
- prosthesis to bypass the tumor or prevent aspiration
- esophagectomy—removal of all or part of the esophagus (the resected esophagus is replaced with a dacron graft)
- esophagogastrostomy—resection of the lower portion of the esophagus and anastomosis of the remainder to the stomach
- esophagoenterostomy—resecting the esophagus and replacing it with a segment of the descending colon
- gastrostomy or jejunostomy tube placement as needed for nutrition

Nursing Management

Medical

- Monitor nutritional status and caloric intake.
- Obtain daily weights.
- Monitor intake and output.
- Provide tube feedings.
- Maintain skin integrity around the gastrostomy feeding tube:
  — wash area with gentle soap and water and dry thoroughly twice a day
  — apply protective ointments, such as zinc oxide or Karaya
- Keep in upright position to prevent aspiration of secretions.
- Provide receptacle for saliva and mucous secretions when client unable to swallow.
- Assist with frequent oral care.
- Provide emotional support to assist with coping with poor prognosis and change in body image.
- See "Chemotherapy," p. 149.

Surgical

Preoperative Care

In addition to routine preoperative care:
- Provide hyperalimentation or tube feedings for nutritional support for 2–3 weeks preoperatively.
- Perform oral care four times per day.
- Perform bowel preparation as ordered if esophagoenterostomy will be performed.

Postoperative Care

In addition to routine postoperative care:
- See "Mechanical Ventilation," p. 467, if client on mechanical ventilation.
- Administer analgesics as ordered to assist with effective turning, coughing, and deep breathing.
- Place in semi-Fowler's to prevent reflux.
- Maintain chest tube patency; assess for amount and color of drainage.
- Monitor intake and output (client will be NPO for 4–5 days).
- Monitor nasogastric drainage (bloody for the first 24 hours, then a greenish-yellow color).

- Monitor anastomosis site (leakage is common for 5–7 days after surgery).
- Assess all wounds for signs of bleeding, drainage, or separation of the suture lines.
- Reinitiate oral intake with sips of water as ordered. Position upright and monitor for signs of leakage at the anastomosis site. If client tolerates sips, slowly advance to pureed and semi-solid foods.
- Instruct on importance of small, frequent feedings, sitting upright for meals and for 1 hour after meals.

COMMUNITY AND SELF-CARE

Instruct client/significant other regarding:
- nutritional support
- wound care and healing
- respiratory care
- wound and respiratory complications and when to contact physician

Refer to home health agency as needed.

Refer to support groups (American Cancer Society, Hospice) as appropriate.

(For more information, see pp. 1743–1746 of Black and Matassarin-Jacobs: *Medical-Surgical Nursing: Clinical Management for Continuity of Care,* 5th ed.)

Extracellular Fluid Volume Deficit (ECFVD)

OVERVIEW

- An extracellular fluid volume deficit (ECFVD) is a decrease in intravascular and interstitial fluids. Extracellular fluid volume deficit is a serious fluid imbalance. ECFVD can lead to cellular fluid loss owing to fluid shifting from the cells to the vascular fluid to restore fluid balance.
- The pathophysiologic changes related to ECFVD are usually related to changes in sodium levels and fluid balance. Serum sodium concentration is in-

creased with ECFVD due to insufficient water intake or water loss. The increased serum sodium concentration causes a shifting of water from the cells to the vascular space to decrease the hyperosmolality that occurs with water loss. This shift causes cells to shrink and cellular dehydration to occur.

- There are three major types of ECFVD: (1) hyperosmolar fluid volume deficit — water loss is greater than electrolyte loss, (2) iso-osmolar fluid volume deficit — equal proportions of water and electrolyte loss, and (3) hypotonic fluid volume deficit — loss of electrolytes is greater than water loss.
- ECFVD commonly occurs with severe vomiting, diaphoresis, or diarrhea, traumatic injuries with excessive blood loss, third space fluid shifts, and insufficient water or fluid intake.
- Risk factors include fever, nasogastric suction, ileostomy, fistula, burns, diuretic use, hyperventilation, and diabetes insipidus.

CLINICAL MANIFESTATIONS

- thirst (thirst mechanism may be depressed in elderly or debilitated client)
- decreased skin turgor
- dry mucous membranes
- dry, cracked lips or tongue
- soft and sunken eyeballs
- apprehension and restlessness; coma with severe deficit
- elevated temperature
- tachycardia
- postural hypotension
- narrowed pulse pressure (difference between systolic and diastolic pressure readings)
- flattened neck veins in supine position
- weight loss
- muscle weakness
- oliguria (less than 30 ml/hr)
- laboratory findings:
  — increased osmolality
  — increased or normal serum sodium
  — hyperglycemia (due to hemoconcentration)

— elevated hematocrit
— increased urine specific gravity

ACUTE AND SUBACUTE CARE

Medical Management

- fluid and electrolyte replacement
- blood replacement
- measures to control fluid/electrolyte loss as indicated:
  - — antidiarrheal agents
  - — antiemetics
  - — nasogastric tube placement

Nursing Management

- Administer fluid/electrolyte replacement.
- Encourage oral fluid intake.
- Monitor vital signs including orthostatic blood pressure.
- Assess for signs of fluid overload—cerebral edema, congestive heart failure (may occur if replacement fluids are given too rapidly).
- Assess intake and output.
- Daily weights.
- Administer antiemetics or antidiarrheals as ordered.
- Monitor for signs of increasing fluid loss (increased drainage from NG tube, chest tube or wound site, etc.).
- Provide frequent oral care.
- Implement measures to maintain skin integrity.
- Initiate appropriate safety measures (postural hypotension).
- Monitor laboratory findings—BUN, hematocrit, serum sodium, serum osmolality, specific gravity.

COMMUNITY AND SELF-CARE

Discharge care is based on the etiologic factor(s) causing extracellular fluid volume deficit.

(For more information, see pp. 277–284 of Black and Matassarin-Jacobs: *Medical-Surgical Nursing: Clinical Management for Continuity of Care,* 5th ed.)

Extracellular Fluid Volume Excess (ECFVE)

OVERVIEW

- Extracellular fluid volume excess (ECFVE) is increased fluid retention in the intravascular and interstitial spaces (fluid overload). ECFVE usually results from an increase in total body sodium content.
- With a fluid volume excess, the fluid pressure is greater than usual at the arterial end of the capillary. Fluid is pushed into the tissue spaces. Peripheral and pulmonary edema may result. As fluid pressure increases in the tissues, it also increases in the left ventricle, which can result in heart failure.
- Causes of ECFVE include:
  - heart failure—impaired pumping action
  - renal disorders—decreased sodium and water excretion
  - cirrhosis of the liver—decreased serum protein and albumin levels, therefore, oncotic pressure is decreased, resulting in less fluid reabsorption from the tissue spaces
  - lymphatic obstruction—blocked lymph channels, increasing tissue oncotic pressure
  - tissue injury—increased movement of plasma protein into tissue, increasing oncotic pressure
  - increased ingestion of foods containing high amounts of sodium—increased water retention
  - excessive amounts of IV fluids containing sodium—increased water retention
  - Cushing's syndrome (hyperaldosteronism)—increased sodium and water retention
  - syndrome of inappropriate secretion of antidiuretic hormone (SIADH)

CLINICAL MANIFESTATIONS

- dyspnea
- crackles in the lungs
- cyanosis

- constant irritating cough (due to fluid accumulation in the alveolar sacs)
- neck vein engorgement in semi-Fowler's position
- hand vein engorgement
- bounding pulse
- elevated blood pressure
- S_3 gallop
- pitting edema of the lower extremities
- sacral edema
- weight gain
- malaise, confusion, headache, and lethargy (secondary to cerebral edema)
- laboratory findings:
  — decreased serum osmolality (indicates there are fewer solutes in proportion to the fluid volume)
  — serum sodium may be normal, decreased, or elevated (depending upon the amount of sodium retention or water retention)
  — decreased hematocrit (hemodilution)
  — decreased urine specific gravity

ACUTE AND SUBACUTE CARE

Medical Management

- diuretic therapy
- digitalis (to improve myocardial function)
- fluid restriction
- low-sodium diet
- management of underlying disorder—heart failure, cirrhosis, renal disease, etc.

Nursing Management

- Administer diuretics as ordered and monitor effectiveness.
- Assess for signs/symptoms of congestive heart failure—neck vein distention, S_3 gallop, shortness of breath, rales, etc.
- Assess for signs/symptoms of cerebral edema—malaise, confusion, lethargy, etc.
- Monitor vital signs.
- Monitor laboratory values—electrolytes, osmolality, specific gravity, arterial blood gases, renal profile, liver enzymes.

- Monitor intake and output.
- Daily weights.
- Maintain fluid restriction.
- Maintain low sodium diet.
- Frequent skin care to edematous areas.

COMMUNITY AND SELF-CARE

Instruct client regarding:

- dietary modifications — low sodium
- importance of medication regime
- signs of fluid overload and need to report to physician:
  - — weight gain
  - — increased edema
  - — increased shortness of breath
- importance of follow-up appointments

(For more information, see pp. 284–289 of Black and Matassarin-Jacobs: *Medical-Surgical Nursing: Clinical Management for Continuity of Care,* 5th ed.)

Extracellular Fluid Volume Shift (Third-Spacing)

OVERVIEW

- A fluid volume shift is a change in the location of extracellular fluid between the intravascular and the interstitial spaces.
- There are two types of fluid shift: (1) vascular fluid to interstitial space leading to a fluid volume deficit (hypovolemia), and (2) interstitial fluid to vascular fluid space leading to fluid volume excess (hypervolemia).
- Fluid that shifts into the interstitial space due to increased capillary permeability or increased vascular fluid volume and remains there, is referred to as third-space fluid. Third-space fluid is physiologically useless because it does not circulate to provide nutrients. Common sites for third-spacing are the abdomen, pleural cavity, peritoneal cavity, and pericardial sac.

- Clinical causes of fluid shift include:
  — increased capillary permeabililty
    - crushing injuries
    - major surgery
    - extensive burns
    - sepsis
  — increased fluid pressures
    - large venous thrombosis
    - lymphatic obstruction
    - intestinal obstruction
  — inflammatory responses to infectious, noninfectious, or autoimmune disorders cause pleural and pericardial fluid shifts
  — conditions that promote hypoalbuminemia
    - malnutrition
    - alcoholism

CLINICAL MANIFESTATIONS

Fluid shift from vascular to interstitial (resembles shock)

- skin pallor
- cold extremities
- weak, rapid pulse
- hypotension
- oliguria
- decreased level of consciousness

Fluid shift from interstitial to vascular (resembles fluid overload)

- bounding pulse
- crackles
- neck vein engorgement
- elevated blood pressure

ACUTE AND SUBACUTE CARE

Medical Management

- determination/treatment of the cause of the fluid shift
- management of hypovolemia
  — fluid replacement
  — vasoactive agents
- albumin administration if protein deficit present
- management of overload
  — diuretics
  — fluid restriction

Nursing Management

- Monitor vital signs.
- Administer ordered treatments for hypovolemia or hypervolemia.
- Measure abdominal girth daily, if ascites is present.
- Daily weights.
- Monitor intake and output.
- Assess neurological status.
- Provide frequent skin care to edematous areas.
- Monitor laboratory findings—electrolytes, renal profile, serum ammonia levels.
- Provide frequent oral care

COMMUNITY AND SELF-CARE

Discharge care is based on the etiologic factor(s) causing fluid shift.

(For more information, see pp. 289–291 of Black and Matassarin-Jacobs: *Medical-Surgical Nursing: Clinical Management for Continuity of Care,* 5th ed.)

F

Fatty Liver

- Lipid infiltrations of the liver cause enlargement, increased firmness, and possible decreased function of the liver. Triglycerides are the lipid usually causing fatty liver, although cholesterol or phospholipid also may infiltrate the liver.
- Major causes include: chronic alcoholism, protein malnutrition in early life, obesity, diabetes mellitus, Cushing's syndrome, prolonged IV hyperalimentation, and Reye's syndrome.
- Clients may be asymptomatic, but anorexia, abdominal pain, and jaundice may be seen with massive infiltration.
- Treatment involves removal of the source of the problem and return to metabolic balance.
- Nursing care involves preparing for diagnostic procedures; providing emotional support and supportive physical care and promoting proper diet to prevent recurrence.

(For more information, see p. 1895 of Black and Matassarin-Jacobs: *Medical-Surgical Nursing: Clinical Management for Continuity of Care,* 5th ed.)

Flail Chest

- A flail chest consists of fractures of two or more adjacent ribs on the same side, and possibly the sternum, with each bone fractured into two or more segments.
- The flail segment no longer has bony or cartilaginous connections with the rest of the rib cage. Lacking attachment to the thoracic skeleton, the flail section "floats," moving independently of the chest wall during ventilation, and causes a paradoxical motion.

- During paradoxical motion, the flail portion of the chest and its underlying lung tissue are "sucked in" with inspiration and ballooned out with expiration. This diminishes the ability to achieve an adequate tidal volume and to cough adequately. Hypoventilation and hypoxemia may result without prompt intervention.
- Paradoxical motion also causes mediastinal flutter (movement of the mediastinal structures [heart, trachea, esophagus] in a swinging, back and forth motion), which may affect circulatory dynamics, causing elevated venous pressure, impaired filling of the right side of the heart and decreased arterial pressure.
- Signs and symptoms of flail chest are excruciating pain; cyanosis; severe dyspnea; rapid, shallow grunting respirations, and obvious paradoxical movement of the chest wall.
- Treatment is usually intubation and mechanical ventilation.

(For more information, see p. 2527 of Black and Matassarin-Jacobs: *Medical-Surgical Nursing: Clinical Management for Continuity of Care,* 5th ed.)

Fracture, Femur (Femoral Shaft / Femoral Neck)

OVERVIEW

- Femoral shaft fractures occur most often in young or middle-aged people. Fractures of the proximal femur are more common in the elderly.
- Femoral neck fractures occur in persons who fall from significant heights or are involved in automobile accidents in which the knee strikes the dashboard.

CLINICAL MANIFESTATIONS

- marked displacement and deformity
- extensive soft tissue damage
- swelling
- pain

ACUTE AND SUBACUTE CARE

Medical Management

- splint application
- traction

Surgical Management

- placement of internal fixation devices (rods, nails, plates, or screws)
- hemiarthroplasty or total hip arthroplasty (femoral head fracture)

Nursing Management

- See "Fracture, General Information," below
- See "Fracture, Hip," p. 283
- See "Traction," p. 708.

COMMUNITY AND SELF-CARE

Discharge instructions will be determined by the type/location of fracture and selected treatment regime.

(For more information, see pp. 2159–2160 of Black and Matassarin-Jacobs: *Medical-Surgical Nursing: Clinical Management for Continuity of Care,* 5th ed.)

Fracture, General Information

OVERVIEW

- A fracture is a disruption of normal bone continuity that occurs when more stress is placed on a bone than it is able to absorb. Surrounding soft tissue (skin, muscle, blood vessels, nerves, ligaments, tendons, and subcutaneous tissues) injury often also occurs.
- About 25 per cent of the population suffers some type of musculoskeletal injury yearly.
- Classification of fractures:
  - — Closed (simple)—uncomplicated with intact skin over the fracture site

- Open (compound)—a break in the skin is present over the fracture site
- Avulsion—bone fragments are torn away from the body of the bone
- Greenstick—one side of the bone is broken and the other side is bent
- Stress (fatigue)—results from repeated stress on a bone when there is no evidence of bone disease or trauma
- Comminuted—more than one fracture line and bone fragments are crushed or broken into several pieces
- Impacted—one bone fragment is forcibly driven into another adjacent bone fragment
- Pathologic—fracture occurs due to underlying bone disorders, such as osteoporosis or tumor; usually occurs with minimal trauma
- Compression—produced by force applied to the long axis of the bone

- At the time of the fracture, muscles that are attached to the ends of the now fractured bone are no longer suspended across the length of the bone. The muscles can then spasm and pull the loose bony ends into various positions.
- When a bone is broken, the periosteum and blood vessels are disrupted. Bleeding occurs from the damaged ends of the bone and nearby soft tissue. A hematoma forms in the medullary canal between the fractured ends of the bone and beneath the periosteum.

CLINICAL MANIFESTATIONS

Clinical manifestations vary with site, severity, type of fracture, and amount of damage to other structures.

- deformity
- swelling
- bruising (from subcutaneous bleeding)
- muscle spasm (involuntary muscle contraction near the fracture)
- tenderness
- pain
- impaired sensation (numbness)
- loss of normal function
- crepitus

- hypovolemic shock (from blood loss or other injuries)
- abnormal mobility of the affected part

ACUTE AND SUBACUTE CARE

Medical Management

- traction—to align bone fragments
- closed reduction—manual application of traction to restore bone alignment
- cast application
- management of shock

Surgical Management

- open reduction—an incision is made and the fracture is aligned under direct vision
- internal fixation device placement (insertion of screws, plates, pins, wires, nails, or rods)
- external fixation—pins placed through the skin into the fractured bone and connected to a rigid external frame

Nursing Management

- Apply traction as ordered. See "Traction," p. 708.
- Administer PRN analgesics.
- Assess for signs/symptoms of arterial damage
  - — variable or absent pulse
  - — swelling
  - — pallor or patch cyanosis distal to the fracture
  - — pain
  - — poor capillary return
  - — coolness of the extremity
  - — paralysis or sensory loss distal to fracture
- Assess for signs/symptoms of compartment syndrome (caused by bleeding or edema within a compartment that consists of muscles, bones, nerves and blood vessels wrapped by fibrous membrane):
  - — ischemic pain
  - — pain with elevation (due to increased arterial inflow)
  - — paresthesias
  - — diminished or absent pulses

— coolness or pallor

- Assess for signs/symptoms of fat embolism (may occur 24–48 hours after injury)
  — altered mental status
  — tachypnea
  — tachycardia
  — hypoxemia
  — petechiae
  — fever
- Assess for signs/symptoms of nerve injury
  — paresthesia
  — paralysis
  — pallor
  — coolness of the extremity
  — increasing pain
  — changes in ability to move the extremity
- Assess for signs/symptoms of infection
  — increased temperature
  — rapid pulse
  — pain
  — drainage
- Monitor for signs/symptoms of shock and administer ordered therapy.
- Monitor for DVT and pulmonary embolism.
- Consult with Physical/Occupational Therapy for prescribed exercises, ambulation techniques, and adaptive devices.

See "Casts," p. 131. See "Traction," p. 708.

COMMUNITY AND SELF-CARE

Discharge instruction will be determined by type/location of fracture and selected treatment regime.

See "Casts," p. 131.

(For more information, see pp. 2129–2137 of Black and Matassarin-Jacobs: *Medical-Surgical Nursing: Clinical Management for Continuity of Care,* 5th ed.)

Fracture, Hip

OVERVIEW

- Each year more than 250,000 Americans suffer hip fractures; 90 per cent of these fractures occur in clients older than 65 years. Women outnumber men by a 2:1 ratio.
- Intertrochanteric fractures are the most common hip fracture.
- Two contributing factors seen in the elderly are loss of postural stability with increased incidence of falls and decreased bone mass.

CLINICAL MANIFESTATIONS

- shortened, externally rotated hip
- ecchymosis
- inability to bear weight
- pain, tenderness

ACUTE AND SUBACUTE CARE

Medical Management

- Buck's traction (skin traction)—realigns fracture and reduces muscle spasms until surgery can be performed
- analgesia

Surgical Management

- placement of internal fixation device (screw, pin, plate)
- total hip arthroplasty—joint replacement

Nursing Management

Medical

- Apply Buck's traction.
- Administer PRN analgesics.
- Monitor skin for signs of breakdown.
- Initiate measures to prevent complications of immobility.

In addition to routine postoperative care:

- Maintain repaired limb so it is internally rotated and in a neutral or abducted position.
  - — Place a pillow or an A-frame between the client's legs to maintain abduction.
  - — Place a trochanter roll beside the external aspect of the thigh to prevent external rotation.
  - — Never adduct the operated leg past the body's midline.
- Encourage client to perform in-bed exercises for upper and lower extremities.
  - — Place trapeze to facilitate upper arm and shoulder strength.
- Implement passive and active range of motion exercises.
- Consult Physical Therapy for assisted ambulation, exercises, transfer techniques, and adaptive devices as prescribed.
- Monitor for signs/symptoms of hip dislocation.
- Turn the client only with a physician's order.
  - — When helping the client turn:
    - avoid adduction and excessive movement of the operated limb
    - prevent strain on the hip
    - keep the leg and hip in proper alignment
- Avoid acute flexion of the operated hip by not elevating the head of the bed greater than 40 degrees.
- Keep operated limb extended, well supported ,and elevated when client is allowed to sit in a chair. Follow prescribed amount of weight bearing.
- Remind client not to cross legs.
- Administer PRN analgesics.
- Monitor for signs/symptoms of deep vein thrombosis (redness, warmth, pain in calf, positive Homan's sign).
- Provide meticulous skin care and monitor for signs of skin breakdown.
- Monitor for clinical manifestations of compartment syndrome (caused by bleeding or edema into a compartment that consists of muscle, bone, nerves, and blood vessels wrapped by a fibrous

membrane); pallor, pulselessness, paresthesias, pain, and paralysis.

COMMUNITY AND SELF-CARE

These types of clients benefit most when transferred to an extended care facility where they can complete their rehabilitation.

(For more information, see pp. 2153–2159 of Black and Matassarin-Jacobs: *Medical-Surgical Nursing: Clinical Management for Continuity of Care,* 5th ed.)

Fracture, Pelvis

OVERVIEW

- Pelvic fractures occur in nearly 30 per cent of all multiple trauma injuries.
- Pelvic fractures are associated with injuries to the major arteries, lower urinary tract, uterus, bowel and rectum, abdominal wall, spine, and testes.

CLINICAL MANIFESTATIONS

- hypotension—resulting from hemorrhage (the pelvis can contain up to four liters of blood)
- pain

ACUTE AND SUBACUTE CARE

Medical Management

- bedrest and traction (less severe fracture)
- analgesia

Surgical Management

- open reduction with internal fixation

Nursing Management

- See "Traction," p. 708.

(For more information, see p. 2160 of Black and Matassarin-Jacobs: *Medical-Surgical Nursing: Clinical Management for Continuity of Care,* 5th ed.)

Fracture, Ribs

- Rib fractures usually are associated with a blunt injury, such as a fall, blow to the chest, or the impact of a steering wheel during an automobile accident.
- Clinical manifestations include:
  — localized pain and tenderness over the fracture area on inspiration and palpation
  — shallow respirations
  — guarding of the chest
- Fractured ribs predispose the client to atelectasis and pneumonia due to shallow breathing and ineffective coughing.
- Bone splinters from fractured ribs may cause a pneumothorax or hemothorax.
- Treatment involves rest, local heat, and analgesics. (Strapping the ribs is not recommended because it increases the incidence of atelectasis and pneumonia.)
- Intercostal nerve blocks may be used if ventilation is significantly impaired.
- The pain from fractured ribs lasts 5–7 days. Healing is complete in approximately 6 weeks.

(For more information, see p. 2526 of Black and Matassarin-Jacobs: *Medical-Surgical Nursing: Clinical Management for Continuity of Care,* 5th ed.)

Fracture, Specific Sites

Also see, "Fracture, General Information," p. 279.

FRACTURE OF THE TIBIA AND FIBULA

- Most commonly casted after reduction.
- Complex fractures may require traction or internal fixation.

FRACTURE OF THE PATELLA

- The patella (kneecap) can fracture during falls from heights, or direct blows to the patella.
- The bone fragments may be wired or require total joint athroplasty.

FRACTURE OF THE FOOT

- Minimally displaced fractures are treated with open walking shoes, casts, or braces.
- Open reduction and casting may be necessary.

FRACTURE OF THE HUMERUS

- Common fracture in the elderly.
- Impacted fractures of the proximal humerus are treated with a sling.
- Displaced fractures of the proximal humerus are treated with surgical open reduction and fixation with pins.
- Fractures of the shaft of the humerus are usually managed with traction via a hanging arm cast or splint. Sometimes the fracture is surgically reduced and repaired with rods, plates, or screws.
- Nonunion is a common complication of humeral shaft fractures, and bone grafting may be required.
- Fractures of the condyles of the humerus are usually treated with open reduction and internal fixation devices.

FRACTURE OF THE RADIUS AND ULNA

- Colles' fracture is a fracture of the distal radius from a fall on an outstretched hand. It is treated with open reduction and internal fixation, splints, casts, or external fixation, depending upon severity.
- The radius and ulna usually fracture together. Closed reduction with casting is the most common form of treatment.

FRACTURE OF THE OLECRANON

- Usually results from a fall onto the elbow.
- Treatment includes closed reduction and long arm casting for 6–8 weeks.

FRACTURE OF THE WRIST AND HAND

- Closed reduction and casting are the most common treatment for 6–12 weeks.
- Fractures of the metacarpals and phalanges are seldom displaced. They are immobilized with splints.

See "Casts," p. 131.
See "Traction," p.708.
See "Fracture, General Information," p. 279.

(For more information, see pp. 2160–2161 of Black and Matassarin-Jacobs: *Medical-Surgical Nursing: Clinical Management for Continuity of Care,* 5th ed.)

Fracture, Sternum

- Sternal fractures usually result from blunt deceleration injuries, such as the impact from the steering wheel in a motor vehicle accident.
- Other injuries typically accompany sternal fractures, such as flail chest; hemothorax; pneumothorax; ruptured aorta, trachea, bronchus or esophagus; and pulmonary or myocardial contusions.
- Clinical manifestations include sharp, stabbing pain; crepitus; and tenderness, swelling and discoloration over the fracture site.
- Treatment is aimed at the associated injuries. Analgesics and possibly nerve blocks are given for pain. Surgical fixation may be performed for severe sternal fractures.

(For more information, see pp. 2526–2527 of Black and Matassarin-Jacobs: *Medical-Surgical Nursing: Clinical Management for Continuity of Care,* 5th ed.)

Frostbite

- Frostbite is damage to tissues and blood vessels as a result of prolonged exposure to cold. The fingers, toes, nose, and ears are most often affected.

- There may be initial numbness, paresthesia, and pallor of the affected part. Severe pain, swelling, erythema, and blistering may occur once the client is in a warm environment. Necrosis and gangrene may develop in severe cases.
- Treatment is rewarming of the affected part with tepid water (about 105° F.). Massage never is used as it may result in further tissue damage. Bulky dressings are applied and a bed cradle may be needed.
- Vasodilators or nerve blocks may be prescribed.

(For more information, see p. 2536 of Black and Matassarin-Jacobs: *Medical-Surgical Nursing: Clinical Management for Continuity of Care,* 5th ed.)

G

Gastric Cancer

OVERVIEW

- Gastric cancer refers to malignant neoplasms in the stomach, usually adenocarcinoma.
- Stomach cancer is twice as common in men as in women, more common in whites, and in clients with pernicious anemia.
- The incidence in the United States has been declining, but it is still the sixth most common cause of death from cancer.
- Risk factors include Helicobacter pylori (H. pylori) infection, pernicious anemia, wood or tobacco smoke, chronic gastritis, nitrite food preservatives and carcinogens in the diet, such as pickled foods and salted fish. There may also be a genetic factor.

CLINICAL MANIFESTATIONS

Early symptoms are vague and indefinite. Other symptoms occur late, so diagnosis is usually at a late stage.

- weight loss, vague indigestion, anorexia
- blood in stool, anemia
- palpable mass, ascites, bone pain from metastasis

ACUTE AND SUBACUTE CARE

Medical Management

- chemotherapy—combinations of Fluorouracil, mitomycin C, and doxorubicin
- radiation

Surgical Management

- partial or complete gastrectomy (removal of the stomach) and removal of associated lymph nodes
- palliative gastroenterostomy—surgical creation of a passage between the stomach and small intestine

Nursing Management

- See "Chemotherapy," p. 149, and "Radiation Therapy," p. 605.
- Administer analgesics and assess effectiveness.
- Administer total parenteral nutrition (TPN) or jejunostomy tube feedings.
- See "Peptic Ulcer Disease," p. 543, for information on surgical procedures.

COMMUNITY AND SELF-CARE

- Instruct client/significant other regarding:
  - — pain management
  - — TPN therapy
  - — jejunostomy feedings
  - — wound care
  - — signs/symptoms of infection
  - — signs/symptoms of complications and to report to physician
- Make home health care referral for TPN therapy/ jejunostomy feedings.
- Refer to support groups, e.g., I Can Cope, Hospice.

(For more information, see pp. 1781–1784 of Black and Matassarin-Jacobs: *Medical-Surgical Nursing: Clinical Management for Continuity of Care,* 5th ed.)

Gastritis, Acute

OVERVIEW

- Acute gastritis is inflammation of the gastric mucosa caused by ingestion of a corrosive, erosive, or infectious substance.
- Common causes include ingestion of excessive amounts of tea, coffee, mustard, paprika, cloves, and pepper. Aspirin, nonsteroidal anti-inflammatories, digitalis, steroids, acute alcoholism, and food poisoning may also cause this disorder.
- Incidence is highest in the fifth and sixth decades of life.
- Risk factors include ingestion of the above substances, cigarette smoking, and heavy drinking.

CLINICAL MANIFESTATIONS

- epigastric discomfort, abdominal tenderness, cramping, eructation, severe nausea and vomiting, hematemesis, and gastrointestinal bleeding
- diarrhea, if due to food poisoning

ACUTE AND SUBACUTE CARE

Medical Management

- phenothiazines to treat vomiting
- antacids or H_2 antagonists
- Cytotec to protect the stomach mucosa and suppress gastric acid secretion
- NPO status, then slow introduction of simple bland substances

Nursing Management

- Assist to assess factors that increase symptoms (e.g., stress, fatigue) and ways to reduce these.
- Administer antacids as ordered.
- Maintain NPO status if nausea and vomiting present; slowly initiate a bland diet.

COMMUNITY AND SELF-CARE

- Instruct client regarding:
  - — signs/symptoms of gastrointestinal bleeding and to report these to physician
  - — foods and beverages to avoid
  - — stress reduction
  - — use of antacids
- Refer to smoking cessation program.

(For more information, see pp. 1761–1762 of Black and Matassarin-Jacobs: *Medical-Surgical Nursing: Clinical Management for Continuity of Care,* 5th ed.)

Gastritis, Chronic

OVERVIEW

- Chronic gastritis is inflammation of the gastric mucosa in one of three forms:

(1) Superficial gastritis—causes a reddened, edematous mucosa with hemorrhages and small erosions.
(2) Atrophic gastritis—occurs in all layers of the stomach; characterized by a decreased number of parietal and chief cells.
(3) Hypertrophic gastritis—causes a dull and nodular mucosa with irregular, thickened, or nodular rugae.

- Risk factors include ingestion of excessive amounts of tea, coffee, mustard, paprika, pepper, cloves, and alcohol. Aspirin, nonsteroidal anti-inflammatories, digitalis, steroids, cigarette smoking, and acute alcoholism also may cause this disorder. Infection with the Helicobacter pylori organism and advanced age are also risk factors.

CLINICAL MANIFESTATIONS

Symptoms are vague and may be absent.

- anorexia, dyspepsia, belching, nausea, and vomiting
- a feeling of fullness, vague epigastric pain, and intolerance of spicy or fatty foods

ACUTE AND SUBACUTE CARE

Medical Management

- bland diet, small frequent meals
- antacids, anticholinergics, sedatives
- avoidance of foods that cause symptoms
- H_2 receptor antagonists, mucosal protectants such as Carafate and Cytotec
- corticosteroids
- Vitamin B_{12} if pernicious anemia is present
- treatment for H. pylori bacteria if present

Surgical Management

- partial gastrectomy, pyloroplasty, vagotomy, or total gastrectomy (see p. 546 for discussion of these procedures)

Nursing Management

- Maintain NPO status if nausea and vomiting are severe.

- Administer antacids (Gaviscon is antacid of choice) and other medications as above.
- Assist to assess factors that increase symptoms (e.g., stress, fatigue) and explore ways to reduce these.

COMMUNITY AND SELF-CARE

- Instruct client regarding:
  — avoidance of aggravating foods and beverages
  — use of medications/antacids
  — signs/symptoms of gastrointestinal bleeding
  — methods to reduce stress
  — need for follow-up and periodic testing for development of gastric cancer (clients are at increased risk for cancer following Helicobacter pylori [H. pylori] infection or atrophic gastritis)
- Refer to smoking cessation program.

(For more information, see pp. 1762–1764 of Black and Matassarin-Jacobs: *Medical-Surgical Nursing: Clinical Management for Continuity of Care,* 5th ed.)

Gastroenteritis

OVERVIEW

- Gastroenteritis is an inflammation of the stomach and intestinal tract usually caused by a virus or bacteria.
- This disorder can be serious in infants, the elderly, and debilitated people.

CLINICAL MANIFESTATIONS

- abdominal cramps
- diarrhea
- vomiting
- fever
- fluid and electrolyte loss
- may have blood in the stool

ACUTE AND SUBACUTE CARE

Medical Management

- rest the GI tract and replace fluids
- antibiotics for specific organisms
- antidiarrheals and antispasmodics are controversial (not given with *C. difficile*)

Nursing Management

- Assess the stools for consistency, frequency, color, and odor.
- Assess for accompanying symptoms.
- Inquire about recent foreign travel, eating habits, and antibiotic use.
- Examine the abdomen and auscultate bowel sounds.
- Monitor electrolytes.
- Assess for dehydration.
- Assess for weakness and fatigue.
- Administer medications to treat symptoms.
- Monitor intake and output, daily weights.
- Administer IV fluids as ordered.
- NPO until vomiting stops then start on a small amount of clear liquids as tolerated—advance the diet in 24 hours.

COMMUNITY AND SELF-CARE

Instruct client regarding:

- good handwashing techniques
- symptom management
- increased fluids
- monitoring stools
- need to notify the physician for worsening symptoms

(For more information, see pp. 1788–1790 of Black and Matassarin-Jacobs: *Medical-Surgical Nursing: Clinical Management for Continuity of Care,* 5th ed.)

Gastroesophageal Reflux Disease

OVERVIEW

- Gastroesophageal reflux disease (GERD) is a term used to describe a syndrome resulting from esophageal reflux. Esophageal reflux is the backward flow of gastric contents into the esophagus.
- Reflux exposes the esophageal mucosa to the gastric contents and gradually breaks down the esophageal mucosa (this is referred to as reflux esophagitis).
- The exact cause of GERD seems to be an inappropriate relaxation of the lower esophageal sphincter (LES).
- Risk factors include: obesity; pregnancy; nicotine; high-fat foods; theophylline; caffeine; chocolate; and high levels of estrogen and progesterone.

CLINICAL MANIFESTATIONS

- heartburn, dysphagia, acid regurgitation, water brash (the release of salty secretions in the mouth) and eructation
- burning sensation in the epigastric region that moves up and down
- pain that may radiate to the back, neck, or jaw
- pain after meals relieved by antacids or fluids
- pain worsened with supine position or when stomach is distended

ACUTE AND SUBACUTE CARE

Medical Management

- antacid therapy—1 hour before and 2-3 hours after a meal
- histamine receptor antagonists, e.g., ranitidine (Zantac) or famotidine (Pepcid)
- bethanecol (Urecholine) to increase lower esophageal sphincter pressure and prevent reflux
- metoclopramide (Reglan) to increase the rate of gastric emptying

- cisapride (Propulsid) to increase lower esophageal tone, improve esophageal peristalsis, and promote gastric emptying
- omeprazole (Prilosec) is a proton pump inhibitor that suppresses secretion of gastric acid
- dietary changes (see Nursing Management below)

Surgical Management

- Nissen fundoplication—the fundus of the stomach is wrapped 360° around the lower esophagus. An increase in pressure or volume in the stomach closes the cardia and blocks reflux.
- Hill's operation—involves narrowing the esophageal opening and anchoring the stomach and distal esophagus to the median arcuate ligament. It reinforces the sphincter and recreates the gastroesophageal valve (180° esophageal wraparound).
- Belsey's repair—plicating the anterior and lateral aspects of the stomach onto the distal esophagus (280° esophageal wraparound).

Nursing Management

Medical

- Instruct on use of medications/antacids.
- Provide pain medications; monitor effectiveness.
- Instruct on dietary management:
  - — Eat four to six small meals/day.
  - — Drink adequate fluids at meals to promote food passage.
  - — Eat slowly and chew food thoroughly.
  - — Avoid extremely hot or cold foods, spices, coffee, alcohol, fats, citrus juices, and chocolate.
  - — Avoid eating and drinking for 3 hours before retiring to prevent nocturnal reflux.
  - — Elevate the head of bed 6 to 8 inches to prevent nocturnal reflux.
  - — Lose weight (if overweight).
  - — Avoid tobacco, salicylates, or phenylbutazone.

Surgical

In addition to routine postoperative care:

- Maintain patent chest tube (if the thoracic approach was used).
- Assess for signs/symptoms of wound infection.
- Assist to turn, cough, and deep breathe (may be painful). Medicate for pain prior to performing.
- Maintain NG tube patency to prevent distention.
- Slowly advance diet as ordered (fluids are resumed in 24 hours).

After fundoplication:

- Monitor for gas-bloat syndrome (occurs if the fundus wrap is too tight, causing bloating and the inability to eructate).
- Avoid carbonated beverages and drinking with a straw.
- Instruct to report to physician dysphagia, epigastric fullness, bloating, or excessive rumbling.

COMMUNITY AND SELF-CARE

Instruct client regarding:

- substances to avoid (alcohol, aspirin, chocolate, and caffeine)
- diet (see Nursing Management above)
- keeping head of bed elevated for sleeping
- signs/symptoms of recurrence and to report to physician (nausea, vomiting, hematemesis, or symptoms of obstruction)
- ambulating after meals

Surgical

- avoidance of straining the incision for at least 6 weeks after surgery
- avoidance of lifting heavy objects
- signs/symptoms of infection to report to physician

See also "Hiatal Hernia," p. 353.

(For more information, see pp. 1737–1740 of Black and Matassarin-Jacobs: *Medical-Surgical Nursing: Clinical Management for Continuity of Care,* 5th ed.)

Genital Herpes

OVERVIEW

- Genital herpes is one of the most common sexually transmitted diseases (STD).
- Peak incidence is in the adolescent and young adult.
- It is caused by herpes simplex virus type II.
- The herpes simplex virus organism is in the exudate of the lesion. The disease can be transmitted while a lesion is present and for 10 days after it has healed.
- Genital herpes usually is transmitted by direct contact during sexual activity, but transmission is possible by fomites, such as towels used by an infected client.
- Newborns can be infected during vaginal delivery when acute lesions are present.
- Potential complications include aseptic meningitis, transverse myelitis, and spontaneous abortion.

CLINICAL MANIFESTATIONS

Symptoms generally occur 3–7 days after contact.

- Acute phase
  — paresthesia/burning at site of exposure
  — painful genital vesicles that ulcerate, crust and heal with a scar in 2–4 weeks
  — fever, chills, muscle aches
- Latent phase—herpes virus lies dormant, probably in the sacral ganglion until triggered by stress, infection, trauma, etc.
  — asymptomatic
- Recurrent phase
  — symptoms similar to acute phase, although usually less severe
  —vesicles rupture in 24–48 hours, and the syndrome genrerally lasts 7–10 days

ACUTE AND SUBACUTE CARE

Medical Management

Genital herpes is a chronic disease; there is no cure.

- acyclovir (Zovirax) orally for 5 to 10 days

Nursing Management

- Administer acyclovir as ordered.
- Maintain medical asepsis to prevent spread from highly contagious exudate.
- Provide palliative measures—sitz baths, cool applications, and analgesics.

COMMUNITY AND SELF-CARE

Instruct client regarding:

- importance of completing acyclovir regime
- information about the disease, transmission, treatment, and follow-up
- the need to evaluate all sexual contacts and, if symptomatic, the need to be treated
- the use of condoms in latent phases as there is a risk of transmission even though symptoms are not present
- if pregnant, the possibility of infecting the newborn
- annual pelvic examinations and Pap smears because of the association of herpes simplex virus with cervical cancer

(For more information, see pp. 2472–2473 of Black and Matassarin-Jacobs: *Medical-Surgical Nursing: Clinical Management for Continuity of Care,* 5th ed.)

Genital Warts

OVERVIEW

- Genital warts are caused by the human papillomavirus (HPV).
- Genital warts are the fourth most common sexually transmitted disease (STD).

- Warts occur 1-2 months after exposure.
- HPV can cause laryngeal papillomatosis in infants born to mothers with vaginal warts.
- Clients with genital warts are at an increased risk for genital malignancy, such as cancer of the vulva, cervix, or penis.

CLINICAL MANIFESTATIONS

- Warts occur in multiple, painless clusters on the vulva, vagina, cervix, perineum, anorectal area, urethral meatus, or glans penis.
- Oral and pharyngeal lesions can also occur.

ACUTE AND SUBACUTE CARE

Medical Management

Recurrence is high and there is no cure.
- topical application of podophyllin in compound with tincture of benzoin.

Sexual partners also must be treated if symptomatic on evaluation.

Surgical Management

- cryotherapy with liquid nitrogen or a cryoprobe
- carbon dioxide laser, electrocautery, or surgical excision for extensive warts

Nursing Management

- Apply topical treatment as ordered.

COMMUNITY AND SELF-CARE

Instruct the client regarding:
- information about the disease, transmission, and treatment
- need to treat all sexual partners if symptomatic
- if pregnant, the possibility of infecting the baby
- importance of annual Pap smear and follow-up due to increased risk of genital malignancy

(For more information, see p. 2473 of Black and Matassarin-Jacobs: *Medical-Surgical Nursing: Clinical Management for Continuity of Care,* 5th ed.)

Glaucoma

OVERVIEW

- Glaucoma includes a group of ocular disorders characterized by increased intraocular pressure, optic nerve atrophy, and visual field loss.
- Intraocular pressure is determined by the rate of aqueous production in the ciliary body and the resistance of outflow of aqueous from the eye. Increased intraocular pressure (usually greater than 23 mm Hg) may result from hyperproduction of aqueous or obstruction of the outflow. As aqueous fluid builds up in the eye, the increased pressure inhibits blood supply to the optic nerve and retina. These tissues become ischemic and gradually lose function.
- The terms open (wide) and closed (narrow) describe the width of the angle between the cornea and iris. Narrow anterior chamber angles predispose clients to an acute onset of angle-closure glaucoma.
- Types of glaucoma:
  - primary open-angle glaucoma
    - bilateral
    - insidious in onset
    - slow to progress
    - cause—degenerative changes resulting in decreased outflow of aqueous
  - angle-closure glaucoma
    - acute onset
    - develops only in an eye in which the anterior chamber is anatomically narrowed
    - cause—sudden blockage of the anterior angle by the base of the iris
  - low-tension glaucoma
    - similar to primary open-angle glaucoma in all respects except that intraocular pressure is normal
  - secondary glaucoma
    - etiologic factors
      - postoperative edema
      - trauma
      - lens displacement

- hemorrhage into the anterior chamber
- tumor encroachment

- It is estimated that over 50,000 people in the United States are blind as a result of glaucoma. The incidence is about 1.5 per cent and in blacks between the ages of 45 and 65, the prevalence is five times that of whites.

CLINICAL MANIFESTATIONS

- primary open-angle glaucoma—visual changes include blind spots in periphery, decreased visual acuity, loss of contrast sensitivity
- angle-closure glaucoma—severe pain, blurred vision or vision loss, rainbow halos around lights, nausea and vomiting
- increased intraocular pressure
- cupping or indentation of optic nerve disc

ACUTE AND SUBACUTE CARE

Medical Management

- topical miotics—constrict pupils and increase outflow (pilocarpine hydrochloride)
- topical epinephrine—increase outflow
- topical beta-blockers—suppress secretion of aqueous humor (timolol maleate)
- oral carbonic anhydrase inhibitors—reduce production of aqueous humor (acetazolamide [Diamox])
- oral osmotic agents—glycerin (Osmoglyn), isosorbide (Ismotic)—diuretic action lowers intraocular pressure
- IV osmotic agents—mannitol (glaucoma crisis)

Surgical Management

- laser trabeculoplasty—creation of an opening in the trabecular meshwork to facilitate outflow
- filtering procedures (trephination, trabeculectomy, thermal sclerostomy, sclerectomy)—creation of an outflow channel from the anterior chamber into the subconjunctival space where the aqueous is absorbed through the conjunctival vessels

- cyclocryotherapy (application of a freezing tip)—damages the ciliary body, thus decreasing the production of aqueous

Nursing Management

Medical

- Administer eye drops and oral medications as ordered.
- Implement appropriate safety measures.

Surgical

Postoperative Care

In addition to routine postoperative care:

- Maintain eye pad and shield in place.
- Instruct client not to lie on operative side.
- Observe for signs of increased intraocular pressure (pain, nausea).
- Assist with ambulation and activities of daily living.

COMMUNITY AND SELF-CARE

Instruct client regarding:

- disease process and importance of medications in preventing loss of vision
- technique for instilling eye drops
- signs/symptoms of increased intraocular pressure (pain, nausea, decreased vision)
- rationale for eye protection (shield or glasses at all times)
- measures to provide a safe home environment
- measures to prevent intraocular pressure increase:
  - — no bending at the waist
  - — no lifting of heavy objects
  - — no straining during bowel movements
  - — avoidance of coughing and vomiting
- Postoperative
  - — signs/symptoms of infection (redness, swelling, drainage, blurred vision or pain)
  - — how to cleanse the eye with warm water
  - — instruct not to rub or apply pressure over closed eye (could damage healing tissue)
- importance of follow-up visits

(For more information, see pp. 952–958 of Black and Matassarin-Jacobs: *Medical-Surgical Nursing: Clinical Management for Continuity of Care,* 5th ed.)

Glomerulonephritis, Acute

OVERVIEW

- Glomerulonephritis is a term that encompasses a wide variety of diseases, most of which are caused by an immunologic reaction that results in proliferative and inflammatory changes in the glomerular structure.
- Damage occurs due to trapping of circulating antigen-antibody complexes within the glomerulus or by the fixing of antibodies to the glomerular basement membrane.
- There are two forms of acute glomerulonephritis:
  (1) Postinfectious glomerulonephritis—usually caused by a beta-hemolytic streptococcal infection elsewhere in the body. It occurs about 21 days after a respiratory or skin infection.
  (2) Infectious glomerulonephritis—caused by a beta-hemolytic streptococcal infection or another bacterial, viral, or parasitic infection in the body. It occurs during or within a few days of the original infectious process.

CLINICAL MANIFESTATIONS

- sudden onset of hematuria and proteinuria
- fever, chills, weakness, pallor, nausea, and vomiting
- generalized edema, ascites, pleural effusion, congestive heart failure
- headache, hypertension
- oliguria or anuria for several days
- signs/symptoms also may be insidious or mild with reports of anorexia, vague weakness, lethargy

ACUTE AND SUBACUTE CARE

Medical Management

Interventions aim to eliminate antigens, alter the immune balance, and inhibit or alleviate inflammation to prevent further renal damage.

- plasmapheresis in conjunction with immunosuppressive therapy
- antibiotic therapy
- diuretics, antihypertensives, and restriction of dietary sodium and water to treat volume overload and hypertension
- corticosteroids and immunosuppressive agents

Nursing Management

- Monitor for complications: congestive heart failure with pulmonary edema, increased intracranial pressure, or renal failure.
- Obtain daily weights.
- Monitor intake and output.
- Maintain fluid restriction and provide hard candies or ice chips for thirst.
- Measure edematous areas daily.
- Monitor laboratory results: BUN, creatinine.
- Monitor vital signs.
- Maintain bedrest or activity restrictions.
- Provide good skin care and change position frequently.
- Protect the client from infection since the client has increased susceptibility due to an altered immune response.

COMMUNITY AND SELF-CARE

- Instruct client regarding:
  - — high calorie, low protein, low sodium diet to avoid protein catabolism and to rest the kidney
  - — avoidance of infection
  - — avoidance of stressors on the kidneys
  - — need for follow-up testing of renal function.
- If client develops renal failure and requires dialysis, see "Renal Failure, Chronic," p. 618, and "Dialysis," p. 225.
- Also see "Glomerulonephritis, Chronic," p. 307.

(For more information, see pp. 1630–1632 of Black and Matassarin-Jacobs: *Medical-Surgical Nursing: Clinical Management for Continuity of Care,* 5th ed.)

Glomerulonephritis, Chronic

OVERVIEW

- Chronic glomerulonephritis is an insidious disease, progressing over extended periods as long as 30 years.
- All forms of acute glomerulonephritis can progress to a chronic state.
- Glomeruli and tubules are destroyed by the pathologic process with fibrous and scar tissue replacing functioning renal tissue.

CLINICAL MANIFESTATIONS

- hypertension, malaise, weight loss, mental cloudiness, metallic taste in the mouth, polyuria, and nocturia
- headache, dizziness, and digestive disturbances
- advanced disease—generalized edema, respiratory difficulty, angina, hematuria, and anemia
- signs/symptoms of end stage renal failure requiring dialysis

ACUTE AND SUBACUTE CARE

Medical Management

- dialysis, transplant, and control of symptoms, such as edema and hypertension
- chemotherapy with anti-inflammatory agents and anticoagulants
- diet management and reduced fluid intake

Nursing Management

- Monitor for signs/symptoms of complications.
- Assess for relief of symptoms.
- Instruct on disease and management.
- Provide support; discuss coping strategies to deal with long-term illness.

COMMUNITY AND SELF-CARE

Also see "Glomerulonephritis, Acute," p. 305; "Dialysis," p. 225; "Renal Failure, Chronic," p. 618; and "Renal Transplantation," p. 621.

(For more information, see pp. 1632–1633 of Black and Matassarin-Jacobs: *Medical-Surgical Nursing: Clinical Management for Continuity of Care,* 5th ed.)

Gonorrhea

OVERVIEW

- Gonorrhea is caused by the gram-negative diplococcus Neisseria gonorrhoeae.
- This disease continues to be one of the most common sexually transmitted diseases (STD). It is almost always transmitted by sexual contact. There is a large carrier population (i.e., people who have no symptoms but carry the organism and can transmit the disease).
- Teenagers and young adults are at highest risk; the highest rates occur in the 20–24 year-old age group.
- Gonorrhea may be divided into two groups:
  - local—can involve the mucosal surfaces of the urethra, cervix, and rectum; pharynx; vestibular glands; or conjunctiva
  - systemic (disseminated gonococcal infection) involves bacterimia with polyarthritis, dermatitis, endocarditis, and meningitis. Systemic infection is more common in women than in men.
- There is no lasting immunity that prevents reinfection.
- The most common complication in women is salpingitis (inflammation of the fallopian tubes), which can progress to pelvic inflammatory disease (PID), both of which can cause infertility. In men, complications include epididymitis and prostatitis.

CLINICAL MANIFESTATIONS

- Female
  - may be asymptomatic

— thick, purulent vaginal discharge
— cervical erythema
— dysuria and frequency
— abnormal menstrual bleeding
— red, swollen vulva
— pharyngeal infection

- Male
  — may be asymptomatic
  — urethral discharge
  — dysuria, frequency
  — pharyngeal infection
- Disseminated (systemic), either sex
  — bacteremia
  — arthritis
  — dermatitis

ACUTE AND SUBACUTE CARE

Medical Management

All sexual contacts within 30 days before diagnosis should be treated.

- ceftriaxone sodium (Rocephin)—one intramuscular dose, or a single oral dose of cefixime (Suprax), ciprofloxacin (Cipro), or ofloxacin (Floxin) followed by oral doxycycline (Vibramycin) for 7 days
- disseminated gonococcal infection—hospitalization and administration of ceftriaxone IM or IV every 24 hours and continued 24-48 hours after clinical manifestations begin to improve. This is followed by cefixime or ciprofloxacin orally for 1 week.
- repeat cultures after therapy completed

Nursing Management

- Administer antibiotics as ordered.
- Monitor temperature.

COMMUNITY AND SELF-CARE

Instruct client regarding:

- importance of taking the complete course of antibiotics and follow-up culture
- information about the disease, how it spreads, and treatment regime
- importance of identifying and treating sex partners

- importance of abstinence or use of a male or female condom until infection is cured
- the possibility of reinfection and infection of sexual partners
- if client is pregnant, possibility of infecting the baby during delivery
- avoidance of oral sexual activity if there is pharyngeal infection
- medication administration:
  — take 1–2 hours after meals
  — avoid iron, dairy products, and antacids

(For more information, see pp. 2465–2469 of Black and Matassarin-Jacobs: *Medical-Surgical Nursing: Clinical Management for Continuity of Care,* 5th ed.)

Gout and Gouty Arthritis

OVERVIEW

- Gout is a metabolic disorder in which purine (protein) metabolism is altered and the by-product, uric acid, accumulates.
- Gout is classified as primary or secondary. Primary gout is caused by an inherited defect of purine metabolism. Primary gout accounts for 80 per cent of all cases, of which 95 per cent are males. The initial attack of gout occurs in the third or fourth decade. Secondary gout is an acquired condition, following hematopoietic or renal disorders. Multiple myeloma, polycythemia vera, and leukemia are disorders that cause an increase in cell turnover and thus uric acid production. Gout may also develop secondary to rapid induction of chemotherapy or radiation therapy when there is massive destruction of cells. Renal disorders that decrease the excretion of uric acid may lead to gout. Hyperuricemia may also result from use of aspirin, thiazide, and mercurial diuretics. Alcohol intoxication and starvation increase serum urate levels by inhibiting renal excretion of uric acid.

- When uric acid levels reach a certain level they crystallize and the crystals, called tophi, are deposited in connective tissue.

CLINICAL MANIFESTATIONS

Stage I

- asymptomatic hyperuricemia

Stage II

- acute attack with redness, swelling, and tenderness in one joint (toes, fingers, wrists, ankles, or knees), the great toe is the most common site
- fever, tachycardia
- malaise, anorexia

The acute episode usually subsides within a week. Following the inital attack the affected joint returns to normal and the client may be asymptomatic for years.

Stage III

- permanent changes in multiple joints with restricted movement
- tophi on the ears, hands, elbows, feet, and knees
- uric acid, renal stones

ACUTE AND SUBACUTE CARE

Medical Management

- colchicine and nonsteroidal anti-inflammatory agents
- allopurinol and probenecid (lower uric acid level)
- ice therapy
- dietary management—avoid foods high in purine (liver, kidney, sweet breads, mussels, etc.)
- increased fluid intake to promote uric acid excretion
- weight control

Nursing Management

- Administer colchicine and anti-inflammatory agents.
- Restrict activity until pain subsides.
- Encourage increased fluid intake.

- Consult Physical Therapy for assistive devices for ambulation as indicated.
- Initiate Dietary consult for purine restricted diet.

COMMUNITY AND SELF-CARE

Instruct the client/family regarding:

- disease process and treatment regime
- medication regime and possible side effects
- dietary restrictions
- safety measures for the home environment

(For more information, see pp. 2107–2108 of Black and Matassarin-Jacobs: *Medical-Surgical Nursing: Clinical Management for Continuity of Care,* 5th ed.)

Guillain-Barré Syndrome

OVERVIEW

- Guillain-Barré syndrome (GBS) is an inflammatory disease of unknown etiology that involves degeneration of the myelin sheath of peripheral nerves.
- GBS affects people of all ages and races.
- In one-half to two-thirds of cases, an upper respiratory or gastrointestinal infection precedes the onset of the syndrome by 1–4 weeks.
- The characteristic feature of GBS is ascending weakness, usually beginning in the lower extremities and spreading, sometimes rapidly to the trunk, upper extremities, and face with maximal deficit by 4 weeks in 90 per cent of cases.
- Improvement and recovery occur with remyelination. If nerve axons are damaged, some residual deficits may remain. Recovery is usually maximal at 6 months with 85–90 per cent of clients recovering completely.

CLINICAL MANIFESTATIONS

- weakness
- muscle paralysis
- paresthesia (tingling sensation) of the limbs
- loss of deep tendon reflexes

- deep, aching muscle pain in shoulder girdle and thighs
- respiratory compromise or failure—dyspnea, decreased breath sounds, decreased tidal volume
- autonomic dysfunction—orthostatic hypotension, hypertension, pupillary disturbances, sweating dysfunction, cardiac dysrhythmias, paralytic ileus, and urinary retention

ACUTE AND SUBACUTE CARE

Medical Management

- supportive therapy
- plasmapheresis—to remove circulating antibodies
- intravenous IgG therapy

Nursing Management

- Monitor cardiac and respiratory status.
- Monitor laboratory arterial blood gas results.
- Monitor results of pulmonary function studies.
- Assure respiratory support equipment is maintained at bedside (oxygen, ambu bag).
- Assess ability to perform self care and provide assistance based on level of client's ability.
- Collaborate with Physical and Occupational Therapy for adaptive devices and exercises.
- Monitor for signs of deep vein thrombosis or pulmonary embolism while on bedrest.
- Initiate appropriate safety measures.
- Provide measures to prevent skin breakdown.

COMMUNITY AND SELF-CARE

- Instruct the client/family regarding:
  - — disease process and prognosis
  - — use of adaptive devices
  - — prevention of skin breakdown
  - — exercise regime
  - — need for clinic follow-up visits
- Refer to available community resources (e.g., home health care agency).

(For more information, see pp. 877–878 of Black and Matassarin-Jacobs: *Medical-Surgical Nursing: Clinical Management for Continuity of Care,* 5th ed.)

H

Hallux Valgus

OVERVIEW

- The hallux valgus (bunion) deformity is the most common disorder of the foot. It is defined as a painful swelling of the bursa mucosa when the great toe deviates laterally at the metatarsophalangeal joint.
- Hallux valgus may be congenital or caused by wearing ill-fitting shoes.
- There is a female predominance.

CLINICAL MANIFESTATIONS

- pain
- deformity of great toe
- callous formation on bottom of the feet

ACUTE AND SUBACUTE CARE

Medical Management

- metatarsal pads
- corticosteroid injections
- analgesics

Surgical Management

- bunionectomy (bone resection of first metatarsal) and insertion of Kirschner wires vertically through the toe that remain in place 3 weeks

Nursing Management

Treatment is generally done on an outpatient basis.

(For more information, see p. 2124 of Black and Matassarin-Jacobs: *Medical-Surgical Nursing: Clinical Management for Continuity of Care,* 5th ed.)

Headaches, Cluster (Histamine Headaches)

- Cluster headaches sometimes are classified as a form of migraine. They are excruciatingly painful, unilateral, and tend to occur in clusters.
- Numerous episodes may occur over a few days or weeks, followed by a remission with no symptoms for months or years.
- Men are affected five times more often than women. Episodes usually begin during mid-life.
- Cluster headaches begin suddenly and may last only a few minutes or as long as 2–3 hours. There may be excruciating, throbbing or steady pain arising high in the nostril and spreading to one side of the forehead, around and behind the affected eye. The nose and affected eye may water, and the skin reddens on the affected side.
- Indomethacin (the medication of choice) and tricyclic antidepressants may be used to prevent the occurrence of cluster headaches. Once the headache occurs, applying cold may help, but most interventions are ineffective because of the shortness of the episodes.
- Supportive care is important because clients may feel depressed over their condition and fearful of another episode.

(For more information, see pp. 819–820 of Black and Matassarin-Jacobs: *Medical-Surgical Nursing: Clinical Management for Continuity of Care,* 5th ed.)

Headaches, Migraine

OVERVIEW

- Migraine headaches are episodic headaches that are unilateral or bilateral, pulsating in nature, moderate to severe in intensity, and exacerbated by activity.

- The early neurologic symptoms are due to constriction of intracranial vessels. The later, throbbing headache is due to dilation of branches of the external carotid artery. The underlying mechanism causing this spasm and dilation is unknown.
- Migraine episodes begin during puberty or ages 20–40 years and generally decrease in frequency and severity with advancing years.
- There are many factors that can precipitate migraines:
  — perfectionist tendencies
  — fatigue
  — excess sleep
  — hunger
  — stress
  — bright lights
  — emotional excitement
  — excessive smoking
  — drinking alcoholic beverages
  — menstruation
  — chocolate, cheese, citrus fruits, coffee, dairy products, and pork products
- Migraines affect about 5–10 per cent of the population. Women are more susceptible than men.

CLINICAL MANIFESTATIONS

Classic or Typical Migraine

- an aura or prodromal phase precedes the headache with depression, irritability, restlessness, or transient neurologic disturbances. It may last several minutes or several hours.
- headache pain, which may be vise-like, dull, pressing, boring, throbbing, or hammering—it is usually unilateral and may be localized to the front, back or side of the head
- hypersensitivity of all sensory organs (client withdraws from light and sound)
- photophobia
- vertigo, tremor
- nausea, vomiting, diarrhea
- arteries of the head become prominent, and the amplitude of their pulsation increases

Atypical or Common Migraine

- sudden headache with or without prodromal phase—may be unilateral or generalized
- nausea and vomiting may or may not be present

ACUTE AND SUBACUTE CARE

Medical Management

- ergot preparations, only effective if taken 30–60 minutes after headache onset
- codeine sulfate, acetaminophen, or acetylsalicylic acid for pain
- prophylactic beta-adrenergic blockers (propranolol) or calcium-channel blockers (nifedipine) to reduce frequent episodes
- medication adjustment during menstrual cycles (menstruation and ovulation can trigger migraines)
- elimination of tyramine in diet

Nursing Management

- Instruct client/significant other regarding:
  - — factors that trigger migraines
  - — use of pressure on the common carotid artery and the affected superficial artery to reduce pain
  - — identifying and avoiding dietary triggers
  - — stress reduction
  - — use of ice on the back of the neck and lying in a dark, quiet room to reduce the pain
- Refer to appropriate resources for relaxation training and biofeedback, if desired.

(For more information, see pp. 818–819 of Black and Matassarin-Jacobs: *Medical-Surgical Nursing: Clinical Management for Continuity of Care,* 5th ed.)

Head Injury

OVERVIEW

- Head injury is any trauma to the scalp, skull, or brain. Traumatic brain injury is an insult to the brain capable of producing physical, intellectual, emotional, social, and vocational changes.

- In the United States, a head injury is experienced approximately every 15 seconds. Head injuries occur in about two million Americans every year.
- Motor vehicle accidents are the main cause of head injuries. Other causes are assaults, falls, and accidents.
- Males ages 15–30 years are three times more likely to succumb to a traumatic head injury than females.

Mechanisms of Injury

Head trauma may be categorized by describing the injury:

— blunt trauma—complex injuries involving several cranial structures, including brain parenchyma and vessels. Because the brain is able to move within the skull, movement of the brain can result in injuries at different locations.

— penetrating injuries—those made by foreign bodies, such as a knife or bullet, or those made by bone fragments from a skull fracture.

— coup injury—injury at the point of impact because of movement within the skull. The same blow may cause injury on the opposite side of the brain, that is, a contrecoup.

Types of Primary Injuries

— scalp injuries can cause lacerations, hematomas, and contusions or abrasions to the skin. They may bleed profusely.

— skull fractures are classified as:
  - linear skull fractures, which appear as thin lines radiographically and usually do not require treatment
  - depressed skull fractures, which are palpable and can be seen radiographically. They may require surgery.
  - basilar skull fractures, which occur in bones over the base of the frontal and temporal lobes

— brain injuries include:
  - open head injuries, which penetrate the skull

- closed head injuries, which are caused by blunt trauma
- concussions, which are head injuries that may result in retrograde amnesia and loss of consciousness for 5 minutes or less. There is no break in the skull or dura, and no damage seen on CT or MRI.
- contusions, which cause more damage than concussions. There is damage to the brain substance itself, causing multiple areas of petechial and punctate hemorrhage and bruised areas.

CLINICAL MANIFESTATIONS

Skull Fractures

- cerebrospinal fluid or other drainage from the ear or nose
- blood behind the eardrum
- periorbital ecchymosis (bruising around the eyes)
- bruise over the mastoid (Battle's sign)
- signs of cranial nerve damage

Concussions

- loss of consciousness for 5 minutes or less
- retrograde or post-traumatic amnesia
- headache and dizziness
- nausea and vomiting

Cerebral Contusions

- findings vary depending upon the area of injury

Brain Stem Contusions

- unresponsive or comatose—an altered LOC continues for at least several hours and usually days or weeks
- respiratory, pupillary, eye movement, and motor abnormalities may occur
- high temperature, tachycardia, tachypnea, and profuse diaphoresis secondary to damage to the hypothalmus

Scalp Injuries

- lacerations, hematomas, contusions, abrasions

ACUTE AND SUBACUTE CARE

Medical Management

- prompt recognition and treatment of hypoxia and acid-base imbalances that, if left untreated, contribute to further cerebral edema
- airway management and adequate oxygenation
- management of shock
- osmotic diuretics to reduce intracranial pressure (ICP)
- management of nutrition and gastrointestinal function
- management of fluid and electrolyte balance
- antiseizure medications
- histamine antagonists to prevent stress ulcers
- antibiotic therapy

Surgical Management

Severe Head Injury

- conditions that may require surgery include subdural and epidural hematomas, depressed skull fractures, and penetrating foreign bodies

Simple Skull Depressions

- elevation of the depressed bone fragment and repair of the dura

Compound Depressed Skull Fractures

- debridement of the scalp, skull and devitalized brain and cleansing of the wound

Nursing Management

- Maintain patent airway and support ventilatory function.
- Document baseline neurologic assessment.

After initial stabilization:

- Monitor neurologic status every hour until stable:
  — assess level of consciousness, responsiveness

— assess pupillary size, position, direct and consensual responses
— assess extraocular movements
— note verbalization and response to verbal commands by checking hand grip and release, leg movement, dorsiflexion and plantar flexion
— assess muscle strength, spontaneous activity.

- Monitor for complications:
  — hematoma formation—assess for signs/symptoms of increasing ICP
  — acute hydrocephalus—assess for signs/symptoms of increasng ICP
  — neurogenic pulmonary edema (similar to ARDS)—assess for signs/symptoms of hypoxemia, pulmonary congestion, atelectasis, and ventricular failure.
- Monitor temperature and maintain normothermia with antipyretic agents or hypothermia blanket.
- Elevate head of bed 30 degrees or as ordered; keep head in neutral position (use sandbags).
- Monitor the client for diabetes insipidus:
  — high urine output (over 200ml/hr for 2 consecutive hours)
  — electrolytes and serum osmolality
  — urine osmolality and specific gravity
- Avoid extreme hip flexion (increases ICP).
- Monitor hemoglobin and hematocrit (loss of blood will result in decreased cerebral perfusion).
- Monitor for cardiac dysrhythmias.
- Initiate seizure precautions.
- Begin early range of motion as ordered.
- Reposition every 2 hours.
- Use footboard or high top tennis shoes.
- Use splints to maintain functional position of hands, arms, legs, and feet.
- Facilitate referral to Physical/Occupational Therapy.
- Assess and maintain skin integrity.
- Observe for otorrhea or rhinorrhea.
- Test clear, watery fluid for glucose using a test strip.
- Observe blood-tinged fluid for halo sign.
- Suction oropharynx and trachea as needed.
- Do not suction nasally if anterior fossa fracture is present or if basilar fractures are suspected.

- Instruct not to blow nose, cough, or inhibit sneeze; sneeze through an open mouth.
- Provide mouth care every 4 hours; assess for thrush.
- Administer antibiotics and monitor for signs of meningitis—fever, severe headache, photophobia, nuchal rigidity.
- Monitor daily caloric and protein intake.
- Monitor daily weights.
- Administer enteral feeding as ordered.
- Assess client for pain if restless.
- Reduce environmental stimuli.
- Orient to person, time, and place.
- Devise alternative methods of communicating as needed.
- Assist with gradual progression of activity.
- Encourage to discuss concerns/fears.

COMMUNITY AND SELF-CARE

If the client has mild head injury or is not hospitalized, instruct client/significant other to monitor client for 24 hours and take client to hospital if any of the following occur:

- increased drowsiness or confusion
- inability to be awakened
- vomiting, convulsions
- bleeding or drainage from the nose or ears
- weakness in either arm or either leg
- blurring of vision, slurred speech
- enlargement or shrinkage of one pupil

If the client is hospitalized longer than 48 hours and requires rehabilitation:

- facilitate referral to rehabilitation program
- communicate with rehabilitation facility to ensure continuity of care

(For more information, see pp. 820–830 of Black and Matassarin-Jacobs: *Medical-Surgical Nursing: Clinical Management for Continuity of Care,* 5th ed.)

Hearing Impairment

OVERVIEW

- Hearing impairment ranges from difficulty in understanding words or hearing certain sounds to total deafness.
- Hearing impairment affects one of every 15 Americans.
- Hearing loss may be classified as conductive and/or sensorineural.
- Factors that may cause hearing loss are: hereditary diseases, toxic substances, noise exposure, trauma to the head or ear, age, and infectious diseases (measles, mumps, and meningitis). Arteriosclerosis, neuromas of the 8th cranial nerve, otospongiosis, and degeneration of the organ of corti are causes for hearing loss in the elderly.
- Tympanosclerosis can cause conductive hearing loss, which is caused by repeated infections that create collagen and calcium deposits within the middle ear.
- Preventive measures include:
  - — early, adequate treatment of diseases
  - — prevention of trauma to the ear
  - — early detection of hearing loss
  - — monitoring effects of ototoxic drugs
  - — monitoring and prevention of noise pollution
  - — periodic ear examinations.

CLINICAL MANIFESTATIONS

- loss of discrimination (the ability to understand what is spoken)
- tinnitus (hearing a roaring, cricket-like or musical sound)
- hearing distorted or abnormal sounds
- excessively loud speech
- constant need for clarification of conversation
- constant requests to repeat information
- tilted head when listening
- facial expressions
- failure to respond or inappropriate response to communication.

ACUTE AND SUBACUTE CARE

Medical Management

- aural rehabilitation to teach the client more effective use of vision, touch, and vibration, plus maximizing the use of any remaining hearing ability
- hearing aids
- implantable hearing devices
- assistive listening devices (for use with a television, radio, or telephone)
- hearing education for speech (lip) reading and sign language
- antibiotics for infections
- steroids and vasodilators
- hearing education

Surgical Management

- rare, but may be used to alleviate a conductive hearing loss component or to stop progressive hearing loss

Nursing Management

- Be aware that hearing aids usually amplify all sounds including background noise.
- Facilitate communication with client:
  - — minimize background noise
  - — gain the client's attention by raising an arm or hand
  - — stand so that your face is in light to assist client to speech read
  - — speak facing the client
  - — speak clearly in a normal tone
  - — do not smile, chew gum, or cover the mouth when talking
  - — use phrases to convey meaning rather than one word answers; state the major topic of discussion first and then give details
  - — encourage use of hearing aid
  - — in a group, repeat important statements and avoid asides to other members in the group
  - — do not avoid conversation with a client who has a hearing loss
- Encourage client to remain socially active.

- Assist client in care of hearing aid, if needed:
  — turn off when not in use
  — open the battery compartment at night
  — keep an extra battery available
  — behind-the-ear hearing aids—wash the ear mold with soap and water every 2 weeks or once a month as needed. Dry the ear mold completely before connecting it to the hearing aid.
  — do not wear hearing aids during an ear infection
  — if the hearing aid does not work:
    - check the on-off switch
    - check the earmold for cleanliness
    - replace battery, if necessary
  — if the hearing aid whistles, the ear mold is not inserted properly into the ear canal, or the client needs to have a new ear mold made.

COMMUNITY AND SELF-CARE

Instruct client on avoidance of noisy or crowded areas (hearing aid will amplify).

- Make referrals to home health care, support groups and hearing impaired agencies and associations as needed.

(For more information, see pp. 993–1001 of Black and Matassarin-Jacobs: *Medical-Surgical Nursing: Clinical Management for Continuity of Care,* 5th ed.)

Heart Failure

OVERVIEW

- Heart failure is defined as a physiologic state in which the heart is unable to pump enough blood to meet the metabolic needs of the body (determined as oxygen consumption) at rest or during exercise, even though filling pressures are adequate. Heart failure is not a disease itself; instead, the term denotes a group of manifestations related to inadequate pump performance from either the cardiac valves or myocardium. Pump failure results in hypoperfused tissue, followed by pulmonary and systemic venous congestion. Because heart failure causes vascular congestion, it is often called congestive heart failure, although this term is no longer advised by most cardiac specialists. Other terms used to denote heart failure include cardiac decompensation, cardiac insufficiency, and ventricular insufficiency.

- The healthy heart can meet the demands of life though the use of cardiac reserve (the ability to increase output in response to stress). The failing heart, even at rest, is pumping near its capacity and has lost much of its reserve. The heart in failure has three compensatory mechanisms: (1) ventricular dilation, (2) ventricular hypertrophy, and (3) sympathetic nervous system stimulation (tachycardia). Cardiac decompensation occurs when the heart, despite these mechanisms, fails to meet the demands put upon it, and symptoms of heart failure develop. Right ventricular failure usually follows left ventricular failure.
- The causes of heart failure can be divided into three subgroups: (1) abnormal loading conditions, (2) abnormal muscle function, and (3) conditions or diseases that precipitate or exacerbate heart failure. Causes of congestive heart failure include:
  — congenital heart defects
  — systemic hypertension
  — pulmonary hypertension
  — myocardial infarction
  — myocarditis
  — valvular stenosis or regurgitation
  — cardiac tamponade
  — constrictive pericarditis
  — hypervolemia
  — cardiomyopathy
  — conditions that precipitate heart failure—dysrhythmias, physical or emotional stress, pregnancy, infection, anemia, thyroid disorders, pulmonary disease, etc.
- Estimates from the American Heart Association indicate that three million Americans have heart failure and are alive. The incidence of new cases is about four hundred thousand annually. The incidence of heart failure approaches 10 in 1,000 people after age 65.

CLINICAL MANIFESTATIONS

Left Ventricular Failure

- dyspnea
- weakness, fatigue
- mental confusion
- insomnia
- anorexia
- diaphoresis
- anxiety
- orthopnea or paroxysmal nocturnal dyspnea (PND)
- tachycardia, premature atrial contractions
- S_3, S_4
- pulmonary crackles
- enlarged point of maximal impulse
- elevated pulmonary artery wedge pressure
- cough
- nocturia
- signs of acute pulmonary edema—severe dyspnea; orthopnea; pallor; tachycardia; frothy, blood-tinged sputum; cyanosis; etc.

Right Ventricular Failure

- weight gain
- ankle or pretibial swelling
- abdominal distention
- anorexia, nausea, gastric distress
- pitting edema in dependent areas
- ascites
- jugular vein distention
- hepatomegaly
- increased central venous pressure
- subcostal pain

ACUTE AND SUBACUTE CARE

Medical Management

- oxygen administration
- digitalis therapy to improve contractility
- diuretics—furosemide (Lasix), ethacrynic acid (Edecrin), chlorothiazide (Diuril)
- high Fowler's position
- vasodilators—nitroprusside, nitroglycerin, hydralazine, isosorbide dinitrate, prazosin

- physical and emotional stress reduction
- inotropic agents (facilitate myocardial contractility and enhance stroke volume)—dopamine, dobutamine, amrinone)
- angiotensin-converting enzyme (ACE) inhibitors—suppress renin-angiotensin-aldosterone system (captopril)
- dietary modifications—low sodium, high potassium, water restriction

Surgical Management

- cardiac transplantation or use of an artificial heart
- venoarterial bypass—diverts blood to a pump that returns the blood to the arterial tree
- counterpulsation—adjusts the aortic blood pressure either by changing the volume of blood in the aorta (with use of an external pump) or the capacity of the aorta (with use of an internal balloon)

Nursing Management

Medical

- Monitor intake and output.
- Maintain fluid restriction.
- Provide frequent oral care.
- Daily weights.
- Monitor laboratory results—electrolytes, digoxin level.
- Assess for signs/symptoms of decreased cardiac output.
- Assess heart rate and rhythm, and hemodynamic readings.
- Auscultate heart sounds.
- Assess for changes in mental status.
- Monitor blood pressure closely with diuretic and vasodilator therapy.
- Assess for jugular vein distention, peripheral or sacral edema, hepatic engorgement, or pain in right upper quadrant.
- Administer oxygen therapy and monitor arterial blood gas results and oxygen saturations.
- Assess lung sounds.
- Maintain high-Fowler's positioning with legs in a dependent position as much as possible.

- Monitor for digitalis toxicity—bradycardia, first-degree heart block, "colored vision," headache, fatigue, anorexia, etc.
- Maintain sodium restricted diet. Provide small meals and rest periods after eating.
- Promote adequate rest, quiet environment.
- Monitor response to diuretic therapy—increased urinary output, decreased peripheral edema, clear lung sounds.
- Monitor for signs of hypokalemia due to diuretic therapy—lethargy, hypotension, muscle cramping.
- Monitor response to inotropic and vasodilator therapy—increased activity tolerance, increased urinary output, improved respiratory status.
- Monitor cardiopulmonary response to progressive exercise program.

COMMUNITY AND SELF-CARE

Instruct the client regarding:

- importance of medication regime
- dietary modifications—low sodium, high potassium, and possible fluid restriction
- importance of potassium supplement if taking non-potassium sparing diuretics (furosemide, thiazides, ethacrynic acid) to prevent dysrhythmias and digitalis toxicity
- signs/symptoms of increasing heart failure
- activity restrictions
- need for adequate rest
- importance of follow-up visits

(For more information, see pp. 1276–1291 of Black and Matassarin-Jacobs: *Medical-Surgical Nursing: Clinical Management for Continuity of Care,* 5th ed.)

Heat Exhaustion

OVERVIEW

- Heat exhaustion occurs after sustained exposure to heat and results from dehydration.

CLINICAL MANIFESTATIONS

- headache
- dizziness
- anorexia, nausea
- prostration
- weakness
- collapse
- cool, clammy skin

ACUTE AND SUBACUTE CARE

Medical Management

- oral or IV fluids

Nursing Management

- Administer fluids.
- Monitor body temperature.
- Monitor intake and output.
- Ensure adequate rest.
- Implement safety measures.

COMMUNITY AND SELF-CARE

Instruct client regarding:
- measures to prevent recurrence

(For more information, see pp. 2534–2535 of Black and Matassarin-Jacobs: *Medical-Surgical Nursing: Clinical Management for Continuity of Care,* 5th ed.)

Heatstroke

- Heatstroke is an emergency and requires immediate treatment for survival.
- There are two forms of heatstroke: classic heatstroke and exertional heatstroke.
  — Classic heatstroke is usually seen in the poor, the elderly, the chronically ill, clients with heart disease, the obese, and alcoholics. Hot humid weather lasting three or more days increases the risk of heatstroke in these clients. The

mechanism for classic heatstroke is not known but involves the failure of the heat regulating mechanism with cessation of sweating.

— Exertional heatstroke is more common in laborers, farmers, athletes, and clients who work in boiler rooms or foundries. Symptoms are similar to classic heatstroke except sweating occurs. Clients with exertional heatstroke tend to develop more lactic acidosis and severe bleeding problems than clients with classic heatstroke.

ACUTE AND SUBACUTE CARE

Nursing Management

Immediate nursing management involves rapidly reducing body temperature via immersion in cool water, if possible, for classic heatstroke. Sponging with cold water or a hypothermia blanket may be used for exertional heatstroke or as a secondary treatment for classic heatstroke if a cool water bath is not available.

- The client should be placed in a cool place with adequate circulation of cool air and with most of the clothing removed.
- Insert an intravenous line.
- Monitor cardiac rhythm continuously.
- Obtain frequent vital signs.
- Administer chlorpromazine or diazepam as ordered to reduce shivering.
- Insert urinary catheter.
- Provide supplemental oxygen as ordered.

(For more information, see pp. 2534–2435 of Black and Matassarin-Jacobs: *Medical-Surgical Nursing: Clinical Management for Continuity of Care,* 5th ed.)

Hemochromatosis

- Hemochromatosis is a disorder of iron metabolism often associated with portal hypertension, which eventually causes hepatomegaly.

- Clients with hemochromatosis often have total body iron levels of 20 grams or higher (normal range 2–5 grams). The excess iron travels to parenchymal cells and damages the liver and pancreas. These organs become fibrotic and lose function.
- Hemochromatosis may be primary (caused by a recessive inherited metabolic defect) or secondary (caused by alcoholism, excessive dietary intake of iron or conditions that require repeated blood transfusions).
- The most common problems associated with this disorder are: diabetes, enlarged liver, cirrhosis, cardiac disease, increased skin pigmentation, and arthritis.
- Treatment may include phlebotomy (gradually reduced to a maintenance level of 2 to 3 times per year) and administration of desfer–rioxamine mesylate (a chelating agent), which facilitates removal of iron from the body.

(For more information, see p. 1902 of Black and Matassarin-Jacobs: *Medical-Surgical Nursing: Clinical Management for Continuity of Care,* 5th ed.)

Hemophilia

OVERVIEW

- Hemophilia is a genetically transmitted coagulation disorder.
- There are three major types of hemophilia: Hemophilia A (classic hemophilia), Hemophilia B (Christmas disease), and von Willebrand's disease.
  - — Hemophilia A—factor VIII deficiency
  - — Hemophilia B—factor IX deficiency
  - — von Willebrand's disease—factor VIII deficiency and defective platelet function.
- Classic hemophilia makes up 80 per cent of the hemophilias.
- In the United States an estimated 25,000 people are affected with a form of hemophilia.

CLINICAL MANIFESTATIONS (HEMOPHILIA A)

- slow, persistent bleeding from cuts or scratches
- delayed bleeding that follows minor injuries
- bleeding into deep subcutaneous and intramuscular tissue
- easy bruising
- joint pain—secondary to hemorrhage into joints
- platelet function, platelet count, bleeding time, and prothrombin time are normal

ACUTE AND SUBACUTE CARE

MEDICAL MANAGEMENT (HEMOPHILIA A)

- factor VIII concentration transfusion
- packed red blood cell replacement if severe blood loss
- topical bleeding control—applying pressure, packing area with fibrin foam, topical hemostatics, such as thrombin
- joint immobilization and/or aspiration
- analgesics and corticosteroids for joint pain
- desmopressin—increases plasma factor VIII activity

NURSING MANAGEMENT (HEMOPHILIA A)

- Administer factor VIII replacement.
- Institute ordered measures to control topical bleeding.
- Assess all body systems for signs of bleeding.
- Administer analgesics.
- Immobilize affected joints until swelling subsides, then begin range of motion exercises.
- Monitor daily laboratory findings—CBC, factor VIII level.
- Institute bleeding precautions:
  - — no intramuscular or subcutaneous injections
  - — soft toothbrush
  - — electric razor
  - — hold venipuncture sites
  - — safety measures for ambulation
- Provide emotional support.

COMMUNITY AND SELF-CARE

- Instruct client regarding:
  - — disease process and treatment regime
  - — factor VIII administration (life-long therapy)
  - — precautions to prevent bleeding:
    - no contact sports
    - soft toothbrush
    - electric razor
    - care when preparing food
    - care when doing yard work
    - safety precautions
  - — emergency administration of factor VIII and methods to control bleeding if injury occurs
  - — signs/symptoms of complications and when to call physician
  - — importance of laboratory and clinic follow-up visits
- Refer to available community resources.

(For more information, see pp. 1515–1518 of Black and Matassarin-Jacobs: *Medical-Surgical Nursing: Clinical Management for Continuity of Care,* 5th ed.)

Hemorrhoids

OVERVIEW

- Hemorrhoids are perianal varicose veins. They may be internal or external.
- Hemorrhoids may result from the many anastomoses between the plexuses or from the lack of valves in the veins of the superior hemorrhoidal plexus, which leads into the portal vein.
- Enlargement of hemorrhoids is caused by increased intra-abdominal pressure.
- Pregnancy, congestive heart failure, prolonged sitting or standing, cirrhosis with portal hypertension, constipation, diarrhea, and prolonged straining with defecation contribute to hemorrhoid development and enlargement.

CLINICAL MANIFESTATIONS

- enlarged mass at the anus (external hemorrhoids)
- bright red bleeding, prolapse, rectal itching and constipation (internal hemorrhoids)
- pain may be present if associated with thrombosis

ACUTE AND SUBACUTE CARE

Medical Management

- treatment of constipation (fiber, increased fluids, stool softeners, hydrophilic psyllium preparations)
- heat application and astringent lotions to relieve pain
- topical anesthetic or steroid preparations

Surgical Management

- sclerotherapy—injection of a sclerosing agent between and around the veins
- ligation—placement of a rubber band around the neck of the hemorrhoid through an anoscope (for internal hemorrhoids only)
- cryosurgery—freezing of the hemorrhoids, performed infrequently
- laser removal—burning off the hemorrhoid with a laser
- hemorrhoidectomy—excision of the vein with the area left open to heal by granulation (high success rate) or sutured closed

Nursing Management

Surgical

Postoperative Care

In addition to routine postoperative care:
- Monitor for urinary retention.
- Monitor for hemorrhage.
- Provide warm sitz baths 3–4 times daily after a hemorrhoidectomy.
- Apply zinc oxide ointment for perianal irritations.
- Instruct to wipe area very gently.
- Warn that fainting can occur due to pain and vagal stimulation during the first postoperative bowel movement.

- Administer analgesics for pain.

COMMUNITY AND SELF-CARE

Instruct client regarding:

- measures to avoid constipation
- monitoring stool for blood
- high fiber diet
- adequate fluid intake
- use of bulk laxatives or mineral oil
- warm sitz baths 3–4 times per day
- good cleansing of the perianal area

(For more information, see pp. 1825–1828 of Black and Matassarin-Jacobs: *Medical-Surgical Nursing: Clinical Management for Continuity of Care,* 5th ed.)

Hemothorax

- Hemothorax is the presence of blood in the pleural space. Hemothorax may be present in clients with chest injuries.
- A small amount of blood (less than 300 ml) may cause no symptoms and require no treatment (the blood will be reabsorbed spontaneously).
- A large amount (1400–2500 ml) may be life-threatening because of resultant hypovolemia and compression of the lung. Clinical manifestations may include dullness to percussion on the affected side, tachycardia, hypotension, and shock.
- For severe distress, the physician may insert a 16-gauge needle into the fifth or sixth intercostal space at the mid-axillary line to aspirate the blood.
- A chest tube catheter may be inserted and connected to a closed drainage system.
- An initial drainage of 500–1000 ml is considered moderate. Continued large amounts of drainage (200 ml or more per hour) may indicate a need for emergency thoracotomy.

(For more information, see p. 2526 of Black and Matassarin-Jacobs: *Medical-Surgical Nursing: Clinical Management for Continuity of Care,* 5th ed.)

Hepatic Encephalopathy

OVERVIEW

- Hepatic encephalopathy encompasses a spectrum of central nervous system (CNS) disturbances. These may appear in conjunction with severe liver injury, liver failure, or a portocaval shunt.
- Hepatic encephalopathy is characterized by elevation of ammonia levels in the blood and cerebrospinal fluid. Ammonia is produced in the gastrointestinal tract when protein is broken down by bacteria, in the liver, and in lesser amounts by gastric juices. Normally, the liver converts ammonia into glutamine, which is stored in the liver and later converted to urea and excreted through the kidneys. Blood ammonia rises when the liver cells are unable to perform this function due to liver cell damage or necrosis. With a portal shunt, serum ammonia levels may rise since the blood bypasses the liver and is directly shunted into the systemic venous circulation.
- Mental status changes occur with high ammonia levels because ammonia is a CNS toxin, causing altered CNS metabolism and function.
- In clients with impaired liver function, any process that increases protein in the intestine, such as increased dietary protein or gastrointestinal bleeding, causes elevated blood ammonia levels.

CLINICAL MANIFESTATIONS

- fatigue, restlessness, irritability
- impaired memory, decreased attention span, impaired concentration, decreased rate of response
- personality changes, sleep pattern reversal
- deterioration in handwriting
- asterixis (rapid extension and flexion of the fingers and wrists when the arms are extended and the hands dorsiflexed—also called liver flap)
- drowsiness, confusion
- lethargy
- hyperventilation with respiratory alkalosis (high ammonia levels stimulate the respiratory center)

- severe confusion, inability to follow commands
- coma, unresponsiveness to painful stimuli
- absence of reflexes
- decerebrate or decorticate posturing

ACUTE AND SUBACUTE CARE

Medical Management

- dietary protein restriction
- neomycin to reduce bacteria in the intestinal tract
- lactulose to bind ammonium ions in the bowel, which are then eliminated
- prevention of gastrointestinal bleeding, or if it occurs, quick removal of the blood with lactulose enemas
- fluid and electrolyte replacement
- respiratory support for hypoxia
- hemodialysis or exchange transfusion to reduce toxic levels of ammonia

Nursing Management

- Discuss need for low-protein diet.
- Monitor for signs/symptoms of gastrointestinal bleeding: bright red blood in stools or dark tarry stools (bleeding increases protein in the gastrointestinal tract, which will produce ammonia when it is broken down).
- Monitor for therapeutic effect of lactulose (usual goal is 2–4 soft stools daily).
- Maintain adequate fluid volume (hypovolemia may precipitate hepatic encephalopathy).
  - — Monitor intake and output.
  - — Monitor vital signs.
  - — Measure central venous pressure hourly.
  - — Administer IV fluids as ordered.
- Monitor electrolyte and pH levels (electrolyte or acid-base disturbances may precipitate encephalopathy).
- Monitor neurologic status and perform neurologic checks frequently.
- Assess for possible side effects of diarrhea and vitamin K deficiency with neomycin therapy, due to depletion of intestinal flora.

- Maintain safety precautions (especially if confused/agitated).
- Prevent and treat hypoxia, which may precipitate encephalopathy.
- Protect from infection.
- Avoid use of depressants, which may precipitate coma.
- Review medications and avoid use of medications solely metabolized by the liver (metabolism by the kidney preferred). Discuss with physician.
- Provide good skin care and good pulmonary hygiene for the client with decreased level of consciousness.

COMMUNITY AND SELF-CARE

- Instruct client/significant other regarding:
  - — signs/symptoms of encephalopathy/worsening encephalopathy and to call physician
  - — medications—action and side effects
  - — need for low-protein diet
  - — signs/symptoms of gastrointestinal bleeding and other complications of cirrhosis
  - — safety precautions
- Refer to chemical dependency group or support group such as Alcoholics Anonymous.

See also, “Cirrhosis,” p. 174.

(For more information, see pp. 1891–1895 of Black and Matassarin-Jacobs: *Medical-Surgical Nursing: Clinical Management for Continuity of Care,* 5th ed.)

Hepatitis, Alcoholic

- Alcoholic hepatitis is an acute or chronic inflammation of the liver caused by parenchymal necrosis from heavy alcohol ingestion.
- This condition is the most frequent cause of cirrhosis.
- Clinical manifestations usually follow a recent bout of heavy drinking: anorexia, nausea, abdominal

pain, splenomegaly, hepatomegaly, jaundice, ascites, fever, and encephalopathy.

- Nursing intervention includes a high-vitamin, high-carbohydrate diet; folic acid and thiamine supplements and parenteral fluids.
- The prognosis is poor, particularly if the client continues to use alcohol.

(For more information, see p. 1872 of Black and Matassarin-Jacobs: *Medical-Surgical Nursing: Clinical Management for Continuity of Care,* 5th ed.)

Hepatitis, Chronic

- Chronic hepatitis exists when liver inflammation continues beyond a period of 3–6 months. It may be manifest as chronic persistent hepatitis (CPH) or chronic active hepatitis (CAH).
- CPH is benign and seldom progressive. CAH is more serious and leads to hepatic inflammation, hepatic necrosis, and progressive fibrosis.
- CPH may follow hepatitis B and hepatitis C. Recurrent episodes are not acute in nature and extrahepatic involvement seldom occurs. Prognosis is generally excellent.
- CAH may be due to an autoimmune response, from the hepatitis B virus, or follow cytomegalovirus infection. It also may follow acute hepatitis C or post-transfusion hepatitis. Certain medications also cause inflammatory changes consistent with CAH (methyldopa, dantrolene, isoniazid).
- Clinical manifestations of CPH are: nausea, anorexia, fatigue, abdominal pain. Most clients are asymptomatic, however.
- Clinical manifestations of CAH are: jaundice, fever, bleeding tendencies, abdominal pain, severe weakness, arthralgias, and extrahepatic abnormalities (such as thyroiditis, hemolytic anemia, amenorrhea, arthritis, urticaria, or glomerulonephritis).
- Treatment of symptomatic CAH may include steroids with or without azathioprine (Imuran). Bedrest is encouraged during the active phase of disease.

- Nursing management includes:
  - — supportive care
  - — instructing client on steroid therapy, possible side effects and not to abruptly stop medication
  - — instructing client/significant others on signs and symptoms to report to physician
  - — discussing importance of compliance with follow-up (untreated chronic hepatitis has a high mortality rate)
- See also, "Hepatitis, Viral," p. 341.

(For more information, see pp. 1867–1871 of Black and Matassarin-Jacobs: *Medical-Surgical Nursing: Clinical Management for Continuity of Care,* 5th ed.)

Hepatitis, Viral

OVERVIEW

- Hepatitis is inflammation of the liver. Hepatocytes are damaged and become inflamed and necrosed by the body's immune response to the virus. This alters cellular function. The degree of impairment depends on the amount of hepatocellular damage. Typically, persons with viral hepatitis completely recover in 3–16 weeks. Mortality from hepatitis A is low. Persons with hepatitis B tend to develop more complications. One of ten persons develop chronic hepatitis as a result of hepatitis B. Cirrhosis may follow a severe case of hepatitis B or chronic hepatitis. There are five types of viral hepatitis:

  (1) Hepatitis A (also called short incubation hepatitis, infectious hepatitis, and MS hepatitis)—caused by an enterovirus, it is transmitted primarily by the fecal-oral route, although parenteral transmission can occur, though rarely. It also may be transmitted through contaminated shellfish or via the airborne route if there are copious secretions. Causes of epidemics include infected water, milk, food, or raw shellfish from contaminated waters. The

client excretes the virus in the stool before the onset of manifestations, increasing the risk to close contacts. The incubation period is 2–6 weeks. Hepatitis A is endemic in areas of poor sanitation. It is common in fall and early winter.

(2) Hepatitis B—transmitted via the blood of an infected client, but also may be spread through semen, saliva, sexual contact, or the fecal-oral route. It may be spread by carriers. The virus can survive on surfaces up to 1 week. The incubation period is 6 weeks to 6 months. The incidence of hepatitis B is worldwide especially in drug addicts, homosexuals, and people exposed to blood products. It occurs year round.

(3) Hepatitis C—transmitted parenterally through the blood, by personal contact, and possibly by the fecal-oral route. In contrast to hepatitis A, but similar to hepatitis B, hepatitis C may be spread by carriers. The incubation period is 6–7 weeks.

(4) Hepatitis D (Delta agent)—transmitted only through blood contact. It is a defective RNA virus that must coexist with hepatitis B. The incubation period is 6 weeks to 6 months.

(5) Hepatitis E—is a waterborne virus that primarily affects young adults. There is no evidence that it becomes chronic. The incubation period is 2–9 weeks.

- Risk factors for each type of hepatitis are:

(1) Hepatitis A
— handling feces or contaminated articles
— working with animals imported from areas where hepatitis A is endemic

(2) Hepatitis B
— health care workers
— multiple blood transfusions or dialysis
— homosexually active males
— morticians
— persons who undergo tattooing
— parenteral drug abusers

(3) Hepatitis C
— similar risk factors as for hepatitis B

(4) Hepatitis D
— same risk factors as for hepatitis B

(5) Hepatitis E

- travel to countries with a high incidence
- eating or drinking food or water contaminated with the virus

- Preventive measures include:
  (1) Hepatitis A
  - good personal hygiene and handwashing
  - avoidance of shellfish or polluted fishing waters
  - monitoring of eating establishments by local health authorities
  - isolating newly imported animals for 2 months
  - prophylactic immune globulin (protects for 3 months) before and after exposure

  (2) Hepatitis B
  - using universal precautions when handling blood or body fluids
  - screening donors' blood
  - use of volunteers rather than paid donors for blood products
  - encouraging clients who are having elective surgery to donate their own blood
  - good personal hygiene by clients with hepatitis B or carriers
  - vaccination with specific hepatitis B immune globulin after exposure (passive immunization)
  - use of hepatitis B vaccine (active immunization) before exposure

  (3) Hepatitis C
  - similar measures as for hepatitis B
  - immune globulin for post-exposure passive immunization

  (4) Hepatitis D
  - similar measures as for hepatitis B

  (5) Hepatitis E
  - personal hygiene and sanitation

CLINICAL MANIFESTATIONS

Symptoms vary from client to client. Hepatitis B and hepatitis D usually produce the most severe symptoms, although some clients may be asymptomatic.

- jaundice, lethargy, irritability, fatigue, weakness
- myalgia, arthralgia, anorexia

- nausea, vomiting, abdominal pain in right upper quadrant, diarrhea, constipation
- flu-like symptoms, fever
- pruritus
- dark urine, clay-colored stools
- bleeding tendencies
- anemia
- drowsiness
- hepatic encephalopathy
- asterixis (rapid extension and flexion of the fingers and wrists when the arms are extended and the hands are dorsiflexed, also called "liver flap")
- spider angiomas, palmar erythema

Fulminant Viral Hepatitis

This life-threatening form resembles acute liver failure and has a poor prognosis.

- encepalopathy (increased excitability, insomnia, somnolence, impaired mentation)
- decreased liver size
- other problems develop such as gastrointestinal bleeding, DIC, leukocytosis
- oliguria
- edema and ascites
- hypotension
- respiratory failure

ACUTE AND SUBACUTE CARE

Medical Management

- rest
- proper diet high in carbohydrates and low in fat
- standard immune globulin—can prevent hepatitis A if given early to close contacts
- hepatitis B vaccine for active immunization
- antiemetics for nausea and vomiting
- cholestyramine or ursodiol for pruritus (binds with bile salts in the intestine)
- vitamin K therapy if prothrombin time is prolonged

Nursing Management

- Monitor mental status and assess for early signs of hepatic encephalopathy (ask patient to write name every shift—deterioration of handwriting is an early sign of encephalopathy).

- Consider possible effects of medications on liver function before administering.
- Assess for asterixis.
- Monitor hemoglobin, hematocrit, and prothrombin time.
- Monitor for signs/symptoms of bleeding.
- Encourage a reasonable activity level and frequent rest periods.
- Assist with activities of daily living as needed.
- Implement measures to prevent complications of immobility.
- Encourage adequate nutrition.
  - — Avoid heavy, greasy foods.
  - — Provide good breakfast (usually best tolerated meal).
  - — Devise dietary plan high in protein (unless encephalopathic), high in carbohydrates and low in fat.
  - — Suggest multiple small meals.
  - — Instruct to avoid alcohol (hepatotoxic agent).
- Discuss disease and its treatment, and how to prevent recurrence and spread.
- Provide opportunities for discussion of feelings/concerns regarding duration and cost of illness and effects of illness on future health.
- Administer oral cholestyramine as ordered for pruritus.
- Administer oral antihistamines for itching as ordered.

COMMUNITY AND SELF-CARE

Instruct client regarding:

- slowly returning to former activity levels to avoid a relapse
- obtaining adequate rest
- diet
- how to avoid reinfection or infecting other family members
- avoidance of alcohol and medications such as aspirin or sedatives that are hepatotoxic
- avoidance of sexual activity until physician permits
- need for follow-up visits

See also "Hepatitis, Chronic," p. 340.

(For more information, see pp. 1861–1871 of Black and Matassarin-Jacobs: *Medical-Surgical Nursing: Clinical Management for Continuity of Care,* 5th ed.)

Herniated Intervertebral Disc

OVERVIEW

- Displacement of intervertebral disc material may be referred to as prolapse, herniation, rupture, or extrusion of the disc. These interchangeable terms indicate loss of integrity of the disc between two vertebrae. Ruptured intervertebral discs may occur at any level of the spine; however, lumbar discs are the most likely to rupture.
- Compression of spinal nerve roots may result from herniation of the disc. When the disc impinges on the sciatic nerve, the condition and resulting pain is called sciatica.
- Risk factors include:
  — heavy physical labor
  — strenuous exercise
  — weak abdominal and back muscles
  — use of poor body mechanics.
- It is estimated that 10 per cent of those who seek medical attention for back pain have herniated discs.

CLINICAL MANIFESTATIONS

Ruptured Lumbar Disc

- lower back pain that radiates down the sciatic nerve into the posterior thigh
- muscle spasm
- aggravation of pain by straining (coughing, defecation, bending, lifting, and straight-leg raising)
- depression of deep tendon reflexes
- hyperesthesia in the area of distribution of affected nerve roots

Ruptured Cervical Disc

- stiff neck
- shoulder pain that radiates down the arm into the hand
- paresthesias and sensory disturbances in the hand

ACUTE AND SUBACUTE CARE

Medical Management

- anti-inflammatory agents
- muscle relaxants
- analgesics
- ultrasonic heat treatment
- localized moist heat application
- localized ice application (for the first 48 hours)
- progressive muscle strengthening exercises
- bedrest—initially with progressive activity schedule
- brace, corset, or cervical collar

Surgical Management

- laminectomy—surgical removal of the posterior arch of a vertebra, exposing the spinal cord for removal of the portion of the nucleus pulposus that is protruding or ruptured from a herniated intervertebral disc
- spinal fusion—placement of a bone graft in the disc interspace that grows and fuses the two vertebrae together, thus immobilizing them. The bone graft may be obtained from a bone bank or a region of the client's iliac crest. An anterior or posterior surgical approach may be taken.
- discectomy—microsurgical techniques to remove ruptured discs cause less trauma and preserve tissue integrity.

Nursing Management

Medical

- Administer anti-inflammatory and analgesic agents and muscle relaxants as ordered.
- Apply heat/cold applications as ordered.
- Collaborate with Physical Therapy for a progressive exercise/activity schedule.

Surgical

Postoperative Care

In addition to routine postoperative care:

Cervical Laminectomy or Fusion

- Assess for possible complications:
  (1) posterior approach
    — soft tissue hematoma
    — air embolism
    — wound dehiscence
  (2) anterior approach
    — laryngeal nerve damage
    — injury to neck structures, such as carotid arteries, trachea, or esophagus
- Assess neurologic status:
  — movement of shoulders and extremities
  — presence of numbness or tingling
  — changes in sensation
  (Progressive worsening of motor and sensory function may indicate spinal cord edema or hemorrhage compressing the spinal cord.)
- Maintain soft cervical collar.
- Elevate head of bed to degree ordered. Use a small folded towel or bath blanket under the head to maintain alignment.
- Assist with repositioning, avoid any jarring movements.
- Initiate out-of-bed activities as prescribed with collar in place.
- Implement measures to relieve sore throat (anterior approach) — throat lozenges, viscous lidocaine, humidified air, minimal talking.
- Monitor respiratory status.
- Assure that emergency respiratory equipment is readily available.
- Prevent flexion of the neck.
- Administer PRN analgesics and assess effectiveness.

Lumbar Laminectomy, Fusion, or Discectomy

- Assess for possible complications:
  — epidural hematoma
  — injury to nerve roots
  — injury to nearby structures

— urinary retention
— paralytic ileus

- Assess neurologic status:
  — movement of extremities
  — presence of numbness or tingling
  — changes in sensation
  (Progressive worsening of motor and sensory function may indicate spinal cord edema or hemorrhage compressing the spinal cord.)
- Position as ordered (in immediate postoperative period):
  — laminectomy—client is not turned for 1–2 hours and is left flat
  — spinal fusion—bed is generally kept flat, logrolling side-to-side usually beginning 4 hours after surgery
  — microdiscectomy—head of bed elevated to position of comfort
- Reposition side-to-side using log-rolling technique.
- Initiate out-of-bed activities as ordered.
- Administer PRN analgesics and muscle relaxants as ordered. Assess effectiveness.
- Collaborate with Physical Therapy regarding progressive activity/exercise program and adaptive devices (braces, corsets, etc.).
- Assess for urinary retention.
- Assess for paralytic ileus.

COMMUNITY AND SELF-CARE

Instruct client regarding:

- signs/symptoms to report
- walking restrictions
- driving restrictions
- lifting restrictions
- work restrictions
- use of adaptive devices
- wound care

(For more information, see pp. 917–924 of Black and Matassarin-Jacobs: *Medical-Surgical Nursing: Clinical Management for Continuity of Care,* 5th ed.)

Herniations

OVERVIEW

- A hernia is the abnormal protrusion of an organ, tissue, or part of an organ through the structure that normally contains it.
- Hernias occur due to defects in the integrity of the muscular wall and increased intra-abdominal pressure.
- The most common hernias are:
  — inguinal
    - indirect—occurs through inquinal ring and follows the inguinal canal
    - direct— occurs through the abdominal wall in an area of muscular weakness

  — femoral—occurs through the femoral ring and gradually pulls the peritoneum and urinary bladder into the sac

  — umbilical—due to increased abdominal pressure, as with obese or multiparous women

  — incisional (ventral)—occurs at a site of previous surgical incision that healed inadequately

ACUTE AND SUBACUTE CARE

Medical Management

- mechanical reduction, if the hernia is not strangulated or incarcerated
- truss—a firm pad held in place by a belt; worn daily and applied before arising

Surgical Management

- hernia repair—excision of the hernia sac, returning the herniated contents (usually intestine) back to their normal position and closing the muscle tightly over the area

Nursing Management

Surgical

Postoperative Care

In addition to routine postoperative care:

- Instruct the client to splint incision when coughing or sneezing to provide incisional support.
- Ensure the client voids after surgery.
- Assure the client that the hernia will not recur in the immediate postoperative period.
- Inguinal hernia repair:
  — apply an ice pack to the incisional area.
  — assess scrotal area for swelling in male clients:
    - elevate scrotum and instruct to wear a scrotal support when the client is out of bed.

COMMUNITY AND SELF-CARE

Medical

- Ensure client knows how to wear truss or binder.
- Instruct client on signs/symptoms of hernia strangulation and to report immediately to physician.
- Encourage weight reduction program for obese clients.
- Instruct client to assess for any skin irritation under binder.

Surgical

- Instruct client regarding:
  — no heavy lifting for 4–6 weeks after surgery
  — signs/symptoms of infection
  — wound care
- If binder will be worn at home, instruct how to assess skin for irritation and to evaluate the effectiveness of the system.

(For more information, see pp. 1816–1818 of Black and Matassarin-Jacobs: *Medical-Surgical Nursing: Clinical Management for Continuity of Care,* 5th ed.)

Herpes Zoster

- Herpes zoster (or shingles) is an infection caused by the same virus that causes varicella (or chicken pox).

- After 1–2 days of pain, itching, and hyperesthesia, clusters of grouped vesicles appear unilaterally along cranial or spinal nerve dermatomes. Because they follow nerve pathways, the lesions do not cross the body's midline; however, the nerves of both sides may be involved.
- The eruption clears in about 2 weeks, unless the period between the pain and the eruption is longer than 2 days. In the latter case, a prolonged convalescence may be expected.
- Residual pain, post-herpetic neuralgia, and itching are the major problems with herpes zoster. The pain may last weeks or months to years (especially in the elderly).
- A potential complication is herpes involvement of the facial nerve, acoustic, and ophthalmic nerve, which requires close medical attention.
- Medical management:
  — use of the antiviral agent, acyclovir (Zovirax)
  — analgesics and sedatives
- Nursing management:
  — administer and assess affectiveness of ordered analgesics
  — provide other measures for pain relief: application of cool compresses, use of cooling antipruritic preparations
  — instruct client and significant other on mode of transmission and ways to prevent
  — instruct client and significant other on measures to prevent secondary infection
  — provide emotional support and discuss with client and significant others that continued intervention and long-term support will be needed

(For more information, see p. 2223 of Black and Matassarin-Jacobs: *Medical-Surgical Nursing: Clinical Management for Continuity of Care,* 5th ed.)

Hiatal Hernia

OVERVIEW

- A hiatal hernia (diaphragmatic hernia) is a condition in which the cardiac sphincter becomes enlarged allowing the stomach to pass into the thoracic cavity.
- There are two types:
  - — sliding hernias—the upper stomach and the gastroesophageal junction are displaced upward into the thorax (most common)
  - — rolling or paraesophageal hernias—the gastroesophageal junction stays below the diaphragm, but all or part of the stomach pushes through to the thorax.
- Risk factors include obesity, pregnancy, or ascites.

CLINICAL MANIFESTATIONS

Sliding

- heartburn 30–60 minutes after meals
- substernal pain

Rolling

- no symptoms of reflux
- fullness after a meal
- chest pain, worse when recumbent

ACUTE AND SUBACUTE CARE

Medical Management

See "Gastroesophageal Reflux Disease," p. 296.

Nursing Management

See "Gastroesophageal Reflux Disease," p. 296.

COMMUNITY AND SELF-CARE

See "Gastroesophageal Reflux Disease," p. 296.

(For more information, see pp. 1740–1741 of Black and Matassarin-Jacobs: *Medical-Surgical Nursing: Clinical Management for Continuity of Care,* 5th ed.)

Hodgkin's Disease

OVERVIEW

- Hodgkin's disease is a chronic, progressive, neoplastic disorder of lymphoid tissue characterized by the painless enlargement of lymph nodes with progression to extralymphatic sites such as the spleen and liver. The involvement of tissues and organs throughout the body follows.
- Hodgkin's disease involves the proliferation of abnormal histiocytes.
- Lymphomas are classified as either (1) Hodgkin's—containing the Reed-Sternberg cell, or (2) non-Hodgkin's—without Reed-Sternberg cell.
- Hodgkin's staging classifications are:
  - — Stage I—involves a single lymph node region
  - — Stage II—involves two or more lymph node regions on the same side of the diaphragm
  - — Stage III—involves lymph node regions on both sides of the diaphragm
  - — Stage IV—involvement of one or more extra-nodal site(s)
- Hodgkin's is a disease of young adults, primarily occurring between the ages of 20 and 40 years. It affects men more than women.
- The complete remission rate for Hodgkin's is 75–90 per cent. There is a 10–20 per cent recurrence rate that varies with the stage of the disease.

CLINICAL MANIFESTATIONS

- painless, enlarged lymph nodes
- fevers and night sweats
- weight loss
- pruritus
- hepatosplenomegaly
- pain over enlarged lymph nodes after ingesting alcohol

- nonproductive cough, dyspnea (mediastinal involvement)
- edema of the face, neck, right arm (superior vena cava syndrome secondary to lymph node enlargement and compression)
- renal failure (ureteral obstruction by enlarged lymph nodes)
- bone pain (vertebral compression)
- paraplegia (spinal cord compression)

ACUTE AND SUBACUTE CARE

Medical Management

- chemotherapy—Mechlorethamine, Oncovin, procarbazine, prednisone (MOPP); adriamycin, bleomycin, vinblastine, decarbazine (ABVD)
- radiation therapy

Surgical Management

- lymph node biopsy or laparotomy with liver and lymph node biopsy to stage the disease
- splenectomy

Nursing Management

- Administer ordered chemotherapy.
- See "Chemotherapy," p. 149.
- See "Radiation Therapy," p. 605.
- Monitor laboratory findings—CBC, BUN, creatinine, platelet count.
- Administer antiemetics as ordered.
- Encourage balanced diet.
- Encourage rest.

COMMUNITY AND SELF-CARE

- Instruct client regarding:
  — disease process and treatment regime
  — see "Chemotherapy," p. 149.
  — see "Radiation Therapy," p. 605.
  — signs/symptoms to report to physician
  — importance of follow-up visits
- Refer to available community resources.

(For more information, see pp. 1500–1503 of Black and Matassarin-Jacobs: *Medical-Surgical Nursing: Clinical Management for Continuity of Care,* 5th ed.)

Human Immunodeficiency Virus (HIV) Infection

OVERVIEW

- Human immunodeficiency virus is the causative agent in the development of acquired immunodeficiency syndrome (AIDS), an advanced stage of disease along a continuum that ranges from asymptomatic HIV infection to the development of this most serious and debilitating condition.
- Once the initial HIV infection takes place, the virus may remain latent inside the cell for an undetermined amount of time. The main target of HIV infection is the T_4 or $CD4^+$ cell. Once these cells are infected, either they are changed and rendered nonfunctional or their actual number is depleted. The normal number of T_4 cells is between 700 and 1300 T_4 cells/mm^3. Opportunistic infections most commonly occur when the T_4 cell count drops below 200. HIV-related malignancies and neurologies can occur at a higher count.
- The disease has grown to epidemic proportions since 1981. By late 1994, 411,000 cases of AIDS in the United States had been reported to the Centers for Disease Control (CDC) with over 284,000 AIDS deaths. By the year 2000, it is projected that 1 million people will be HIV positive in the United States alone.
- HIV infection has an extremely high mortality rate; over 90 per cent of clients who develop the most severe form of the disease will die within 4 years of an AIDS diagnosis. Most clients affected are between the ages of 20 and 49 years.
- Transmission of HIV occurs through horizontal transmission (from either sexual contact or parenteral exposure to blood and blood products) or through vertical transmission (from HIV-infected

mother to infant). HIV is not transmitted by casual contact. Transmission always involves exposure to some body fluid of an infected client. The greatest concentrations of the virus have been found in blood, semen, cerebrospinal fluid, and cervical/vaginal secretions. Risk factors include:

- — homosexual activity
- — heterosexual activity associated with multiple sex partners, receptive anal intercourse, presence of open lesions in the genital area, and sexual exposure without protection
- — direct blood to blood contact
  - sharing contaminated needles
  - transfusion of blood or blood products
  - accidental needlestick
  - blood exposure to non-intact skin or mucous membrane
  - babies born to mothers who are HIV positive
  - babies breastfed by HIV-positive mothers

CLINICAL MANIFESTATIONS

The first stage of HIV infection is the process of being exposed to HIV and becoming antibody-positive (seroconversion). Some clients experience a mononucleosis-like illness consisting of fever, malaise, lymphadenopathy, rash, and at times, aseptic meningitis; others remain asymptomatic throughout this phase. Once the client is HIV positive, the continuum begins with a period of remaining asymptomatic. Although the length of this phase varies, it commonly ranges from 7 to 10 years. HIV disease begins to develop as the immune system becomes depleted or ineffective as a result of the virus' effect on the T-helper cell.

- lymphadenopathy
- skin rashes
- fevers
- fatigue
- drenching night sweats
- persistent diarrhea, weight loss
- oral thrush
- vaginal yeast infection
- pain related to peripheral neuropathies, myalgias, or malignancies
- evidence of opportunistic infections
  - — Pneumocystis carinii pneumonia (PCP)

- number one killer of clients with AIDS
- clinical manifestations:
    - fever
    - fatigue
    - weight loss
    - cough and dyspnea
    - clear lung sounds
    - chest x-ray reveals bilateral diffuse interstitial infiltrates
    - decreased oxygen saturation levels

— Cytomegalovirus infection (CMV)
- almost 90 per cent of AIDS clients develop CMV during the course of their illness
- (1) CMV chorioretinitis
    - — clinical manifestations:
        - mild visual impairment and deficits of peripheral vision
        - blindness
- (2) CMV colitis
    - — clinical manifestations
        - watery diarrhea
        - weight loss
- (3) CMV pneumonitis
    - — clinical manifestations
        - dyspnea, increased respiratory rate
        - hypoxemia

— Herpes simplex virus (HSV)
- clinical manifestations:
    - tingling and burning at the site of the vesicle (mouth, esophagus, genital, or perirectal areas) and later blister formation
    - severe pain at the site of the lesion
    - dysphagia

— Toxoplasmosis
- major opportunistic infection of the central nervous system
- clinical manifestations:
    - headaches
    - seizures
    - hemiparesis
    - lethargy
    - personality changes
    - change in cognitive ability

— Cryptosporidium infection (intestinal protozoan infection)

- clinical manifestations:
  - watery diarrhea
  - malaise
  - nausea and abdominal cramps
- Isospora Belli infection
  - clinical manifestations:
    - watery diarrhea
    - malaise
    - nausea and abdominal cramps
- Mycobacterium tuberculosis (MTB)
  - is often extrapulmonary involving the kidneys, liver, spleen, lymph nodes, and bone marrow
  - clinical manifestations:
    - fever
    - weight loss
    - night sweats
    - fatigue
    - lymphadenitis
- Candida albicans infection
  - fungus that causes infection of the mouth, esophagus, and vagina
  - clinical manifestations:
    - white, thick, cottage cheese-like exudate on the affected mucosa
    - atrophic form—smooth red patch on affected mucosa
    - difficulty and pain with swallowing
    - retrosternal burning
- Cryptococcus neoformans infection
  - can cause meningitis or disseminated disease
  - clinical manifestations:
    - fever
    - headache
    - subtle mental changes
    - focal neurologic signs
    - seizures
    - coma
- Histoplasmosis
  - fungal infection
  - clinical manifestations:
    - fever
    - weight loss
    - skin lesions

- HIV associated malignancies:
  - — Kaposi's sarcoma (KS)
    - most common neoplasm affecting AIDS clients
    - is often aggressive and disfiguring
    - clinical manifestations:
      - purplish-red, nonpainful lesion appearing anywhere on the skin and may include lymph nodes, mucous membranes, and viscera
      - lesion is flat or indurated and frequently progresses to a nodule
  - — Non-Hodgkin's lymphoma
    - clinical manifestations:
      - painless, enlarged lymph nodes
      - fever
      - malaise
      - night sweats
- HIV neurologic disease (AIDS dementia complex)
  - — can involve the central and peripheral nervous systems
  - — clinical manifestations:
    - decreased ability to concentrate
    - memory loss
    - slowed thought processes
    - personality changes
    - irritability
    - depression
    - withdrawal
    - loss of coordination
    - peripheral neuropathies
- HIV wasting syndrome
  - — greater than 10 per cent loss of body weight
  - — clinical manifestations:
    - cachexia
    - chronic weakness
    - persistent fever
    - diarrhea

ACUTE AND SUBACUTE CARE

Medical Management

Medical management is aimed at controlling replication of the virus, thereby delaying further destruction of the immune system.

- antiretroviral therapy—zidovudine (also known as Retrovir, ZDV, and formerly AZT)
- blood and blood product replacement therapy
- Dideoxyinosine (ddI) and Dideoxycytidine (ddC)—antiretroviral agents for clients with intolerance to zidovudine or significant disease progression despite treatment with these drugs
- opportunistic infection treatment:
  - — Pneumocystis carinii pneumonia (PCP)

    Because PCP affects 80–90 per cent of clients with AIDS, it is important to prevent either the first episode or recurrences. PCP prophylaxis is indicated for any HIV-infected client with fewer than 200 $CD4^+$ lymphocytes.
    - trimethoprim-sulfamethoxazole (Bactrim or Septra)
    - pentamidine
    - dapsone
  - — Cytomegalovirus infection
    - gangcyclovir
    - foscarnet
  - — Herpes simplex
    - acyclovir
  - — Toxoplasmosis
    - combination of sulfadiazine and pyrimethamine
  - — Cryptosporidium infection
    - alleviation of symptoms associated with dehydration, fluid and electrolyte imbalance, and weight loss
  - — Isospora Belli infection
    - trimethoprim-sulfamethoxazole
  - — Mycobacterium tuberculosis
    - ethambutol
    - isoniazid
    - rifampin
    - pyrazinamide
  - — Candida albicans
    - clotrimazole (Nystatin); topical for oral lesions
    - miconazole; topical for vaginal candidiasis
    - fluconazole and ketoconazole; systemic antifungals
  - — Cryptococcus neoformans infection
    - amphotercin B

    - Histoplasmosis
        - amphotericin B
- HIV-associated malignancies treatment
    - radiation therapy
    - chemotherapy
    - interferon alpha
- HIV neurologic disease treatment
    - zidovudine
- complete blood counts at frequent intervals
- oral and enteral nutritional supplements

Nursing Management

- Administer antiretroviral and opportunistic infection therapy as ordered
- Monitor for side effects and effectiveness of medication therapy.
- Monitor laboratory findings—complete blood count, platelet count, culture reports, arterial blood gases.
- Assess respiratory status—rate, rhythm, use of accessory muscles.
- Administer supplemental oxygen.
- Monitor oxygen saturation levels at rest and with activity.
- Initiate a progressive activity program and monitor client's response.
- Provide frequent rest periods and a restful environment.
- Administer anti-inflammatory, anti-anxiety, or analgesics for pain control.
- Monitor intake and output.
- Daily weights.
- Provide dietary supplements.
- Institute appropriate safety measures for client with neurologic involvement.
- Inspect skin and oral, vaginal, and rectal areas closely and provide meticulous hygiene.
- Facilitate/provide counseling and support regarding the issues of social stigma, potential losses to body image and child-bearing potential, changes in sexuality, and premature loss of life.

COMMUNITY AND SELF-CARE

- Instruct the client regarding:

- — importance of medication regime
- — strategies aimed at reducing the risk of transmission:
  - safe sex counseling
  - avoidance of sharing needles
  - care of household items
  - proper disposal of items soiled with body fluids
- — health maintenance:
  - maintaining adequate nutrition
  - weight management
  - exercise
  - smoking cessation
  - stress reduction
- — basics of routine skin care and inspection
- — proper oral, vaginal, and rectal hygiene
- — importance of drug and/or alcohol abuse counseling
- — importance of follow-up appointments

- Refer to available community resources.

(For more information, see pp. 614–636 of Black and Matassarin-Jacobs: *Medical-Surgical Nursing: Clinical Management for Continuity of Care,* 5th ed.)

Huntington's Disease

OVERVIEW

- Huntington's disease (HD) is a genetically transmitted degenerative neurologic disease.
- The disease is autosomal dominant, meaning that offspring of an affected person have a 50 per cent chance of inheriting the disease.
- The pathology of Huntington's disease involves degeneration of the striatum (caudate and putamen) in the basal ganglia. This leads to a reduction of some neurotransmitters and relatively higher concentrations of other neurotransmitters (dopamine and norepinephrine). The excess of dopamine in Huntington's disease, a disorder of excessive movement, can be contrasted to the lack of dopamine in Parkinson's disease, a disorder of lack of movement.

- The disease is characterized by abnormal movements (chorea), intellectual decline, and emotional disturbance.
- Signs and symptoms usually begin in the third and fourth decades. Women and men are equally affected.
- The disease is relentlessly progressive, leading to disability and death within 15 to 20 years, usually from respiratory complications.

CLINICAL MANIFESTATIONS

- restless and fidgety appearance
- rapid, jerky choreiform movements involving all muscles (appears to be constantly in motion)
- dysphagia
- hesitant, explosive speech
- bowel and bladder incontinence
- emotional disturbance—becomes negative, suspicious, and irritable
- depression
- psychosis
- temper outbursts, sexual promiscuity
- dementia

ACUTE AND SUBACUTE CARE

Medical Management

There is no known treatment to cure or alter the course.

- dopamine blocker—Haloperidol (Haldol), to control abnormal movements and some behavioral manifestations
- anti-anxiety medications—diazepam (Valium)
- antidepressants

Nursing Management

- Assess client's ability to do self-care activities and provide care as indicated.
- Collaborate with Physical and Occupational Therapy for exercises and adaptive devices for ambulation and self care.
- Determine strategies to optimize communication.
- Initiate aspiration precautions.

- Maintain high caloric intake (required because of excessive movement).
- Initiate appropriate safety measures.
- Provide quiet, restful environment.
- Conserve client energy by spacing activities and allowing rest periods.

COMMUNITY AND SELF-CARE

- Instruct the client regarding:
  - — disease process and prognosis
  - — need to use good posture and swallowing techniques while eating and drinking to prevent aspiration
  - — use of adaptive devices
  - — home environment safety measures
- Refer to available community resources (e.g., Home Health Care).

(For more information, see p. 883 of Black and Matassarin-Jacobs: *Medical-Surgical Nursing: Clinical Management for Continuity of Care,* 5th ed.)

Hydronephrosis

OVERVIEW

- Hydronephrosis is distention of the renal pelvis and calices by an obstruction of normal urine flow. The kidney dilates and eventually nephron destruction may occur from the pressure.
- The obstruction may be due to a calculus, tumor, scar tissue, or a kink in the ureter.
- Treatment involves relieving the obstruction and preventing pyelonephritis from urinary stasis.
- After removal of the obstruction, diuresis occurs, which can lead to dehydration and electrolyte disturbances.

ACUTE AND SUBACUTE CARE

Nursing Management

The nurse performs the following interventions after relief of the obstruction:

- Monitor for potential fluid volume deficit due to increased urine output.
  - Obtain hourly outputs.
  - Monitor vital signs.
  - Obtain urine specific gravities, glucose, and albumin.
  - Monitor serum electrolytes and glucose.

(For more information, see p. 1636 of Black and Matassarin-Jacobs: *Medical-Surgical Nursing: Clinical Management for Continuity of Care,* 5th ed.)

Hypercalcemia

OVERVIEW

- Hypercalcemia is a serum calcium level over 5.5 mEq/L.
- In hypercalcemia, cardiac and smooth muscle activity is decreased. Calcium in the blood stream impairs renal function and precipitates as a salt, forming renal stones.
- Causes of hypercalcemia include:
  - metastatic malignancy—causes bone destruction or increased secretion of ectopic parathyroid hormone (PTH)
  - hyperparathyroidism
  - thiazide diuretic therapy—causes calcium retention
  - prolonged immobilization
  - excessive intake of calcium and Vitamin D
  - hypophosphatemia
  - metabolic acidosis—decreases calcium elimination

CLINICAL MANIFESTATIONS

- anorexia, nausea, vomiting, decreased peristalsis, abdominal distention

- weakness, fatigue
- difficulty concentrating
- lethargy, confusion, coma
- ECG changes—shortened ST segment, prolonged QT interval
- dysrhythmias, heart block
- signs of digitalis toxicity
- cardiac arrest
- polyuria, kidney stones, renal failure
- bone pain and fracture
- serum calcium greater than 5.5 mEq/L

ACUTE AND SUBACUTE CARE

Medical Management

- determination/treatment of underlying cause
- intravenous normal saline with furosemide (Lasix)—promotes urinary calcium excretion
- cardiac monitoring
- antitumor antibiotic therapy—mithramycin C—inhibits action of PTH on osteoclasts in bone tissue reducing decalcification
- calcitonin therapy—inhibits effect of PTH and increases urinary calcium excretion
- corticosteroid therapy—decreases serum calcium by competing with vitamin D, resulting in decreased intestinal absorption of calcium
- phosphate therapy
- etidronate disodium—reduces bone reabsorption of calcium
- aggressive hydration—to flush calcium through the kidneys
- dietary modification—low calcium

Nursing Management

- Administer ordered therapy.
- Assess ECG for rhythm changes.
- Assess bowel sounds every 8 hours.
- Assess neurologic status.
- Encourage fluid intake unless contraindicated.
- Monitor laboratory findings—serum calcium.
- Monitor for signs of digitalis toxicity if on digoxin (calcium enhances the action of digitalis)—bradycardia, nausea, vomiting, blurred vision.
- Strain urine for renal calculi.

- Institute appropriate safety measures.
- Reposition cautiously to prevent pathologic fractures.
- Encourage high fiber foods to prevent constipation.

COMMUNITY AND SELF-CARE

Discharge care is based on the etiologic factor(s) causing hypercalcemia.

(For more information, see pp. 320–322 of Black and Matassarin-Jacobs: *Medical-Surgical Nursing: Clinical Management for Continuity of Care,* 5th ed.)

Hyperglycemia and Diabetic Ketoacidosis

OVERVIEW

- Hyperglycemia and diabetic ketoacidosis are acute complications of diabetes mellitus. Hyperglycemia is an elevated blood glucose over 120 mg/100 ml. Hyperglycemia results when glucose cannot be transported to the cells because of lack of insulin. Due to the lack of carbohydrates for cellular fuel, the liver converts its glycogen stores back to glucose (glycogenolysis) and increases biosynthesis of glucose (gluconeogenesis). This causes blood glucose levels to rise even higher. In insulin dependent diabetes mellitus (IDDM), the need for cellular fuel grows more critical and the body begins to draw on its fat and protein stores for energy. This results in the production of ketone bodies, which accumulate in the blood (ketosis) and are excreted in the urine (ketonuria). Metabolic acidosis develops from the acidic effects of the ketones acetoacetate and betahydroxybutyrate. This condition is called diabetic ketoacidosis. It may cause the client to lose consciousness, a condition called diabetic coma.
- The process of catabolizing fats for fuel gives rise to three pathologic events:

(1) dehydration
(2) ketosis and acidosis
(3) electrolyte and acid-base imbalances

- Diabetic ketoacidosis is primarily a complication of IDDM, although it can occur in non-insulin dependent clients in periods of extreme stress.
- Diabetic ketoacidosis is an emergency.
- Causes of diabetic ketoacidosis and hyperglycemia include:
  — taking too little insulin
  — omitting doses of insulin
  — failing to meet increased need for insulin due to stress, infection, surgery, trauma, pregnancy, or puberty
  — developing insulin resistance due to insulin antibodies.
- Prevention includes:
  — taking insulin as prescribed
  — monitoring blood glucose frequently
  — monitoring urine ketones when blood glucose rises
  — recognizing signs/symptoms of infection and other stressors that may precipitate diabetic ketoacidosis
  — calling physician for anorexia, nausea, vomiting, diarrhea, ketonuria for greater than 8 hours, febrile illness or infection, or any signs/symptoms of acidosis.

CLINICAL MANIFESTATIONS

- warm, dry skin
- nausea, vomiting
- flushed appearance
- dry mucous membranes
- soft eyeballs
- Kussmaul's respirations (deep and rapid respirations) or tachypnea
- fruity or acetone odor of the breath
- abdominal pain
- alteration in level of consciousness
- hypotension
- tachycardia
- polyuria (early sign)
- oliguria (late sign)
- visual disturbances

ACUTE AND SUBACUTE CARE

Medical Management

Goals are to (1) correct fluid and electrolyte imbalances, (2) restore normal circulating blood volume, (3) shift from a state of fat catabolism to carbohydrate catabolism, and (4) identify and correct the factors precipitating the ketoacidosis.

Nursing Management

- Monitor blood glucoses every 1–2 hours.
- Administer low dosage IV insulin as ordered. Never administer subcutaneous insulin to someone in diabetic ketoacidosis. The subcutaneous tissue is dehydrated and poorly perfused.
- Administer fluid replacement (initially isotonic saline) as ordered.
- Monitor hemodynamic readings, vital signs, and level of consciousness every 1–2 hours.
- Maintain nasogastric tube to suction as ordered.
- Assess fluid status:
  - — hematocrit
  - — weight
  - — lung sounds
  - — skin turgor
  - — intake and output.
- Monitor bowel sounds.
- Administer blood, albumin, and plasma volume expanders as ordered for circulatory collapse.
- Monitor for signs/symptoms of hyperkalemia (usually present in first 4 hours of intervention) and hypokalemia (usually develops 4–24 hours after the initial intervention).
  - — signs/symptoms of hyperkalemia include: bradycardia, weakness, flaccid paralysis, oliguria, peaked T waves, loss of P wave, a widened QRS complex, and possible cardiac arrest
  - — signs/symptoms of hypokalemia include: weakness, flaccid paralysis, paralytic ileus, flattening or inversion of the T wave, prolonged QT intervals, and cardiac arrest
  - — do not administer potassium to a client with low urine output (hyperkalemia may result)
  - — encourage foods and liquids high in potassium when able to tolerate eating and drinking.

- Monitor sodium chloride and phosphate levels and replace as ordered.
- Administer sodium bicarbonate as ordered to correct metabolic acidosis (for pH<7.1).
- Monitor level of consciousness and neurologic status and notify physician promptly of any changes (may signal the onset of cerebral edema).
- Administer medications to correct cerebral edema.

COMMUNITY AND SELF-CARE

Instruct client regarding:

- causes and prevention of diabetic ketoacidosis
- monitoring of blood glucose and when to take extra insulin
- monitoring of urine ketones when blood glucose is high
- when to contact physician

See also, "Diabetes Mellitus," p. 218, and "Hyperglycemic, Hyperosmolar, Nonketotic Coma," p. 371.

(For more information, see pp. 1981–1987 of Black and Matassarin-Jacobs: *Medical-Surgical Nursing: Clinical Management for Continuity of Care,* 5th ed.)

Hyperglycemic, Hyperosmolar, Nonketotic Coma (HHNK)

OVERVIEW

- Hyperglycemic, hyperosmolar, nonketotic coma (HHNK) is an acute complication of diabetes. It is a variant of diabetic ketoacidosis and is characterized by extreme hyperglycemia (600–2000 mg/100 ml), mild or undetectable ketonuria and the absence of acidosis.
- It is most often seen in older-aged clients with non-insulin dependent diabetes mellitus (NIDDM). The major difference between HHNK and diabetic ketoacidosis is the lack of ketonuria with HHNK. This is because there is some insulin secretion in NIDDM, so the mobilization of fats for energy is avoided.

- In the absence of adequate insulin, blood glucose levels rise and water moves from the interstitial spaces and cells into the blood by osmosis. Fluid and glucose are lost through the urine. Eventually dehydration results and the client becomes obtunded.
- Precipitating factors for HHNK are stress, infection, dialysis, gastrintestinal bleed, hyperalimentation, pancreatitis, and certain medications (thiazide diuretics, steroids and phenytoin).

CLINICAL MANIFESTATIONS

- polyphagia—excessive hunger
- polydipsia—abnormal thirst
- polyuria—frequent urination
- glucosuria—glucose in the urine
- profound dehydration
- abdominal discomfort
- hyperpyrexia
- hyperventilation
- tachypnea
- changes in sensorium, coma
- hypotension
- shock

ACUTE AND SUBACUTE CARE

Medical Management

- fluid and electrolyte replacement
- insulin therapy

Nursing Management

- Replace fluids as ordered (usually isotonic saline initially).
- Administer potassium, sodium, chloride and phosphates intravenously as ordered.
- Administer IV insulin via an infusion pump.
- Monitor fluid volume and electrolyte levels.
- Monitor blood glucose levels.

COMMUNITY AND SELF-CARE

Instruct client regarding:

- causes of HHNK and how to prevent

- monitoring of blood glucose, and when to call physician or take extra insulin

See also, "Diabetes Mellitus," p. 218, and "Hyperglycemia/Diabetic Ketoacidosis," p. 368.

(For more information, see pp. 1987–1988 of Black and Matassarin-Jacobs: *Medical-Surgical Nursing: Clinical Management for Continuity of Care,* 5th ed.)

Hyperkalemia

OVERVIEW

- Hyperkalemia is an elevated potassium level over 5.0 mEq/L.
- Hyperkalemia increases the cell membrane's excitation threshold, causing the cell to become less excitable. This results in decreased nerve and muscle irritability.
- There are three major causes of hyperkalemia:
  (1) retention of potassium
    — causes:
      - renal insufficiency
      - adrenal insufficiency
      - hypoaldosteronism
      - potassium-sparing diuretics
      - blood transfusion (contains potassium)
  (2) excessive release of cellular potassium
    — causes:
      - crushing injuries
      - severe burns
      - severe infection
      - metabolic acidosis
      - use of a perfusion pump during surgery
  (3) excessive intravenous or oral administration of potassium
- Clients at risk for hyperkalemia are those with insufficient renal function and decreased urinary output (80–90 per cent of potassium is excreted by the kidneys).

CLINICAL MANIFESTATIONS

- initially tachycardia then bradycardia
- ECG changes—peaked, narrow T wave; widened QRS complex; depressed ST segment; widened PR interval; wide flat P wave
- hypotension
- weakened cardiac contraction, cardiac arrest
- nausea
- explosive diarrhea, intestinal colic, hyperactive bowel sounds
- paresthesia
- muscle weakness, paralysis
- muscle cramps
- oliguria and later anuria
- restlessness, convulsions
- serum potassium greater than 5.0 mEq/L

ACUTE AND SUBACUTE CARE

Medical Management

- determination/treatment of underlying cause
- cardiac monitoring
- IV saline or forcing fluids (to improve urinary output)
- sodium bicarbonate administration (promotes potassium uptake by the cell)
- potassium-wasting diuretic therapy
- calcium gluconate infusion—decreases antagonistic effect of excess potassium on the myocardium
- infusion of insulin and glucose—promotes potassium uptake into cells
- albuterol (beta-agonist) given IV—decreases plasma potassium level within 30 minutes and lasts for 6 hours
- cation exchange resin—polystyrene sulfonate (Kayexalate) induces diarrhea and potassium loss
- dietary modification—low potassium, high carbohydrate
- peritoneal dialysis or hemodialysis for marked renal failure

Nursing Management

- Administer ordered therapy.
- Monitor cardiac rhythm and assess for changes.

- Assess neuromuscular status.
- Monitor laboratory findings—potassium level, renal profile.
- Monitor intake and output.
- Daily weights.
- Implement appropriate safety measures.
- Encourage diet low in potassium.

COMMUNITY AND SELF-CARE

Discharge care is based on the etiologic factor(s) causing hyperkalemia.

(For more information, see pp. 310–314 of Black and Matassarin-Jacobs: *Medical-Surgical Nursing: Clinical Management for Continuity of Care,* 5th ed.)

Hypermagnesemia

OVERVIEW

- Hypermagnesemia is a serum magnesium level over 2.5 mEq/L.
- Hypermagnesemia has a sedative effect upon the neuromuscular system, which causes muscle weakness. It blocks the release of acetylcholine from the myoneural junction, thus decreasing cell activity.
- Factors that cause hypermagnesemia include:
  - — renal insufficiency
  - — excessive use of magnesium-containing antacids or laxatives
  - — severe dehydration from ketoacidosis
  - —overuse of IV magnesium for controlling premature labor or pregnancy-induced hypertension
  - — disorders that decrease the synthesis of aldosterone (i.e., Addison's disease or adrenalectomy)
  - —use of potassium-sparing diuretics

CLINICAL MANIFESTATIONS

- hypotension—due to peripheral vessel dilation

- dysrhythmias—premature ventricular contractions, heart block
- ECG changes—prolonged PR interval; prolonged QT interval; widened QRS complex; T wave elevation
- drowsiness, lethargy
- loss of deep tendon reflexes
- muscle weakness
- respiratory paralysis
- loss of consciousness
- serum magnesium greater than 2.5 mEq/L

ACUTE AND SUBACUTE CARE

Medical Management

- saline infusion with a diuretic to increase renal excretion
- calcium salts—antagonize magnesium
- albuterol administration
- respiratory support
- cardiac monitoring

Nursing Management

- Administer ordered therapy.
- Assess cardiac rhythm for ECG changes.
- Assess respiratory status.
- Assess neuromuscular status.
- Monitor magnesium levels.
- Institute appropriate safety measures.

COMMUNITY AND SELF-CARE

Discharge care is based on etiologic factor(s) causing hypermagnesemia.

(For more information, see pp. 324–325 of Black and Matassarin-Jacobs: *Medical-Surgical Nursing: Clinical Management for Continuity of Care,* 5th ed.)

Hypernatremia

OVERVIEW

- Hypernatremia is a serum sodium level over 145 mEq/L. It occurs in approximately 1 per cent of hospitalized clients and carries a high mortality rate. It is usually associated with water loss or sodium gain.
- Hyperosmolality of extracellular fluid (ECF) promotes a shift of water from the cells to the extracellular fluid by osmosis. More sodium is available to move across the excitable membrane, which results in earlier membrane depolarization.
- There are three types of hypernatremia:
  (1) hypovolemic hypernatremia—total body water is greatly decreased relative to sodium
    — causes:
      - severe hyperglycemia
      - osmotic diuresis
      - profuse diaphoresis
      - decreased thirst
      - diarrhea/vomiting without fluid replacement
      - fluid replacement with hyperosmolar solutions
  (2) euvolemic hypernatremia—total body water is decreased relative to sodium
    — causes:
      - excess fluid loss from skin or lungs
      - diabetes insipidus
  (3) hypervolemic hypernatremia—total body water is increased but the sodium gain is in excess of the water gain
    — causes:
      - hypertonic tube feedings
      - administration of concentrated saline solutions
      - excessive salt intake

CLINICAL MANIFESTATIONS

- anorexia, nausea, vomiting
- dry, flushed skin due to decreased interstitial fluid

- dry, sticky mucous membranes
- dry, rough tongue
- elevated body temperature
- restlessness, agitation, irritability due to cerebral cellular dehydration
- lethargy, stupor, coma
- muscle twitching, hyperreflexia
- seizures
- elevated blood pressure (hypervolemic type)
- decreased blood pressure (hypovolemic type)
- erratic heart rate due to myocardial depression as sodium ions compete with calcium ions in the slow channels of the heart
- weight gain
- oliguria, urine dark and concentrated
- edema
- lung crackles, dyspnea
- serum sodium greater than 145 mEq/L
- increased serum osmolality

ACUTE AND SUBACUTE CARE

Medical Management

- determination/management of the underlying cause
- sodium reduction and fluid loss replacement therapy—0.2 per cent or 0.45 per cent NaCl or 5 per cent dextrose in water
- diuretic therapy—furosemide (Lasix)
- dietary management—low sodium
- fluid restriction (hypervolemic)

Nursing Management

- Administer hypo-osmolar electrolyte solution.
- Administer diuretics as ordered.
- Monitor vital signs.
- Assess neurologic status.
- Assess cardiac status.
- Monitor intake and output.
- Monitor laboratory findings — electrolytes, osmolality.
- Encourage oral intake (hypovolemic type).
- Maintain fluid restriction (hypervolemic type).
- Provide frequent oral and skin care.

- Maintain sodium restricted diet.

COMMUNITY AND SELF-CARE

Discharge care is based upon the etiologic factor(s) causing hypernatremia.

(For more information, see pp. 300–304 of Black and Matassarin-Jacobs: *Medical-Surgical Nursing: Clinical Management for Continuity of Care,* 5th ed.)

Hyperparathyroidism

OVERVIEW

- Hyperparathyroidism is a disorder caused by overactivity of one or more of the parathyroid glands.
- The normal function of parathyroid hormone (PTH) is to increase bone resorption, thereby maintaining the proper balance of calcium and phosphorus ions. Excess circulating PTH leads to bone damage, hypercalcemia, renal failure, and decreased phosphate levels.
- Hyperparathyroidism is classified as:
  - Primary—normal regulatory relationship between serum calcium levels and PTH is interrupted secondary to adenoma or hyperplasia.
  - Secondary—glands are hyperplastic from malfunction of another organ system. i.e., renal failure, carcinoma with bone metastasis.
  - Tertiary—PTH production is irrepressible in clients with low or normal calcium levels.
- Hyperparathyroidism usually occurs in clients over 60 years of age and affects women more often than men (about 2 to 1).

CLINICAL MANIFESTATIONS

- backache, joint pain, pathologic fractures of the spine, ribs, and long bones
- polyuria, polydipsia, kidney stones, azotemia, hypertension

- thirst, nausea, anorexia, constipation, ileus, abdominal pain
- listlessness and depression

ACUTE AND SUBACUTE CARE

Medical Management

- hydration to lower serum calcium levels
- loop diuretics to promote renal calcium secretion—furosemide (Lasix)
- plicamycin is a chemotherapy agent that is effective in lowering calcium.
- glucocorticoids
- medications that inhibit bone resorption—mithramycin (Mithracin), gallium nitrate (Ganite), phosphates, calcitonin

Surgical Management

- parathyroidectomy—removal of the gland or glands causing hypersecretion
  - if all four glands are hyperplastic, three and one-half glands are removed
- autotransplantation of the parathyroid gland—taking the healthy gland and placing it somewhere safe in the body

Nursing Management

Medical

- Monitor intake and output.
- Strain all urine for stones.
- Encourage fluid intake up to 3000 ml/day unless contraindicated. Cranberry and prune juice make the urine more acidic and help prevent stone formation.
- Implement safety measures to prevent pathologic fractures.
- Encourage low calcium, low Vitamin D diet.
- Institute measures to prevent constipation and fecal impaction.
- Administer digitalis preparation cautiously, as hypercalcemia increases sensitivity to digitalis.

Surgical

Postoperative Care

In addition to routine postoperative care:

- Monitor for possible complications: airway obstruction, hemorrhage, injury to the recurrent laryngeal nerve, and hypocalcemia.
- Decrease strain on suture line by:
  - — semi-Fowler's positioning
  - — supporting the head and neck with pillows and sandbags
  - — instructing the client not to extend or hyperextend the neck.
- Maintain airway patency by:
  - — instructing client to cough and deep breathe
  - — gentle suctioning of the mouth and trachea
  - — humidified supplemental oxygen.
- Maintain tracheostomy set, endotracheal tube, and laryngoscope at bedside.
- Monitor intake and output.
- Reassure client that symptoms of mild tetany due to drop in serum calcium levels are temporary.
- Ensure that calcium gluconate is readily available.
- Encourage early ambulation as weight-bearing speeds the recalcification process.

COMMUNITY AND SELF-CARE

Instruct client regarding:

- dietary modifications—low calcium, low Vitamin D
- importance of adequate fluid intake
- importance of medications to control hypercalcemia
- safety measures to reduce the risk of injury
- signs of hypocalcemia and hypercalcemia
- if postoperative:
  - — wound care
  - — importance of taking oral calcium preparation (if prescribed)
- importance of follow-up appointments

(For more information, see pp. 2030–2036 of Black and Matassarin-Jacobs: *Medical-Surgical Nursing: Clinical Management for Continuity of Care,* 5th ed.)

Hypersensitivity Disorders

OVERVIEW

- Hypersensitivity is overreaction to a substance. Though widely referred to as allergic reaction, the word "hypersensitivity" is more appropriate as it denotes an increased immune response to the presence of an antigen (allergen) that results in tissue destruction.
- The occurrence and intensity of hypersensitivity responses depend on several factors: host defenses, the nature of the allergen, the concentration of the allergen, the route of allergen entrance into the body, and the exposure to the allergen.
- There are two general categories of hypersensitivity reactions based on the rapidity of the immune response: (1) immediate and (2) delayed. Immune globulins mediate immediate responses, whereas T cells govern delayed responses.
- Types of hypersensitivity reactions are:
  - Type I Anaphylactic Hypersensitivity
    - rapidly occurring reaction
    - mediated by IgE antibodies that cause the release of histamine (causes vasodilation and fluid loss into interstitial space) and leukotrienes (cause spasm of bronchial smooth muscles)
    - Forms of Type I:
      - anaphylactic shock
        - most severe form of Type I
        - clinical manifestations:
          - localized itching and edema
          - sneezing
          - wheezing, dyspnea
          - cyanosis
          - circulatory collapse
      - atopic allergies
        - include hay fever, some types of bronchial asthma, atopic dermatitis, some food and drug allergies
        - clinical manifestations:
          - rash
          - pruritus

        - nasal congestion
        - watery eyes
        - rhinorrhea
        - wheezing
        - urticaria
- Type II Cytolytic or Cytotoxic Cell Hypersensitivity
    - involves IgG or IgM antibodies that attach to antigens forming complexes that bind to cells, usually circulating blood cells, with resultant cell lysis
    - forms of Type II:
        - transfusion reactions (ABO incompatibility)
        - drug-induced hemolytic anemia
            - clinical manifestations of a transfusion reaction:
                - headache and back pain (flank)
                - chest pain similar to angina
                - nausea and vomiting
                - tachycardia and hypotension
                - hematuria
                - urticaria
- Type III Immune Complex Hypersensitivity
    - results from the formation or deposit of antigen-antibody complexes in tissue. Inflammation results and leads to acute or chronic disease of the organ system in which the complexes are deposited.
    - forms of Type III:
        - rheumatoid arthritis
        - glomerulonephritis
        - serum sickness (following injection of a foreign serum)
        - systemic lupus erythematosus
    - clinical manifestations:
        - joint pain and tenderness
        - urticaria
        - lymphadenopathy
        - fever
- Type IV Cell-Mediated or Delayed Hypersensitivity
    - sensitized T cells respond to antigens by releasing lymphokines which direct phagocytic cell activity

- reaction occurs 24–72 hours after exposure to the antigen
- forms of Type IV:
  - intradermal injection of tuberculosis antigen in a client sensitized to tuberculosis
  - graft-versus-host disease (GVHD) and transplant rejection
  - contact dermatitis
- clinical manifestations:
  - tuberculosis testing
    - edema and fibrin deposits that result in induration at the injection site
  - GVHD
    - skin, gastrointestinal, and hepatic lesions
  - contact dermatitis
    - itching
    - erythema
    - vesicular lesions

ACUTE AND SUBACUTE CARE

Medical Management

- anaphylactic shock management:
  - oxygen
  - epinephrine
  - aminophylline
  - IV antihistamines
  - airway management
- transfusion reaction management:
  - immediate discontinuation of infusion
  - IV fluids
  - treat shock with epinephrine, fluids, and oxygen
  - mannitol for renal involvement
- allergy testing
- avoidance of allergens
- antihistamines
- decongestants
- corticosteroids
- anti-inflammatory agents
- immunosuppressant agents
- immunotherapy (desensitization)—precise doses of allergens are injected at intervals over a prolonged period reducing the hypersensitivity reaction

Nursing Management

- Monitor client closely during blood administration for signs/symptoms of transfusion reaction.
- Assess for signs/symptoms of immediate or delayed response when administering the initial or test dose of a new medication.

COMMUNITY AND SELF-CARE

Instruct the client regarding:

- need to wear proper identification, identifying hypersensitivities
- importance of medication regime
- medication injection technique for client and/or household member for self-desensitization or epinephrine administration
- environmental control:
  - — nonallergenic bed linens
  - — replace carpets with throw rugs
  - — launder bed linen frequently
  - — use pull shades rather than venetian blinds
  - — heating and cooling system that humidifies and filters the air
  - — avoid smoking and smoke-filled areas
  - — keep windows at home, in the car, and at work closed; use air conditioner if possible
  - — stay indoors on windy days or when pollen count is high
  - — avoid yardwork (mowing, raking)

(For more information, see pp. 636–641 of Black and Matassarin-Jacobs: *Medical-Surgical Nursing: Clinical Management for Continuity of Care,* 5th ed.)

Hypertension

OVERVIEW

- Arterial hypertension or high blood pressure is generally defined as a persistent elevation of systolic blood pressure above 140 mmHg and diastolic pressure above 90 mmHg.

- The actual pathogenesis of hypertension remains unknown. Arterial blood pressure is a product of cardiac output and total peripheral vascular resistance. Four control systems play a major role in maintaining blood pressure. These include the: (1) arterial baroreceptor system, (2) regulation of body fluid volume, (3) renin-angiotensin system, and (4) vascular autoregulation. Any factor producing an alteration of the above may affect systemic arterial blood pressure. Hypertension causes pathologic changes in blood vessels causing them to become sclerotic, tortuous, and weak.
- Hypertension may be classified according to the following:
  - — systolic hypertension
    - – systolic pressure greater than 140 mmHg
  - — diastolic hypertension
    - – diastolic pressure greater than 90 mmHg
  - — primary (essential, idiopathic) hypertension:
    - – constitutes more than 90–95 per cent of all cases
    - – the etiology is multifactorial; several interacting homeostatic forces are involved
  - — secondary hypertension:
    - – results from an identifiable cause (i.e., renal disease, endocrine disease, stress, etc.)
    - – constitutes less than 10 per cent of the hypertensive population
  - — white coat hypertension:
    - – clients have normal readings except when blood pressure is taken by a health care professional
  - — isolated systolic hypertension
    - – occurs when the systolic blood pressure is 140 mmHg or higher, but the diastolic blood pressure remains below 90 mmHg
    - – thought to occur because of atherosclerotic changes in blood vessel compliance
- — malignant hypertension:
  - – is an emergency condition characterized by diastolic blood pressures above 120 mmHg associated with papilledema (edema and inflammation of the optic nerve at its point of entrance into the eye), acute renal failure, and rapid vascular deterioration

- without treatment, malignant hypertension results in a 90 per cent mortality rate within one year

- Arterial hypertension affects nearly 50 million clients in the United States. Prevalence of hypertension increases with advancing age, and blacks are affected more often than whites. It is the single most important predictor of cardiovascular risk.
- Risk factors include:
  - family history
  - age—incidence increases with age
  - gender—men experience hypertension at higher rates and at an earlier age
  - atherosclerosis
  - ethnic group—more prevalent in blacks
  - stress
  - obesity
  - nutrient imbalance (i.e., high sodium level, low potassium level)

CLINICAL MANIFESTATIONS

- elevation of blood pressure
- morning occipital headache
- fatigue
- dizziness
- palpitations
- flushing
- blurred vision
- epistaxis

ACUTE AND SUBACUTE CARE

Medical Management

- Nonpharmacologic intervention is widely advocated as initial therapy for most clients, at least for the first 3–6 months after initial diagnosis.
  - weight reduction
  - sodium restricted, potassium supplemented diet
  - modification of dietary fat
  - exercise
  - restriction of alcohol
  - caffeine restriction
  - relaxation techniques

— smoking cessation

- Pharmacologic intervention
  - — diuretics:
    - thiazide and sulfonamide diuretics — chlorothiazide (Diuril), hydrochlorothiazide (Esidrex), metolazone (Zaroxolyn)
    - loop diuretics—furosemide (Lasix), ethacrynic acid (Edecrin), bumetanide (Bumex)
    - potassium-sparing diuretics — spironolactone (Aldactone), triamterene (Dyrenium)
  - — vasodilators:
    - hydralazine (Apresoline), minoxidil (Loniten)
  - — beta blockers:
    - propranolol (Inderal), metoprolol (Lopressor), atenolol (Tenormin)
  - — alpha 2 agonists:
    - methyldopa (Aldomet), clonidine (Catapres)
  - — alpha 1 receptor blockers:
    - prazosin hydrochloride (Minipress), terazosin (Hytrin)
  - — calcium antagonists:
    - nifedipine (Procardia), verapamil (Calan, Isoptin), diltiazem (Cardizem)
  - — angiotensin-converting enzyme inhibitors:
    - captopril (Capoten), enalapril (Vasotec)

Malignant Hypertension

- parenteral administration of a combination of vasodilators (nitroprusside, nitroglycerin, hydralazine, enalaprilat) and adrenergic inhibitors (trimethaphan, labetalol) Diuretic, beta blockers

Nursing Management

- Administer antihypertensives as ordered.
- Monitor blood pressure to evaluate effectiveness of therapy.
- Monitor intake and output.
- Daily weights.
- Monitor laboratory results (serum sodium and potassium, BUN and creatinine, cholesterol)

COMMUNITY AND SELF-CARE

Instruct client regarding:

- disease process, factors contributing to its symptoms and risks, and prescribed medication therapy
- techniques for proper home blood pressure monitoring
- dietary modifications—low sodium, low fat, calorie restricted
- importance of consistent exercise regime
- smoking cessation programs
- importance of follow-up visits

(For more information, see pp. 1387–1404 of Black and Matassarin-Jacobs: *Medical-Surgical Nursing: Clinical Management for Continuity of Care,* 5th ed.)

Hyperthyroidism

OVERVIEW

- Hyperthyroidism is the excessive secretion of thyroid hormone secondary to overfunctioning of the thyroid gland.
- The most common form of hyperthyroidism is Grave's disease (toxic, diffuse goiter), which has three hallmarks: (1) hyperthyroidism, (2) thyroid gland enlargement secondary to hyperplasia, and (3) exophthalmus. Grave's disease is thought to be an autoimmune disorder.
- Grave's disease affects women four times as often as men and occurs between the ages of 20 and 40 years.
- The three major complications of Grave's disease are: exophthalmus; heart disease; thyroid storm.
- Ten to 15 per cent of all thyrotoxic clients are elderly.

CLINICAL MANIFESTATIONS

- tachycardia, palpitations, and elevated blood pressure
- congestive heart failure with elderly clients
- increased respiratory rate and depth, shortness of breath
- weight loss despite ravenous appetite

- diarrhea
- heat intolerance, profuse diaphoresis
- hand tremors at rest
- flushed, warm skin
- fine, soft hair
- mood swings ranging from mild euphoria to delirium
- agitation, restlessness, and irritability
- enlarged thyroid gland, bruit over thyroid
- exophthalmus—protruding eyes and fixed stare secondary to fluid accumulation behind the eye
- fatigue and muscle weakness
- amenorrhea, irregular menses
- impotence in males
- thyroid storm (thyroid crisis, thyrotoxicosis)—a medical emergency characterized by high fever, severe tachycardia, delirium, dehydration, and extreme irritability

ACUTE AND SUBACUTE CARE

Medical Management

- antithyroid hormone medication—propylthiouracil (PTU), methimazole (Tapazole)
  - for clients under 18 years of age and pregnant women
- radioiodine therapy with ^{131}I
  - usually used in middle-aged and the elderly
  - contraindicated in pregnancy
- adrenergic blocking agents may also be used to correct tachycardia and lessen tremor and nervousness

Surgical Management

- thyroidectomy—removal of the thyroid gland
- subtotal thyroidectomy—approximately 5/6 of the gland is removed

Nursing Management

Medical

- Monitor vital signs with special attention to tachycardia and/or atrial fibrillation.
- Daily weights, intake and output.

- Assess nutritional status, provide a high-calorie, high-protein diet.
- Limit foods that increase peristalsis.
- Monitor activity level; establish rest periods.
- For exophthalmus—provide eye moisturizers and eye patches as needed to prevent irritation. Diuretics may decrease periorbital edema and glucocorticoids to reduce inflammation.
- Provide a cool and relaxing environment.
- Assure client/significant other that behavioral manifestations should improve with intervention.
- Administer antithyroid hormone therapy.

Surgical

Preoperative Care

Administer antithyroid and iodine preparations to attain a euthyroid state and decrease vascularity of the thyroid gland.

In addition to routine preoperative care:

- Promote optimal nutritional balance.
- Promote rest.

Postoperative Care

In addition to routine postoperative care:

- Monitor for possible complications: respiratory obstruction, hemorrhage, hypocalcemia, and tetany (resulting from accidental removal of one or more parathyroid glands), thyroid storm, and injury to the recurrent laryngeal nerve.
- Decrease strain on suture line by:
  - — maintaining semi-Fowler's positioning
  - — supporting the head and neck with pillows and sandbags
  - — instructing the client not to extend or hyperextend the neck.
- Administer analgesics.
- Maintain airway patency by:
  - — instructing the client to cough and deep breathe
  - — gentle suctioning of mouth and trachea
  - — humidified supplemental oxygen.
- Maintain tracheostomy set, endotracheal tube, and laryngoscope at bedside for emergency treatment of airway obstruction.
- Monitor intake and output.
- Monitor rectal temperature at least every 4 hours

(elevated temperature is one of the first signs of thyroid storm).

- Monitor for hypocalcemia (calcium gluconate should be available).
- Ambulate on day number two.

COMMUNITY AND SELF-CARE

Instruct client regarding:

- importance of taking antithyroid hormone medication daily
- symptoms of thyroid deficiency or excess
- measures to reduce eye discomfort and prevent corneal irritation:
  - — wear dark glasses
  - — avoid getting dust in eyes
  - — wear eye patch(es) if irritated
  - — elevate head of bed
  - — restrict salt intake
- if postoperative, include:
  - — exercises to prevent contractures of the neck
  - — wound care
  - — for total thryroidectomy, importance of taking thyroid replacement medication
- importance of follow-up clinic/laboratory appointments

(For more information, see pp. 2005–2016 of Black and Matassarin-Jacobs: *Medical-Surgical Nursing: Clinical Management for Continuity of Care,* 5th ed.)

Hypocalcemia

OVERVIEW

- Hypocalcemia is a serum calcium level below 4.5 mEq/L.
- Hypocalcemia increases capillary permeability and causes neuromuscular excitability producing hyperactivity of motor and sensory nerves. With hypocalcemia, the bone is stimulated to release calcium, which makes the bone osteoporotic and subject to fracture.

- The causes of hypocalcemia include:
  - — inadequate dietary intake of calcium
  - — Vitamin D deficiency (decreases calcium absorption from the GI tract)
  - — excess intake of phosphorus (inhibits calcium absorption)
  - — malabsorption of fat in the intestine (interferes with Vitamin D absorption)
  - — metabolic alkalosis (decreases ionized calcium)
  - — renal failure (increased loss of calcium)
  - — Cushing's disease
  - — hypoparathyroidism (decreased bone resorption)
  - — inadvertent removal of the parathyroid gland with thyroidectomy
  - — medications:
    - magnesium sulfate, colchicine, and neomycin; inhibit parathyroid hormone secretion
    - aspirin, anticonvulsants, and estrogen; alter Vitamin D metabolism
    - phosphate preparations; decrease serum calcium levels
    - steroids; decrease calcium mobilization
    - loop diuretics; reduce calcium absorption
    - antacids and laxatives; decrease calcium absorption

CLINICAL MANIFESTATIONS

- tetany symptoms—twitching around the mouth, tingling and numbness of the fingers, carpopedal spasms, facial spasms, laryngospasm, and later convulsions
- Trousseau's sign—carpopedal spasm (contraction of the fingers and hand) elicited by inflating a blood pressure cuff on the upper arm for 1–5 minutes, constricting circulation
- Chvostek's sign—spasm of the muscles innervated by the facial nerve, elicited by tapping the client's face lightly (over the facial nerve) below the temple. Spasm of the face, lip, or nose indicates a positive test.
- dyspnea, laryngeal spasm
- increased peristalsis, diarrhea
- prolonged QT interval
- hypotension

- dysrhythmias, palpitations
- pathologic fractures (calcium loss from bones)
- prolonged bleeding times (intrinsic pathway for coagulation is inhibited)
- serum calcium less than 4.5 mEq/L

ACUTE AND SUBACUTE CARE

Medical Management

- determination/treatment of underlying cause
- calcium replacement therapy
- respiratory support
- cardiac monitoring
- dietary modifications—high calcium, low phosphate (if related to parathyroid deficiency)
- Vitamin D supplements

Nursing Management

- Administer calcium replacement therapy.
  - For oral preparations, give 30 minutes before meals for better absorption and with a glass of milk because Vitamin D is necessary in calcium absorption.
- Monitor for cardiac rhythm changes.
- Assess for signs of digitalis toxicity (bradycardia, nausea, vomiting, blurred vision), if administering a calcium supplement that enhances the action of digitalis.
- Monitor IV site if client is receiving intravenous calcium—is irritating to tissue and can cause sloughing if infiltration occurs.
- Assess for positive Chvostek's or Trousseau's signs and respiratory distress.
- Monitor laboratory findings—serum calcium, bleeding times.
- Institute appropriate safety measures.
- Monitor for any signs of bleeding.
- Use caution in turning or moving to prevent pathologic fractures.
- Maintain diet high in calcium, low in phosphorus (if related to parathyroid deficiency).

COMMUNITY AND SELF-CARE

Discharge care is based upon the etiologic factor(s) causing hypocalcemia.

(For more information, see pp. 315–319 of Black and Matassarin-Jacobs: *Medical-Surgical Nursing: Clinical Management for Continuity of Care,* 5th ed.)

Hypoglycemia (Insulin Reaction)

OVERVIEW

- Hypoglycemia is defined as a blood glucose level less than 50-60 mg/100 ml.
- Hypoglycemic reactions result from:
  - — an overdose of insulin, or less commonly, a sulfonylurea
  - — omitting a meal or eating less food than usual
  - — overexertion without additional carbohydrates to compensate
  - — nutritional and fluid imbalances due to nausea and vomiting
  - — alcohol intake.
- Untreated, prolonged hypoglycemia can result in coma and death. When the brain is deprived of glucose, brain cells are destroyed, which can cause permanent brain damage; memory loss, decreased learning ability. Paralysis also can result.

CLINICAL MANIFESTATIONS

- headache, weakness, irritability
- drowsiness, decreased mental acuity
- lack of muscular coordination
- visual disturbances
- apprehension
- diaphoresis
- pallor, hunger
- combative behavior or behavior as if drunk or psychotic
- night hypoglycemia: bizarre nightmares, restlessness, diaphoresis, sleeplessness, or confusion

ACUTE AND SUBACUTE CARE

Nursing Management

Treatment depends upon the severity of the reaction.

Mild Hypoglycemia

- Administer fast-acting sugar, such as orange juice or candy. Instead of orange juice or candy, some clients prefer to purchase glucose tablets or a glucose gel. Follow this with a small snack of carbohydrate or graham crackers and milk (10–15 grams of simple carbohydrates). Perform a blood glucose test at the onset of symptoms. Retest the blood glucose in 15–30 minutes and treat again if the blood glucose is not over 100 mg/100 ml. Continue testing until the blood glucose is over 100 mg/100 ml.

Unconscious or Semiconscious Client

- Glucagon may be administered intramuscularly or subcutaneously. Families should be instructed on how to do this at home. Unconscious or semiconscious clients must never be forced to drink fluids because aspiration may result.
- 50 mls of 50 per cent glucose by intravenous push (10–25 g) over 1–3 minutes may be given in the hospital setting.
- A longer-acting carbohydrate and protein snack should follow either of the above treatments once the client regains consciousness.

COMMUNITY AND SELF-CARE

Instruct client/significant other regarding:

- signs/symptoms of hypoglycemia
- causes of hypoglycemia and preventive measures
- times of peak insulin action
- monitoring blood sugars
- always carrying fast-acting sugar
- following treatment of hypoglycemia with protein and carbohydrate snack
- monitoring blood glucose following hypoglycemic episode until value over 100 mg/100 ml
- administration of glucagon (by significant other)
- documentation of hypoglycemic episode in daily log
- importance of Medic Alert bracelet, necklace, or identification card so that emergency care can be delivered if needed and client will not be mistaken for someone intoxicated or mentally ill

Also see, "Diabetes Mellitus," p. 218.

(For more information, see p. 1988–1990 of Black and Matassarin-Jacobs: *Medical-Surgical Nursing: Clinical Management for Continuity of Care,* 5th ed.)

Hypokalemia

OVERVIEW

- Hypokalemia is a serum potassium level less than 3.5 mEq/L. It is a common electrolyte disorder.
- When serum potassium levels decrease, there is a decreased potassium gradient between the cell and the plasma, causing the resting membrane potential to increase, thus increasing excitability. Therefore, cell membranes are more responsive to stimuli.
- Causes of hypokalemia include:

  (1) gastrointestinal losses:
  - vomiting
  - diarrhea
  - nasogastric suctioning
  - laxative abuse
  - excessive tap water enemas

  (2) dietary changes:
  - malnutrition, starvation
  - potassium-free diet
  - potassium-free intravenous solutions when NPO

  (3) medications (which promote potassium loss):
  - potassium-wasting diuretics (thiazide, osmotic)
  - steroids
  - gentamicin
  - amphotericin B
  - digitalis preparations

  (4) redistribution of potassium
  - insulin moves potassium back into the cell
  - potassium loss from osmotic diuresis in diabetic acidosis
  - alkalosis causes potassium to shift into cells in exchange for hydrogen ions

(5) disorders
  — Cushing's syndrome
  — acute renal failure (diuretic phase)
  — alcoholism

CLINICAL MANIFESTATIONS

- anorexia, vomiting, ileus, abdominal distention (slowed smooth muscle contraction)
- muscle weakness and paralysis
- leg cramps
- ECG changes—depressed ST segment; flat, inverted T waves and a prominent U wave (prolonged repolarization)
- hypotension
- slow, weak pulse (cardiac arrest with severe hypokalemia)
- shallow respirations, shortness of breath
- fatigue, lethargy
- confusion, depression (slowed conduction of nerve impulses)
- polyuria
- decreased serum osmolality
- serum potassium less than 3.5 mEq/L

ACUTE AND SUBACUTE CARE

Medical Management

- determination/management of underlying cause
- cardiac monitoring
- potassium replacement therapy
- dietary modifications—high potassium

Nursing Management

- Administer potassium replacement therapy.
  — Potassium is *not* given intramuscularly and *never* given as an IV push (may cause cardiac arrest).
- Monitor IV sites closely as potassium is irritating to blood vessels.
- Monitor cardiac rhythm and assess cardiac status.
- Monitor respiratory status.
- Monitor bowel function.
- Monitor neurologic status.
- Monitor for signs of digitalis toxicity (bradycardia, nausea, vomiting, blurred vision), potentiated by hypokalemia.

- Implement appropriate safety measures.
- Monitor laboratory findings—serum potassium levels, digoxin levels.
- Encourage foods high in potassium.

COMMUNITY AND SELF-CARE

Discharge care is based on the etiologic factor(s) that caused hypokalemia.

(For more information, see pp. 305–310 of Black and Matassarin-Jacobs: *Medical-Surgical Nursing: Clinical Management for Continuity of Care,* 5th ed.)

Hypomagnesemia

OVERVIEW

- Hypomagnesemia is a serum magnesium level below 1.5 mEq/L.
- The functions of magnesium include the transmission and conduction of nerve impulses and the contraction of skeletal, smooth, and cardiac muscle. It is responsible for the transportation of sodium and potassium across the cell membrane and the synthesis and release of the parathormone. Therefore, a deficit can lead to hypokalemia and hypocalcemia.
- Factors causing hypomagnesemia include:
  - alcoholism—when accompanied by liver disease, due to decreased production of enzymes necessary for the intestinal absorption of magnesium
  - malabsorption syndromes
  - chronic malnutrition
  - prolonged hyperalimentation without magnesium replacement
  - excessive amounts of phosphorus in the intestine (usually from antacids)—will decrease magnesium absorption
  - alkalosis
  - prolonged loss of fluids from the gastrointestinal tract

— medications:
  - osmotic and thiazide diuretics, aminoglycoside antibiotics, amphotericin B, corticosteroids and digitalis—interfere with renal handling of magnesium

CLINICAL MANIFESTATIONS

- anorexia, nausea, abdominal distention
- cardiac dysrhythmias including premature ventricular contractions, atrial or ventricular fibrillation
- ECG changes—prolonged QT intervals; widened QRS complex; flat or inverted T waves; and ST segment depression
- signs of digitalis toxicity (secondary to hypokalemia) (see below)
- vasospasm leading to stroke
- tetany
- positive Chvostek's and Trousseau's signs, see "Hypocalcemia," p. 392.
- convulsions
- depression, psychosis, and confusion
- serum magnesium below 1.5 mEq/L

ACUTE AND SUBACUTE CARE

Medical Management

- determination/treatment of underlying cause
- magnesium replacement therapy
- cardiac monitoring
- dietary modification—high magnesium

Nursing Management

- Administer ordered therapy.
- Assess cardiac rhythm for ECG changes.
- Monitor laboratory findings—magnesium, potassium, calcium.
- Monitor for signs of digitalis toxicity (bradycardia, nausea, vomiting, blurred vision).
- Assess neurologic status.
- Institute appropriate safety measures

COMMUNITY AND SELF-CARE

Discharge care is based upon the etiologic factor(s) causing hypomagnesemia.

(For more information, see pp. 323–324 of Black and Matassarin-Jacobs: *Medical-Surgical Nursing: Clinical Management for Continuity of Care,* 5th ed.)

Hyponatremia

OVERVIEW

- Hyponatremia is a serum sodium level below 135 mEq/L. It is one of the most common electrolyte disorders in adults.
- As the extracellular fluid concentration of sodium decreases, the sodium concentration gradient between extracellular and intracellular fluids decreases. This hypo-osmolality causes water to move into the cell causing intracellular edema. These changes also mean that there is less sodium to move across the excitable membrane, which results in delayed membrane depolarization. Generally, the clinical manifestations reflect this decreased excitability.
- There are four types of hyponatremia:

  (1) hypovolemic hyponatremia—sodium loss is greater than water loss
  - — causes:
    - diuretic use
    - diabetic glycosuria
    - aldosterone deficiency
    - renal disease
    - vomiting
    - diarrhea
    - excessive diaphoresis
    - burns

  (2) euvolemic hyponatremia—total body water is moderately increased and sodium remains at normal level
  - — causes:

- syndrome of inappropriate antidiuretic hormone (SIADH)
- continuous secretion of ADH secondary to pain, medication, or stress

(3) hypervolemic hyponatremia—there is a greater increase in total body water than in sodium
— causes:
- congestive heart failure
- liver cirrhosis
- nephrotic syndrome
- acute and chronic renal failure

(4) redistributive hyponatremia—no change in total body water or sodium, but a water shift occurs between the intracellular and extracellular compartment relative to sodium concentration
— causes:
- hyperglycemia
- hyperlipidemia

CLINICAL MANIFESTATIONS

- nausea, vomiting, abdominal cramps
- hyperactive bowel sounds
- decreased blood pressure, orthostatic hypotension (hypovolemic hyponatremia)
- elevated blood pressure (hypervolemic hyponatremia)
- adventitious lung sounds
- headache, apprehension
- lethargy
- confusion
- decreased muscle tone and deep tendon reflexes
- weakness
- dry skin and mucous membranes
- tremor
- convulsions
- serum sodium below 135 mEq/L

ACUTE AND SUBACUTE CARE

Medical Management

- determination/management of underlying cause
- sodium replacement — 3 per cent saline solution
- fluid replacement (hypovolemic)
- fluid restriction (hypervolemic)—allows sodium balance to be regained

- normal saline in conjunction with furosemide (Lasix)—increases urinary sodium loss and reduces the risk of extracellular fluid volume expansion
- diuretic therapy
- dietary modifications—high sodium, fluid restriction if hypervolemic

Nursing Management

- Administer electrolyte and fluid replacement therapy as ordered.
- Monitor vital signs.
- Monitor neurologic status.
- Monitor cardiac status.
- Daily weights.
- Monitor intake and output.
- Administer PRN antiemetics.
- Monitor laboratory findings—electrolytes, osmolality.
- Promote the intake of fluids containing sodium, such as broths or juices.
- Maintain fluid restriction (hypervolemic).
- Provide appropriate safety measures.

COMMUNITY AND SELF-CARE

Discharge care will be based on the etiologic factor(s) causing hyponatremia.

(For more information, see pp. 296–300 of Black and Matassarin-Jacobs: *Medical-Surgical Nursing: Clinical Management for Continuity of Care,* 5th ed.)

Hypoparathyroidism

OVERVIEW

- Hyposecretion of the parathyroid glands produces a syndrome opposite that of hyperparathyroidism. Serum calcium levels are low and serum phosphate levels are high.

- Parathyroid hormone (PTH) acts to increase bone resorption, which in turn maintains serum calcium levels. When PTH is reduced, bone resorption slows, serum calcium levels decrease, and phosphate levels rise.
- Causes are either:
  - iatrogenic— caused by (1) accidental removal of parathyroid glands during thyroidectomy, (2) infarction of the glands during surgery, or (3) strangulation of one or more glands by postoperative scar tissue.
  - idiopathic—an autoimmune disorder with a genetic basis.
- Risk factors include thyroid and parathyroid surgery.

CLINICAL MANIFESTATIONS

The symptoms of hypoparathyroidism are mainly caused by low serum calcium levels. They are always more severe in clients who have elevated serum pH (alkalosis), as this decreases the amount of ionized calcium, which worsens the symptoms.

- Acute hypoparathyroidism
  - increased neuromuscular irritability resulting in tetany (painful muscle spasms), irritability, grimacing, tingling of the fingers, laryngospasm, and arrhythmias.
  - positive Chvostek's and Trousseau's signs
- Chronic hypoparathyroidism
  - lethargy
  - thin, patchy hair
  - brittle nails, dry, scaly skin
  - personality changes
  - cataract formation

ACUTE AND SUBACUTE CARE

Medical Management

- Acute hypoparathyroidism:
  - IV calcium gluconate infusion—to elevate serum calcium as rapidly as possible
  - anticonvulsant therapy
  - respiratory support
- Chronic hypoparathyroidism:

— oral calcium salts and vitamin D

Nursing Management

- Assess client at risk for acute hypoparathyroidism (i.e., post thyroidectomy) for tetany, positive Chvostek's or Trousseau's sign, or respiratory distress.
- For acute hypoparathyroidism:
  — administer IV calcium as ordered
  — monitor for respiratory distress, have emergency respiratory equipment at hand
  — monitor for convulsions and protect from injury
  — monitor for cardiac arrhythmias.
- Promote adequate rest.
- Administer calcium supplements and vitamin D as ordered.

COMMUNITY AND SELF-CARE

Instruct the client regarding:
- importance of medication regime
- dietary modifications—high in calcium, low in phosphorus
- signs of hypocalcemia and hypercalcemia
- stress the importance of life-long medical care
- follow-up appointments

(For more information, see pp. 2036–2038 of Black and Matassarin-Jacobs: *Medical-Surgical Nursing: Clinical Management for Continuity of Care,* 5th ed.)

Hypopituitarism

OVERVIEW

- Hypopituitarism is a deficiency of one or more of the hormones provided by the anterior lobe of the pituitary gland.
- Some common causes of hypopituitarism are:
  — pituitary tumors, CNS tumors
  — sarcoidosis

— removal of the pituitary gland (hypophysectomy)
— postpartum necrosis
— head trauma
— radiation therapy
— deficiency of an anterior pituitary hormone—growth hormone (GH), thyroid stimulating hormone (TSH), etc.

CLINICAL MANIFESTATIONS

- short stature
- symptoms of adrenocortical insufficiency (due to diminished ACTH synthesis)
- symptoms of hypothyroidism (due to decreased synthesis of thyroid-stimulating hormone [TSH])
- sexual and reproductive disorders (deficiencies of gonadotropins [LH and FSH] can produce sterility, diminished sexual drive, and decreased secondary sex characteristics)

ACUTE AND SUBACUTE CARE

Medical Management

- removal, if possible, of the causative factor (e.g., tumors)
- permanent replacement of the hormones secreted by the target organs (adrenals, thyroid, etc.)

Nursing Management

- Assessment and nursing interventions depend upon type of hormone deficiency. See the appropriate section for specific interventions.

COMMUNITY AND SELF-CARE

Instruct client regarding:

- importance of replacement hormone therapy
- when to seek medical attention

(For more information, see pp. 2065–2066 of Black and Matassarin-Jacobs: *Medical-Surgical Nursing: Clinical Management for Continuity of Care,* 5th ed.)

Hypothermia

OVERVIEW

- Hypothermia is a condition of below normal body temperature (below 34.4° C).
- Hypothermia can occur accidentally through exposure to environmental cold, as a response to illness, or in near drowning victims.

CLINICAL MANIFESTATIONS

- below normal body temperature
- hypotension
- pupils can be fixed and dilated
- somnolence
- loss of muscle coordination, unconsciousness
- ventricular dysrhythmias, cardiac arrest

ACUTE AND SUBACUTE CARE

Medical Management

- if emergency situation—support airway, breathing, circulation
- rewarming measures
- vasoactive therapy
- dysrhythmia management

Nursing Management

- Initiate warming blanket.
- Administer heated oxygen.
- Monitor temperature closely.
- Continuous cardiac monitoring.
- Maintain warm room environment.

COMMUNITY AND SELF-CARE

Hypothermia is resolved before discharge.

(For more information, see pp. 2535–2536 of Black and Matassarin-Jacobs: *Medical-Surgical Nursing: Clinical Management for Continuity of Care,* 5th ed.)

Hypothrombinemia

OVERVIEW

- Hypothrombinemia, a coagulation disorder, refers to a deficient amount of circulating prothrombin.
- Prothrombin is a protein produced in the liver and found in the blood. For prothrombin synthesis to take place, vitamin K must be present in the liver to act as a catalyst. Hypothrombinemia develops from a vitamin K deficiency or an interference with the action of vitamin K.
- Factors causing hypothrombinemia include:
  — vitamin K deficiency due to:
    - improper diet
    - malabsorption syndrome
    - prolonged sulfonamide or antibiotic therapy that sterilizes the bowel removing bacteria that manufacture vitamin K

  — liver disorder
  — overdose of aspirin, coumarin, or coumarin derivative (warfarin) which antagonize the action of vitamin K

CLINICAL MANIFESTATIONS

- ecchymosis after minimal trauma
- epistaxis
- hematuria
- gastrointestinal bleeding
- prolonged bleeding from a venipuncture site

ACUTE AND SUBACUTE CARE

Medical Management

- determination/treatment of underlying cause
- vitamin K therapy
- infusion of prothrombin concentrates or prothrombin factors VII, IX, and X
- dietary modification — high vitamin K

Nursing Management

- Administer vitamin K, prothrombin or factor therapy.

- Assess for signs of bleeding.
- Monitor laboratory findings—CBC, prothrombin time.
- Institute bleeding precautions:
  — soft toothbrush
  — electric razor
  — hold pressure to venipuncture sites
  — no intramuscular or subcutaneous injections
  — no aspirin or nonsteroidal anti-inflammatory drugs
  — stress need to avoid blowing nose
  — stress need to avoid straining with stool
  — safety measures for ambulation

COMMUNITY AND SELF-CARE

Instruct client regarding:

- vitamin K therapy
- signs/symptoms of complications and when to notify physician
- measures to prevent bleeding:
  — soft toothbrush, no flossing
  — electric razor
  — no aspirin or nonsteroidal anti-inflammatory drugs
  — no contact sports
  — avoidance of constipation
- diet high in vitamin K
- need for follow-up appointments

(For more information, see pp. 1509–1510 of Black and Matassarin-Jacobs: *Medical-Surgical Nursing: Clinical Management for Continuity of Care,* 5th ed.)

Hypothyroidism

OVERVIEW

- Hypothyroidism refers to a deficiency of thyroid hormone—thyroxine (T_4) or triiodothyronine (T_3)—resulting in slowed body metabolism (due to decreased oxygen consumption by the tissues) and pronounced personality changes.

- The thyroid gland needs iodine to synthesize and secrete its hormone. If iodine is lacking in the diet or the production of thyroid hormone is suppressed for any other reason, the thyroid enlarges (goiter) in an attempt to compensate for hormonal deficiency.
- Hypothyroidism affects women more than men (about 4 to 1). The highest incidence is between 30 and 65 years of age.
- The three types of hypothyroidism are:
  - — Primary—caused by congenital defects of the thyroid (cretinism), defective hormone synthesis, antithyroid medications, iodine deficiency, surgery, radioactive therapy for hyperthyroidism, or following chronic illnesses.
  - — Secondary—caused by insufficient stimulation of a normal thyroid gland secondary to malfunction of the pituitary or hypothalamus.
  - — Tertiary or Central—caused by failure of the hypothalamus to produce thyroid-releasing hormone (TRH), which stimulates the pituitary to secrete thyroid stimulating hormone (TSH).
- Risk factors include iodine deficient diet, radiation therapy to area of thyroid, surgery for hyperthyroidism, multiple medications, the elderly, and chronic inflammatory diseases.

CLINICAL MANIFESTATIONS

There is a wide range of symptoms depending upon the severity of the disease:

- decreased heart rate, stroke volume, and cardiac output
- hyperlipidemia, hypercholesterolemia
- anemia, easy bruising
- dyspnea, fatigue, lethargy
- fluid retention and possible weight gain
- anorexia, constipation
- sensitivity to cold, decreased ability to sweat
- slowed physical and mental reactions
- forgetfulness, depression, apathy, paranoia
- dry, coarse skin and hair
- normal to enlarged thyroid gland
- expressionless face
- periorbital edema
- slow, deliberate speech

- menorrhagia, irregular menses
- myxedema (dry, waxy, non-pitting type of swelling caused by abnormal deposits of mucin in skin and tissues)
- myxedema coma (drastic decrease in metabolic rate, hypoventilation, hypotension, and hypothermia)

ACUTE AND SUBACUTE CARE

Medical Management

- thyroid hormone preparation
- iodine preparation
- iodine-enriched diet

Surgical Management

- Surgery is done if goiter is very large and not responding to therapy or it is putting too much pressure on other structures in the neck.

Nursing Management

Medical

- Monitor vital signs.
- Assess for signs/symptoms of decreased cardiac output.
- Daily weights.
- Assess nutritional status, encourage well-balanced diet.
- Monitor intake and output.
- Administer thyroid preparations—assess for symptoms of thyrotoxicosis (tachycardia, diarrhea, sweating, agitation, tremors, shortness of breath).
- Establish a progressive exercise/activity program and monitor client tolerance.
- Implement measures to prevent constipation and fecal impaction.
- Provide measures to keep client comfortably warm.
- Assure client/significant other that client's appearance, energy level, affect, and mental capabilities will gradually improve with thyroid hormone therapy.

COMMUNITY AND SELF-CARE

Instruct client regarding:

- importance of taking thyroid hormone daily
- symptoms of thyroid deficiency or excess
- dietary management
- importance of follow-up appointments

(For more information, see pp. 2005–2016 of Black and Matassarin-Jacobs: *Medical-Surgical Nursing: Clinical Management for Continuity of Care,* 5th ed.)

I

Idiopathic Thrombocytopenic Purpura

OVERVIEW

- *Purpura* is the extravasation of small amounts of blood into the tissues and mucous membranes.
- The term *thrombocytopenia* means a reduction of platelets below 100,000/mm^3. The two major problems that characterize thrombocytopenia are spontaneous bleeding into any part of the body and prolonged oozing from sites.
- Idiopathic thrombocytopenia (ITP) refers to thrombocytopenia of unknown cause, possibly an autoimmune reaction. This disorder is characterized by the premature destruction of platelets. Normally, platelets survive 8–10 days. However, platelet survival in ITP is as brief as 1–3 days or less. ITP is characterized by the development of antibodies to one's own platelets, which are then destroyed by phagocytosis in the spleen and liver.
- Ninety per cent of adults with ITP are under 40 years of age; the ratio of women to men is 3 to 1 to 4 to 1.

CLINICAL MANIFESTATIONS

- petechiae
- ecchymosis
- epistaxis
- bleeding gums
- easy bruising
- heavy menses or bleeding between periods
- complications include:
  - — cerebral hemorrhage
  - — gastrointestinal bleeding
  - — bleeding into the diaphragm
  - — nerve pain or paralysis from pressure of hematomas on nerves

ACUTE AND SUBACUTE CARE

Medical Management

- steroid therapy—to suppress phagocytic response of splenic macrophages (rarely produces a permanent cure)
- platelet transfusions
- plasmapheresis—to remove circulating antibodies

Surgical Management

- splenectomy—the effectiveness of splenectomy is believed to be related to the removal of the site of premature destruction of the antibody-sensitized platelets
  - — treatment of choice
  - — 60–80 per cent of cases result in complete and permanent remission

Nursing Management

Medical

- Administer steroids and platelet replacement therapy. See "Blood Component Transfusion," p. 88.
- Monitor laboratory findings—platelet count, CBC.
- Institute bleeding precautions
  - — soft toothbrush
  - — electric razor
  - — no intramuscular or subcutaneous injections
  - — no aspirin or nonsteroidal anti-inflammatory drugs
  - — stress need to avoid blowing nose
  - — stress need to avoid straining with stool
  - — hold pressure to all venipuncture sites
  - — safety measures for ambulation
- Assess for signs of bleeding into other tissues or organs

Surgical

In addition to routine postoperative care:

- Monitor for the development of hemorrhage
  - — vital signs
  - — increased abdominal girth

- Institute measures to prevent the formation of thrombi
  — pressure stockings
  — leg exercises
  — early ambulation

COMMUNITY AND SELF-CARE

MEDICAL

Instruct client regarding:

- importance of long-term steroid therapy
- disease process, signs/symptoms of possible complications, and when to notifiy physician
- measures to prevent bleeding
  — no aspirin or nonsteroidal anti-inflammatory agents
  — no contact sports
  — avoid constipation
  — soft toothbrush, no flossing
  — electric razor
- need for follow-up clinic/laboratory appointments

SURGICAL

Instruct client regarding:

- care of the incision
- need for prophylactic antibiotics
- early signs/symptoms of infection (fever, chills, productive cough) and when to report to physician
- routine immunization against influenza and pneumococci

(For more information, see pp. 1506–1508 of Black and Matassarin-Jacobs: *Medical-Surgical Nursing: Clinical Management for Continuity of Care,* 5th ed.)

Incontinence, Urinary

OVERVIEW

- Incontinence is a condition in which involuntary loss of urine is a social or hygienic problem and is objectively demonstrable.

- There are five categories of incontinence
  - Stress—an immediate, involuntary loss of urine upon an increase in intra-abdominal pressure. Often associated with activities, such as laughing, sneezing, coughing, or running.
  - Urge—inability to hold back the flow of urine when feeling the urge to void.
  - Overflow—urinary retention with overflow of small amounts of urine.
  - Reflex—abnormal activity of the spinal cord reflex leading to involuntary loss of urine. There is no sensation to void.
  - Functional (environmental)—aware of the need to urinate, but unable to reach the toilet unaided.
- Incontinence may be caused by:
  - sphincter weakness or damage
  - urethral deformity
  - alteration of the urethrovesical junction in women
  - weak abdominal and perineal muscle tone
  - dementia, confusion
  - certain medications
- Risk factors include:
  - Stress incontinence
    - women—loss of the correct posterior urethrovesical junction angle
    - men—urethral irritation from infection, radiation damage to the bladder, or after a prostatectomy
  - Urge incontinence
    - multiple sclerosis (due to severe bladder spasms)
    - urinary tract infections
    - strokes
    - medications interfering with mobility, such as hypnotics, tranquilizers, sedatives, and diuretics
  - Overflow incontinence—nervous system lesions, obstruction of the bladder outlet, or fecal impaction
  - Reflex incontinence—spinal cord injury resulting in complete loss of voluntary control of the bladder

CLINICAL MANIFESTATIONS

- involuntary loss of control of voiding
- bladder spasms (associated with urge incontinence)

ACUTE AND SUBACUTE CARE

Medical Management

Treatment for incontinence will depend upon the results of urodynamic evaluation and the specific abnormalities identified for the client.

- pelvic muscle exercises (Kegel's) to strengthen the pubococcygeal muscle. Femina cones (weights placed in the vagina) may be used to enhance effectiveness of these exercises
- bladder training with the client voiding at short intervals (hourly or less) and gradually lengthening time between voidings to intervals up to 3 hours
- behavioral techniques and biofeedback for clients with stress or urge incontinence (may provide significant improvement but requires extensive training)
- medications—used primarily with urge incontinence and sometimes stress incontinence
- mechanical pressure devices to interfere with the outflow of urine
  - — pessaries may be used in females, but are associated with complications
  - — penile clamps for males are controversial, as use may lead to pressure sores and ischemic necrosis of the penis.
- psychotherapy and hypnosis also may help manage incontinence
- weight reduction
- avoiding fluids before bedtime

Surgical Management

- electrical stimulation devices—inhibit the micturition reflex. These include electrodes implanted within the pelvic muscles and intravaginal devices or anal plugs for indirect stimulation
- Marshall-Marchetti-Krantz procedure—involves suturing the bladder neck and urethra to the peri-

chondrium of the symphysis pubis or the periosteum of the superior pubic ramus
- Raz procedure—done transvaginally and involves elevation and suspension of the bladder using tissue or inorganic materials for support
- implantation of an artificial urinary sphincter—as a last resort measure

Nursing Management

Medical

- Instruct the client on Kegel exercises.
- Encourage adequate fluid intake up to 2000–2500 ml/day, instructing the client to avoid caffeine and alcohol, which stimulate the bladder.
- Develop a bladder training program and voiding schedule. Initially, the client should try to void every 30 minutes to 2 hours. As the program progresses, the voiding intervals are lengthened.
- Assist the client with a weight reduction and exercise program.
- Maintain integrity of the skin and instruct the client on the need for good skin care.
- Avoid use of adult diapers as this demeans the client and gives "permission" to be incontinent.
- If above measures fail, provide disposable pads or briefs to increase social mobility and protect the skin.
- External condom catheter—only needed if above measures fail.

Surgical

Postoperative Care

In addition to routine postoperative care:
- Raz procedure
  - — Maintain patency of suprapubic or urethral catheter for 5-8 days (the pressure of a filling bladder inhibits healing).
  - — Encourage high fluid intake to prevent infection.
  - — Initiate clamp and release program after healing occurs to help the detrusor muscle regain tone.

— Obtain and measure residual urine as ordered to determine the effectiveness of bladder emptying.

COMMUNITY AND SELF-CARE

- Instruct the client/family regarding:
  - removing barriers in the home that prevent easy access to toilet facilities
  - obtaining assistive devices or commode as needed
  - providing good skin care
- Instruct the client regarding:
  - Kegel exercises and use of Femina cones
  - bladder training routine
- Refer to continence clinics and support groups.
- Discuss newsletters available from the Simon Foundation for Continence and Help for Incontinent Persons (HIP).

(For more information, see pp. 1604–1616 of Black and Matassarin-Jacobs: *Medical-Surgical Nursing: Clinical Management for Continuity of Care*, 5th ed.)

Increased Intracranial Pressure

OVERVIEW

- Intracranial pressure (ICP) is the pressure exerted in the cranium by its contents: the brain, blood, and cerebrospinal fluid (CSF). The pressure is measured via the CSF in the ventricle or in the subarachnoid space. Normal pressure of CSF is 5–15 mmHg. Pressures over 20 mmHg are called increased ICP (IICP).
- The skull is a hard bony container. Since the skull cannot expand, compensatory mechanisms come into play:
  (1) initial compensation—displacement of CSF into the spinal canal or into venous blood through the arachnoid mater.
  (2) secondary compensation—reduction of blood volume to the brain. This stage of compensa-

tion alters cerebral metabolism and eventually produces brain tissue hypoxia and necrosis.

(3) final compensation—displacement of brain tissue (herniation).

- Increased ICP is most often associated with an expanding lesion (e.g., bleeding or tumor), hydrocephalus (an obstruction to the outflow of CSF), an abscess, or an ingested toxin.
- Clients at risk include those with expanding tumors in the brain, head injury, brain surgery, hydrocephalus, and bleeding (e.g., subarachnoid hemorrhage).

CLINICAL MANIFESTATIONS

- alteration in level of consciousness
- restlessness
- irritability
- confusion
- decrease in Glasgow coma score
- changes in speech
- pupillary reaction changes
- motor or sensory changes
- cardiac rate (bradycardia) and rhythm changes
- headache
- nausea and vomiting
- double vision (diplopia)
- papilledema noted on ophthalmoscopic exam
- hypertension with widened pulse pressure
- irregular respirations
- hyperthermia initially, followed by hypothermia
- seizure activity

ACUTE AND SUBACUTE CARE

Medical Management

- intracranial pressure monitoring—insertion of a subarachnoid or ventricular probe through a hole in the skull to measure ICP
- osmotic diuretics—Mannitol
- fluid restriction
- steroid therapy—dexamethasone (Decadron) to control edema
- antacids and hydrogen blockers; stress ulcer prophylaxis

- barbiturate therapy—pentobarbital to reduce ICP
- blood pressure therapy; to raise or lower BP to maintain cerebral perfusion
- mechanical ventilation; hyperventilation induced by a ventilator or manual ventilation induces a hypocarbic (low carbon dioxide level) state that results in vasoconstriction of cerebral blood vessels and decreased blood flow
- antipyretic therapy
- anticonvulsant therapy
- elevation of the head to promote venous drainage

Surgical Management

A craniotomy may be indicated to:

- place a shunt to allow drainage of CSF
- evacuate a subdural or epidural hematoma
- remove brain tissue (i.e., part of the temporal lobe) to give remaining structures room to expand. If compliance is low at the time of surgery, the bone flap used to gain access to the brain is not replaced or the dura may not be closed. Subsequent surgery is then required to repair the defect.

Nursing Management

Medical

- Monitor for increased ICP readings and accompanying signs and symptoms (posturing or disorientation).
- Manually hyperventilate the client if ICP increases (hypocarbic state decreases cerebral blood volume and ICP).
- Plan nursing interventions so that activities known to increase ICP are not performed when the ICP is elevated (e.g., suctioning, excessive hip flexion, repositioning).
- Monitor for other factors that may increase ICP
  - excess water in ventilator tubing
  - excessive pulmonary secretions (increased pCO_2)
  - endotracheal tube taped too tightly against jugular vein, retarding venous circulation from the head

- Avoid ICP catheter infection by (1) keeping the area around catheter site clean, (2) reporting leakage from catheter, and (3) maintaining a closed system.
- Monitor respiratory status closely.
- Perform suctioning only when necessary to prevent increasing ICP.
  - — never exceed 10 seconds in suctioning time (causes increased ICP)
  - — never suction through the nose (may cause trauma and CSF leak)
- Monitor arterial blood gas results to correct acid-base imbalances promptly.
- Perform complete neurologic assessment using Glasgow coma scale.
- Prevent venous obstruction
  - — raise the head of the bed 30 degrees
  - — avoid turning the head sharply to either side and keep head in alignment with the body to facilitate venous drainage
  - — avoid extreme rotation and flexion of the neck, which may compress the jugular veins and increase ICP
  - — avoid extreme hip flexion, which increases intra-abdominal and intrathoracic pressure that increases ICP
  - — maintain regular bowel program (excessive strain can cause a Valsalva's maneuver, resulting in venous back-up and increased ICP)
- Administer diuretics and steroids as ordered.
- Monitor intake and output.
- Monitor parenteral fluid therapy closely, administering only the minimal volumes ordered.
- Monitor temperature closely.
  - — Increased temperature causes an increased metabolic rate and aggravates ICP. Hyperthermia requires vigorous treatment.
- Monitor hemodynamic parameters closely, if administering barbiturate therapy (may cause cardiac depression).
  - — Monitor daily serum barbiturate level.
- Observe for and report any signs of increasing ICP (see "Clinical Manifestations" listed above).
- Maintain quiet, restful environment.

- Assess for complications of immobility (pulmonary embolism, deep vein thrombosis, skin breakdown).
- Administer stress ulcer prophylaxis.

Surgical

Postoperative Care

In addition to routine postoperative care and the above medical interventions:

- Assure patency of and record output of surgical drains placed.
- Monitor incision for CSF leak.
- Observe and report complications of craniotomy.

See "Intracranial Tumors," p. 431, for postoperative care following a craniotomy.

COMMUNITY AND SELF-CARE

Increased ICP is resolved before discharge.
Instruct the client regarding:

- wound care, if postoperative

(For more information, see pp. 771–783 of Black and Matassarin-Jacobs: *Medical-Surgical Nursing: Clinical Management for Continuity of Care,* 5th ed.)

Infectious Mononucleosis

OVERVIEW

- Infectious mononucleosis is a self-limiting condition characterized by painful enlargement of the lymph nodes.
- The cause of infectious mononucleosis is a herpes virus, the Epstein-Barr virus. The disease may be spread by the oropharyngeal route.
- Primarily a disease of the young, infectious mononucleosis usually strikes children between the ages of 3 and 5 years and young adults between the ages of 15 and 25 years.
- Fever typically lasts 4–6 weeks with a long convalescence until strength is regained.

CLINICAL MANIFESTATIONS

- fatigue
- headache
- malaise, myalgias
- fever
- pharyngitis
- lymphadenopathy
- maculopapular rash
- splenic enlargement with left upper quadrant pain
- possible splenic rupture (secondary to infiltration of the spleen by massive numbers of lymphocytes)

ACUTE AND SUBACUTE CARE

Medical Management

No specific intervention mitigates or shortens the disease process.

- bedrest
- antipyretics

Surgical Management

- splenectomy

Nursing Management

Medical

- Administer antipyretics and implement other cooling measures (tepid bath, light clothing).
- Monitor temperature.
- Monitor intake and output.
- Encourage rest.
- Assess for signs/symptoms of splenic rupture—abdominal pain, shock.
- Administer PRN analgesics.

Surgical

- See "Idiopathic Thrombocytopenic Purpura," p. 413, for postoperative care following a splenectomy.

COMMUNITY AND SELF-CARE

Instruct client regarding:

- need for adequate rest
- signs of splenic rupture

- avoidance of contact sports for a period of at least 1 month (could result in splenic rupture)
- see "Idiopathic Thrombocytopenic Purpura," p. 413, for discharge instructions following a splenectomy.

(For more information, see pp. 1503–1504 of Black and Matassarin-Jacobs: *Medical-Surgical Nursing: Clinical Management for Continuity of Care,* 5th ed.)

Infective Endocarditis

OVERVIEW

- Endocarditis is an inflammatory process of the endocardium, especially the valves. This disorder was once lethal, but morbidity and mortality have been reduced greatly with the use of antibiotics and advanced diagnostic procedures.
- Circulating microorganisms in the bloodstream attach to the endocardium and multiply. Usually this multiplication requires a rough or abnormal endocardial surface. These vegetations can severely damage heart valves by perforation, and deforming the valve leaflets.
- The most common organisms causing endocarditis are streptococci, gram-negative bacilli, or fungi.
- Risk factors include:
  - — rheumatic heart disease
  - — mitral valve prolapse
  - — heart valve replacement
  - — invasive procedures (i.e., minor surgery, dental procedures, indwelling catheter)
  - — chronic debilitating disease
  - — immunosuppression
  - — intravenous drug abuse
- Terms used to classify endocarditis include:
  - — subacute bacterial endocarditis (SBE)—develops gradually over weeks or months. It is usually caused by organisms of low virulence, such as *Streptococcus viridans*, which has limited ability to infect other tissues.
  - — acute bacterial endocarditis—develops over days or weeks with an erratic course. Frequently

caused by *Staphylococcus aureus*, which is capable of infecting other body tissues.
  - native valve endocarditis—an infection of a previously normal or damaged valve
  - prosthetic valve endocarditis —an infection of a prosthetic valve
  - nonbacterial thrombotic endocarditis—caused by sterile thrombotic lesions (frequently aggregates of platelets), which may develop with malignancies or chronic diseases
- The proportion of acute cases of infective endocarditis is rising. Five of every 1000 patients admitted to the hospital have endocarditis. Overall mortality is 20–30 per cent and as high as 70 per cent in the aged.

CLINICAL MANIFESTATIONS

- fever, chills, rigors, sweats, malaise, weakness, anorexia, weight loss, backache, splenomegaly
- dyspnea, chest pain, murmur
- cold, painful extremities
- petechiae
- Roth's spots—visualized on fundoscopic examination as a white or yellow center surrounded by a red irregular halo
- Osler nodes—painful, erythematous nodules on the skin of the extremities, usually on the fingertips
- splinter hemorrhages—linear hemorrhages that appear similar to tiny splinters under the nail
- headaches and musculoskeletal complaints
- symptoms of cardiac failure

ACUTE AND SUBACUTE CARE

Medical Management

- intravenous antibiotic therapy for 4-6 weeks (penicillin and streptomycin are commonly used)

Nursing Management

- Assess for rapid pulse, easy fatiguability, dyspnea, restlessness, signs of heart failure, and embolic manifestations.
- Administer antibiotics as ordered.

- Treat fever with rest, cooling measures, forced fluids, and antipyretics.
- Encourage fluids and a well-balanced diet.
- Administer PRN analgesics.
- Provide rest periods.
- Implement progressive activity schedule.

COMMUNITY AND SELF-CARE

Instruct client regarding:

- cause of infective endocarditis
- purpose of long-term antibiotic administration and the need to comply with the entire course
- need for prophylactic antibiotics when undergoing dental procedures or surgical interventions
- importance of follow-up care. Recently there has been a trend to allow appropriate clients to complete the intravenous therapy at home with the assistance of home health agencies.

(For more information, see pp. 1331–1334 of Black and Matassarin-Jacobs: *Medical-Surgical Nursing: Clinical Management for Continuity of Care,* 5th ed.)

Influenza

- Influenza refers to an acute viral respiratory tract infection.
- The risk factors include: very young children, the institutionalized, the elderly, clients with chronic illnesses, and healthcare workers.
- Clinical manifestations include: fever, myalgias, cough, and complications associated with influenza like viral bronchitis, pneumonia, and superinfections.
- Medical management consists of: symptom management, annual immunizations for high risk clients to help prevent influenza, short-term administration of antiviral agents in institutions with influenza outbreaks.
- Nurses can instruct the public to help prevent the spread of infection by practicing good handwashing

and covering the mouth when sneezing or coughing.

- Nurses should also be aware that clients with an allergy to eggs or a history of Guillain-Barré syndrome should not receive the influenza vaccine.

(For more information, see pp. 1133–1134 of Black and Matassarin-Jacobs: *Medical-Surgical Nursing: Clinical Management for Continuity of Care,* 5th ed.)

Intestinal Obstruction

OVERVIEW

- Intestinal obstruction is the partial or complete impairment of the forward flow of intestinal contents.
- Intestinal obstruction has a high mortality rate if not diagnosed and treated within 24 hours.
- Obstruction of the small intestine may be caused by inflammation, neoplasms, adhesions, hernia, volvulus, intussusception, paralytic ileus, vascular problems, hypokalemia, food blockage, or compression from outside the intestine.
- Obstruction of the large intestine usually is due to cancer but may be caused by diverticulitis and ulcerative colitis.
- Risk factors include: adhesions, hernia, volvulus, intussusception, tumors, neurogenic factors, and obstruction of blood flow to the bowel.

CLINICAL MANIFESTATIONS

- nausea and vomiting (vomiting progresses from semi-digested food to watery material with bile and finally dark fecal material)
- abdominal pain in rhythmically recurring waves
- abdominal distention with high pitched bowel sounds
- visible peristaltic waves
- hypoxia (due to severe abdominal distention raising the diaphragm)

ACUTE AND SUBACUTE CARE

Medical Management

- insertion of an intestinal tube
- gastric suction and rest for adynamic ileus

Surgical Management

Surgery is performed when medical management fails and is aimed at relieving the obstruction by elimination of the cause and removal of any ischemic bowel.

Nursing Management

- Assess presence and quality of bowel sounds.
- Assess for abdominal distention.
- Assess character, duration, and quality of abdominal pain.
- Monitor for dehydration and electrolyte imbalance (especially note serum pH, potassium and sodium).
- Replace fluids and electrolytes as prescribed.
- Maintain intestinal tube to suction and monitor relief of distention and nausea.
- Monitor and document amount, color, odor, and consistency of intestinal tube drainage or any emesis.
- Monitor intake and output.
- Monitor for signs/symptoms of bowel strangulation and report immediately to physician: emesis, increasing distention and pain, and fever.
- Prepare for emergency bowel resection if strangulation occurs.

COMMUNITY AND SELF-CARE

Postoperative discharge teaching depends upon the surgical procedure performed.

Instruct client regarding:

- ways to prevent recurrence and maintain bowel elimination
- ways to regain nutritional status after weight loss

(For more information, see pp. 1820–1823 of Black and Matassarin-Jacobs: *Medical-Surgical Nursing: Clinical Management for Continuity of Care,* 5th ed.)

Intracellular Fluid Volume Excess (ICFVE)—Water Intoxication

OVERVIEW

- Intracellular fluid volume excess (ICFVE) secondary to hypo-osmolar disorders results from either water excess or solute deficit. In water excess, the number of solutes is normal but diluted by excessive water. In solute deficit, the amount of water is normal, but there are too few particles per liter of water. Hypo-osmolality of vascular fluid exists and cellular swelling occurs.
- Hypo-osmolar fluids move by osmosis to maintain fluid equilibrium, forcing fluids to move from lesser concentration (in the vessels) to the higher concentration (in the cells) in ICFVE. Too much fluid accumulates in the cell causing cellular edema. Brain cells are usually involved first resulting in cerebral edema.
- Causes of intracellular fluid volume excess include: administration of excessive amounts of hypo-osmolar intravenous fluids; consumption of excessive amounts of water; or increased secretion of antidiuretic hormone (SIADH) secondary to pain, narcotic use, or stress.

CLINICAL MANIFESTATIONS

- headache, nausea, vomiting (cerebral cellular edema)
- apprehension, irritability, disorientation
- pupillary changes (pressure on third cranial nerve)
- decreased muscle strength
- unequal grasp
- weight gain
- bradycardia, widened pulse pressure (difference between systolic and diastolic pressure readings), altered respiratory patterns, muscle twitching, projectile vomiting, convulsions (increased intracranial pressure)
- low serum sodium level (hypo-osmolality)
- decreased hematocrit (hemodilution)

ACUTE AND SUBACUTE CARE

Medical Management

- identification/management of underlying cause
- solute replacement therapy
- diuretic therapy

Nursing Management

- Administer solute replacement therapy.
- Monitor neurologic status.
- Administer diuretic therapy.
- Monitor vital signs.
- Monitor intake and output.
- Daily weights.
- Institute appropriate safety measures.

COMMUNITY AND SELF-CARE

Discharge care is based upon the etiologic factor(s) causing the cellular fluid excess.

(For more information, see pp. 291–293 of Black and Matassarin-Jacobs: *Medical-Surgical Nursing: Clinical Management for Continuity of Care,* 5th ed.)

Intracranial Tumors

OVERVIEW

- Intracranial tumors may be benign or malignant, but both are potentially fatal. These tumors cause death by infiltration and compression of the brain tissue. The tumors occupy space and also produce cerebral edema. Because the skull is rigid, there is little room for expansion of contents. Brain tumors progressively increase intracranial pressure (ICP), which causes brain stem herniation and death.
- Intracranial tumors may be:
  - — primary tumors that developed from central nervous system tissue
  - — secondary tumors that have metastasized from other locations in the body

— intra-axial tumors originating from glial cells within the cerebrum, cerebellum, or brain stem. These tumors infiltrate and invade brain tissue.
— extra-axial tumors originating from the skull, meninges, cranial nerves, or pituitary gland. These tumors have a compressive effect on the brain.

- Primary brain tumors occur equally in males and in females of all age groups; 36,000 new cases are diagnosed yearly.
- There is no clear etiology for the development of primary tumors, and, therefore, no risk factors.
- Tumors of the lung, breast, kidney, and malignant melanoma are the most common primary sites that metastasize to the brain.
- Primary intracranial tumors do not metastasize to other sites in the body unless the protective barriers are damaged.

CLINICAL MANIFESTATIONS

Symptoms vary according to the area and extent of the brain involved.

- focal weaknesses (i.e., hemiparesis)
- sensory disturbances (i.e., paresthesias)
- language disturbances
- coordination disturbances
- visual disturbances
- visual field deficits
- headaches (intermittent and of increasing duration), most severe in the frontal or occipital region
- nausea and vomiting
- papilledema (edema of the optic disc)
- seizures
- dizziness and vertigo
- mental status changes (lethargy, drowsiness, confusion, disorientation, and personality changes)

ACUTE AND SUBACUTE CARE

Medical Management

Depends upon the type and location of the tumor and the client's condition

- intrathecal chemotherapy (placed within the cerebrospinal fluid [CSF] via an intraventricular reservoir or lumbar puncture)

- systemic chemotherapy
- stereotactic radiation therapy—precise localization of target tissue
- internal radiation—seeds implanted through catheters into the tumor

Surgical Management

- stereotactic radiosurgery—application of ionizing beams of radiation focused with the help of intracranial guiding devices
- craniotomy—removal of the tumor through a surgical opening in the skull. During brain surgery, the brain may become edematous and expand so that the surgeon can not close the dura. A bone flap may be created to permit expansion of the brain.
- craniectomy—permanent removal of the cranium to relieve pressure on the brain by providing space for expansion

Nursing Management

Medical

- Administer chemotherapy as ordered and assess for side effects (see "Chemotherapy," p. 149).
- Assess neurologic status.
- Maintain safety precautions.

Surgical

Preoperative Care

In addition to routine preoperative care:

- Assess and document the following as a baseline for comparison with postoperative assessment findings:
  - vital signs; level of consciousness; orientation to person, place, and time; ability to follow instructions; pupil size, equality, and reaction to light (Glasgow Coma Scale Score)
  - limb movements; limited or exaggerated movements; strength in extremities (grip); any paresis or paralysis; sensory abnormalities; edema
  - manifestations of increasing ICP
  - presence of aphasia, visual or auditory problems
- Provide emotional support to client and significant other.

- Administer parenteral corticosteroids as ordered.
- Discuss scalp preparation (i.e., shaving) and reassurances that hair will grow back.

Postoperative Care

In addition to routine postoperative care:

- Monitor and document the following, comparing to baseline assessment (report abnormals to the physician):
  - — vital signs and neurologic function (include level of consciousness, ability to move extremities, speech, orientation and pupillary response)
- Assess head dressing for any drainage.
- Assess intactness of head dressing — ensure it is not too tight.
- Obtain intake and output every hour.
- Monitor electrolyte levels, serum glucose, osmolarity, and hematocrit.
- Assess for any signs of increasing ICP (headache, vomiting, seizures, visual or speech disturbances, widening pulse pressure, respiratory irregularity, muscle weakness or paralysis, pupillary changes, hypertension, bradycardia).
- Maintain head in midline position to facilitate venous drainage and reduce ICP.
- Position as ordered by physician to prevent increased ICP:
  - — Supratentorial Surgery—elevate head of the bed 30 degrees; do not lower the head of the bed for any procedure without a written order from the neurosurgeon.
  - — Infratentorial Surgery—most common to keep client flat without head elevation to prevent pressure on the brain stem. Turn every 2 hours.
  - — Posterior Fossa Surgery—position on either side but never on the back. A pillow may be placed under the head for support.
  - — Bone Flap (surgically removed for decompression)—place the client only on the unoperated side or back.
- Maintain ventilator function. Monitor oxygen saturations and arterial blood gases.
- Administer osmotic diuretic therapy and steroids as ordered to prevent increased ICP.
- Monitor for CSF leaks.

— Place a gauze pad near the nose, ears, or head dressing to absorb any drainage noted.
— Test any blood or clear fluid for presence of glucose (the presence of glucose indicates CSF).
— Note if any drainage/fluid dries in concentric circles (indicates CSF).

- If CSF leak is present, administer ordered antibiotics.
- Monitor for seizure activity; administer anticonvulsants as ordered.
- Monitor for meningitis (may develop 2–3 days after surgery):
  — headache, nuchal rigidity, chills, fever, decreased level of consciousness, increased sensitivity to light
- Monitor for stress ulcer. Test gastric pH and administer antacids to maintain pH above 4.5.
- Use sterile technique for all dressing changes to prevent meningitis.
- Assess operative site and sites around drains or catheters for edema and signs of infection.
- As the wound heals, remove dry flaky scalp skin by softening the scalp with baby oil or glycerin and washing with soap and water.
- Administer ordered medications for pain (such as acetaminophen or codeine).
- Keep the environment quiet, calm, and dimly lit.
- Provide nasogastric feedings as ordered, once the swallowing reflex and peristalsis are present.
- Monitor respiratory status and oxygenation to ensure cerebral oxygenation and avoid hypercapnia (hypercapnia increases ICP).
- Do not suction through the nose (if the nasal membrane is torn, CSF may leak, and an infection may result). Suction by other routes minimally (suctioning increases ICP).
- Provide method of communicating needs and facilitate communication.
- Prevent complications of immobility by providing frequent position changes (as ordered).
- Begin range of motion exercises as ordered.
- Encourage as much independence with self care as possible.
- Encourage client to discuss concerns or changes in body image or self-esteem disturbances. Make referrals as necessary.

- Assist client/family to develop a plan for managing home care, if residual deficits present.
- Provide emotional support to family. Make referrals as necessary.

COMMUNITY AND SELF-CARE

Needs vary greatly depending upon the amount of brain damage, residual deficits, and whether client is going home or to a long-term rehabilitation center. Referrals may be needed, especially to support groups for family members.

(For more information, see pp. 843–856 of Black and Matassarin-Jacobs: *Medical-Surgical Nursing: Clinical Management for Continuity of Care,* 5th ed.)

Irritable Bowel Syndrome (IBS)

OVERVIEW

- Irritable bowel syndrome (IBS) is a functional disorder of motility in the small and large intestines, causing diarrhea, constipation, or an alternation between the two. The motility can be altered by a number of factors including diet and emotions. It develops without organic disease or anatomic abnormality.
- IBS is the most common gastrointestinal disorder in Western society and is more common in women.
- IBS is also called spastic colon, irritable colon, nervous indigestion, pylorospasm, and spastic colitis.
- Risk factors include:
  — diets high in rich foods such as creams and fats
  — stress
  — fresh fruits
  — gas-producing foods
  — alcohol
  — cigarette smoking.

CLINICAL MANIFESTATIONS

- abdominal pain

- constipation or diarrhea
- hypersecretion of colonic mucous
- flatulence, nausea, anorexia
- left lower quadrant abdominal pain
- cramping in the morning or following eating
- anxiety or depression

ACUTE AND SUBACUTE CARE

Medical Management

Treatment is palliative and supportive.

- sedatives and antispasmodic medications
- vegetable mucilages, such as psyllium hydrophilic mucilloid (Metamucil)
- increased dietary fiber
- reduce stress and encourage exercise

Nursing Management

- Monitor number and characteristics of stools.
- Monitor intake and output.
- Administer antispasmodics as ordered.

COMMUNITY AND SELF-CARE

Instruct client regarding:

- use of fiber to manage constipation and diarrhea
- adequate fluid intake (8 glasses of water daily)
- need for adequate sleep, exercise, and nutrition
- diarrhea:
  — limit gas-producing foods
  — avoid caffeine, alcohol, and foods containing nondigestible carbohydrates (e.g., beans)
  — exclude milk and milk products

(For more information, see pp. 1823–1825 of Black and Matassarin-Jacobs: *Medical-Surgical Nursing: Clinical Management for Continuity of Care,* 5th ed.)

K

Kaposi's Sarcoma

- Kaposi's sarcoma is a vascular malignancy that presents as a skin disorder.
- Kaposi's sarcoma used to be a skin disease common in 50- to 60-year-old men in central or Eastern Europe. Recently, Kaposi's sarcoma has been seen in many clients with acquired immunodeficiency syndrome (AIDS).
- The cause of Kaposi's sarcoma is not known, although the human immunodeficiency virus and cytomegalovirus have been suggested as the cofactors in its development. It is considered to be due to a failure in the immune system.
- Kaposi's sarcoma lesions begin as red, dark blue, or purple macules on the lower legs that coalesce into larger plaques. These plaques frequently ulcerate or open and drain.
- The lesions spread by metastasis to the upper body, then to the face and oral mucosa. About 75 per cent of clients develop lesions of the lymph nodes, gastrointestinal tract, and lungs.
- Clients report pain and itching in the lesions; as the disease progresses, the legs become edematous.
- Treatment involves excision of local lesions with intralesional chemotherapy. Systemic lesions are treated with a combination of interferon-alpha, cytotoxic agents, and radiation.

See also, "Human Immunodeficiency Virus (HIV) Infection," p. 356.

(For more information, see pp. 2230–2231 of Black and Matassarin-Jacobs: *Medical-Surgical Nursing: Clinical Management for Continuity of Care,* 5th ed.)

L

Laryngeal Cancer

OVERVIEW

- Cancer of the larynx is cancer of the voice box. It commonly occurs on the glottis (true vocal cords), the supraglottic structures (above the vocal cords), or the subglottic structures (below the vocal cords).
- Risk factors include cigarette smoking, alcohol abuse, voice abuse, and chronic laryngitis.

CLINICAL MANIFESTATIONS

- hoarseness that persists longer than 2 weeks
- neck masses, pain in throat radiates to ear,
- laryngeal tumors seen on laryngoscopy

ACUTE AND SUBACUTE CARE

Medical Management

Treatment depends upon the stage and site of the tumor.

- Radiation therapy for glottic cancer is limited to the true vocal cords or for supraglottic tumors that have not metastasized.
- Chemotherapy generally is not performed except for prevention of new primary tumors.

Surgical Management

- Laser surgery with irradiation for small tumors.
- Partial laryngectomy is the removal of one-half or more of the larynx. It is performed for cancer involving one true vocal cord and sometimes a portion of the other true vocal cord. A temporary tracheostomy is also performed.
- Supraglottic laryngectomy is a form of partial laryngectomy and is performed for cancer of the supraglottis. The surgeon removes the superior

portion of the larynx from the false vocal cords to the epiglottis. Lymph node dissection and removal of a portion of the base of the tongue may or may not be performed, but the true vocal cords are preserved.

- Total laryngectomy is required for large glottic tumors with fixation of the vocal cords. The larynx is removed and the voice permanently lost. A permanent tracheostomy is always performed with this procedure.
- Radical neck dissection involves the above procedure for total laryngectomy plus removal of the lymphatic drainage channels and nodes, sternocleidomastoid muscle, spinal accessory nerve, jugular vein, and submandibular area. It is performed when there is a risk of metastasis to the cervical lymph nodes.

Nursing Management

Surgical

Partial Laryngectomy

Preoperative Care

In addition to routine preoperative care:

- Assess the client's nutritional status, including usual caloric intake, lymphocyte levels, serum albumin, hemoglobin, and hematocrit.
- Assess the oral mucosa and state of dentition.
- If the client is an active alcoholic, discuss with physician plans for support during the withdrawal period.
- Assess the client's usual coping strategies and available support systems (there will be some disfigurement after surgery).
- Discuss alternate means of communication to be used in the postoperative period.

Postoperative Care

In addition to routine postoperative care:

- Monitor closely for possible complications of airway obstruction, hemorrhage, carotid artery rupture, fistula formation, and tracheostomy stenosis.
- Prevent aspiration by:
  - — maintaining semi-Fowler to high-Fowler's position

- — suctioning or instructing client to cough every hour to remove secretions
- — instructing on swallowing technique (the epiglottis has been removed).

- Maintain a patent tracheostomy tube by cleaning the inner cannula to remove mucous as needed (at least three times/day).
- Prevent tracheostomy tube displacement or accidental decannulation by:
  - — ensuring intactness of sutures
  - — using two nurses to change tracheostomy ties
  - — ensuring snugness of tracheostomy ties
  - — keeping a tracheal dilator and emergency tracheostomy tray in the room
  - — understanding use of stay sutures (if used).
- Reduce the risk of tracheal necrosis or stenosis by:
  - — deflating the tracheostomy cuff (during exhalation) every shift to improve circulation and remove secretions
  - — using the minimal *occlusion* volume technique to reinflate the cuff, never the minimal *leak* technique.
- Monitor for and prevent infection by:
  - — assessing the amount and color of drainage every 4 hours
  - — assessing incisional site, noting any redness, swelling, or tenderness
  - — ensuring that supplemental oxygen is humidified
  - — ensuring patency of wound drains
  - — cleansing suture lines twice daily with hydrogen peroxide, followed by a saline rinse.
- Maintain NG tube to suction for removal of gastric secretions.
- Provide adequate nutrition through tube feedings when ordered, using care to prevent aspiration.

COMMUNITY AND SELF-CARE

Instruct client regarding:

- wound care
- need for follow-up with Speech and Swallowing Therapy
- need for follow-up of potential malignancy
- importance of good nutrition

Total Laryngectomy

Preoperative Care

- Preoperative care is the same as for the partial laryngectomy client, except the tracheostomy is permanent, and the client will need to learn alternative methods to speak. Nasogastric feedings also will be started sooner.

Postoperative Care

Postoperative care is the same as for the partial laryngectomy client with the following added interventions:

- Provide nasogastric feedings when edema has subsided and the client can swallow his own secretions.
- Instruct on and provide an alternative means to communicate in the first few postoperative days, such as a writing board or picture boards where the patient can point to what he needs.
- Reinforce speech techniques taught by speech therapist
  — use of an artificial larynx
  — esophageal speech
  — use of a voice button or trapdoor prosthesis.

COMMUNITY AND SELF-CARE

Instruct client regarding:

- tracheostomy care and dressing changes
- covering stoma lightly with bib, scarf, etc. to prevent entrance of foreign bodies
- need for smoking cessation program
- avoidance of water sports
- importance of wearing Medic-Alert bracelet (to identify need for mouth-stoma breathing if resuscitation needed)
- signs/symptoms to report to physician:
  — hemoptysis
  — difficulty swallowing/breathing
  — change in voice quality
  — persistent cough, sore throat
  — lump in the neck or elsewhere in body
- reinforce nutritional plan
- discuss follow-up with Speech Therapy

Radical Neck Dissection

Preoperative Care

In addition to routine preoperative care:

- Encourage the client to discuss fears and concerns, especially of deformity or diagnosis of cancer.
- Discuss what to expect after surgery (transfer to intensive care unit, drainage tubes, tracheostomy).
- Assess usual coping mechanisms/support systems.
- Discuss alternative means of communication (voice will be lost).

Postoperative Care

In addition to routine postoperative care:

- Monitor closely for patent airway (airway occlusion can occur due to bleeding or edema).
- If musculocutaneous flaps were used for repair, assess perfusion of the flap every hour for the first 24 hours, then every 4 hours.
- Place in semi-Fowler's to reduce edema.
- Monitor patency and drainage of neck catheters. Aspirate the drains with a needle or empty every 4 hours.
- Maintain pressure dressings (except on musculocutaneous flap) — reinforce as needed.
- Instruct on exercises to increase range of motion and muscle strength in affected shoulder.
- See also "Tracheostomy," p. 705.

COMMUNITY AND SELF-CARE

Instruct client regarding:

- increased risk of neck tissue injury because of lack of sensation
- avoidance of temperature extremes or use of heating pads
- wound care
- tracheostomy care

See also "Tracheostomy," p. 705.

(For more information, see pp. 1082–1100 of Black and Matassarin-Jacobs: *Medical-Surgical Nursing: Clinical Management for Continuity of Care,* 5th ed.)

Laryngeal Edema, Acute

- Laryngeal edema may be associated with inflammation, injury, or anaphylaxis.
- Signs and symptoms are hoarseness and severe shortness of breath progressing to respiratory arrest.
- Emergency tracheostomy may be required because endotracheal intubation is difficult due to the edema.
- Subcutaneous epinephrine 1:1000 and intravenous corticosteroids are used if anaphylaxis is the cause.

(For more information, see p. 1100 of Black and Matassarin-Jacobs: *Medical-Surgical Nursing: Clinical Management for Continuity of Care,* 5th ed.)

Laryngeal Edema, Chronic

- Chronic laryngeal edema occurs when lymphatic drainage is obstructed due to infection, tumor, or radiation therapy.
- A tracheostomy or endotracheal tube may be required, depending upon the severity of the edema.

(For more information, see p. 1101 of Black and Matassarin-Jacobs: *Medical-Surgical Nursing: Clinical Management for Continuity of Care,* 5th ed.)

Laryngitis

- Laryngitis is an inflammation of the larynx or hoarseness. It may be due to an inflammatory process, voice abuse, gastroesophageal reflux, abnormal movements of the vocal cords, or a tumor of the vocal cords.
- Treatment of laryngitis is aimed at the causative factors, such as antibiotics for infection; voice rest

for voice abuse; and antacids and histamine receptor antagonists for gastroesophageal reflux.
- Nursing care involves administration of supplemental humidification and mucolytic agents; voice rest; and instructing the client to avoid whispering, which strains the vocal cords.

(For more information, see p. 1081 of Black and Matassarin-Jacobs: *Medical-Surgical Nursing: Clinical Management for Continuity of Care,* 5th ed.)

Laryngospasm

- Laryngospasm is a spasm of the laryngeal muscles due to:
  - — administration of certain general anesthetic agents
  - — repeat and/or traumatic endotracheal intubation attempts
  - — inhaled agents or foreign material
  - — hypocalcemia.
- Treatment is administration of 100 per cent oxygen until the laryngeal spasm stops. If the laryngospasm continues, paralysis with neuromuscular blocking agents may be necessary to allow intubation. Mechanical ventilation follows.
- Emergency cricothyroidotomy or tracheostomy may be required.

(For more information, see p. 1101 of Black and Matassarin-Jacobs: *Medical-Surgical Nursing: Clinical Management for Continuity of Care,* 5th ed.)

Leukemia

OVERVIEW

- Leukemia is a malignant disease of the blood-forming organs. Leukemia accounts for 8 per cent of all human cancers and is the most common malignancy in children and young adults. One-half of all leukemias are classified as acute with rapid onset and progression. The remaining are classified as chronic and have a more indolent course.

- Acute leukemia is caused by the proliferation of large numbers of abnormal immature leukocytes in the bone marrow, lymph nodes, liver, spleen and eventually all body systems. In addition, the production of other blood cells (i.e., red blood cells, platelets, and neutrophils) is inhibited and results in inadequate oxygen transport, thrombocytopenia, and immune system malfunction. For a leukemic process to be termed acute, at least 50 per cent of the marrow cells must be immature.
- Chronic leukemias have a gradual onset and a more protracted course. The white cells produced are more mature and can better defend the body against infection. Chronic leukemia occurs in adulthood.
- There are two major forms of acute leukemia: (1) lymphocytic—involves the lymphocytes and lymphoid organs, and (2) nonlymphocytic—involves the hematopoietic stem cells that differentiate into myeloid cells (monocytes, granulocytes, erythrocytes, and platelets). From these two broad categories leukemias are further classified according to the specific malignant cell line. Ninety per cent of acute leukemia is acute lymphoblastic leukemia (ALL), caused by proliferation of precursor lymphocytes called lymphoblasts. ALL presents most often in children 2–10 years of age. Acute nonlymphocytic leukemia (ANLL), formerly known as acute myelogenous leukemia (AML), is characterized by aberrations in the growth of megakaryocytes, monocytes, granulocytes, and erythrocytes. ANLL is more common in adulthood, with a median age of 67 years.
- Chronic leukemia is classified as chronic myelogenous leukemia (CML) or chronic lymphocytic leukemia (CLL).
  - CML originates in the stem cells, and there is an increased production of granulocytes. After a relatively slow course for a median of 4 years, the CML client invariably enters a blast crisis that resembles acute leukemia. During this

phase, increasing numbers of blasts (immature myeloid precursor cells, especially myeloblasts) proliferate in the blood and bone marrow. Blast crisis is diagnosed when blasts and promyelocytes (another myeloid cell precursor type) exceed 20 per cent in the blood and 30 per cent in the marrow.
- — CLL is characterized by the proliferation of early B lymphocytes. CLL is an indolent form of leukemia most often seen in men over 50 years of age. As the disease progresses, lymphocytes infiltrate the lymph nodes, liver, spleen, and bone marrow. Progression of the disease may take as long as 15 years.

- Although the cause of leukemia is unknown, there are several host factors associated with leukemia. These include exposure to ionizing radiation and chemicals, congenital abnormalities (i.e. Down's syndrome), presence of primary immunodeficiency, and infection with the human T-cell leukemia virus type 1 (HTLV-1).

CLINICAL MANIFESTATIONS

The signs and symptoms of all types of leukemia are similar.

- fatigue, weakness
- easy bruising
- bleeding gums
- epistaxis
- fever
- headache and generalized pain
- feeling of abdominal fullness and early satiety (as a result of splenomegaly)
- pallor
- scattered petechiae and ecchymosis
- generalized lymphadenopathy
- hepatosplenomegaly
- bone and joint pain
- CBC values
  - — WBC may be normal, abnormally low, or extremely high. The differential may reveal that one type of leukocyte is predominant.
  - — Platelet count—usually low.
  - — Hemoglobin—usually low.

ACUTE AND SUBACUTE CARE

MEDICAL MANAGEMENT

Acute Leukemia

- chemotherapy
  - — protocol involves three phases:
    - induction—client receives an intensive course of chemotherapy designed to induce a complete remission (defined as less than 5 per cent of the bone marrow cells are blast cells and peripheral blood counts are normal, and both conditions are sustained for 1 month).
    - consolidation phase—modified courses of intensive chemotherapy are given to eradicate the disease.
    - maintenance phase—small doses of different combinations of chemotherapeutic agents are given every 3–4 weeks and continued for a year or more.
- radiation therapy
- bone marrow transplantation—see "Bone Marrow Transplantation," p. 92.
- blood component replacement therapy
- broad spectrum antibiotics and antifungals for signs/symptoms of infection

Chronic Myelogenous Leukemia (CML)

- leukopheresis—temporary lowering of the white cell count using an automated blood cell separator that returns red cells and plasma to the client
- thrombocytopheresis—operates on same principle as leukopheresis but removes thrombocytes
- chemotherapy
  - — busulfan
  - — hydroxyurea
- blood component replacement therapy
- bone marrow transplantation—see "Bone Marrow Transplantation," p. 92.
- antibiotic therapy

Chronic Lymphocytic Leukemia (CLL)

- radiation therapy

- chemotherapy
  - chlorambucil
  - prednisone
  - fludarabine
  - cyclophosphamide
- blood component therapy
- antibiotic therapy

Surgical Management

Chronic Myelogenous Leukemia

- splenectomy

Chronic Lymphocytic Leukemia

- splenectomy

Nursing Management

Medical

- Administer ordered chemotherapy. See "Chemotherapy," p. 149.
- Administer blood component replacement therapy. See "Blood Component Transfusion," p. 92.
- See "Radiation Therapy," p. 605.
- Monitor temperature and assess for any signs/symptoms of infection.
- Maintain protective isolation or laminar flow if neutrophil count is less than $500/mm^3$.
- Restrict visitors with possible communicable diseases.
- Provide meticulous oral and physical care.
- Maintain a low-bacteria diet that excludes raw fruits and vegetables.
- Avoid rectal suppositories and rectal temperatures (may seed the bloodstream with microorganisms).
- Obtain cultures as ordered.
- Administer antibiotics as ordered.
- Monitor the client for signs/symptoms of bleeding: ecchymosis, petechiae, epistaxis, heme-positive stools, disorientation.
- Test all urine, stool, and emesis for blood.
- Monitor vital signs, noting symptoms of altered tissue perfusion.

- Institute bleeding precautions:
  — soft toothbrush, cotton swabs, or sponges for oral hygiene
  — avoid blowing nose
  — avoid straining with stool
  — electric razor
  — avoid mucosal trauma during suctioning
  — no intramuscular or subcutaneous injections
  — no aspirin products
  — pad side rails and maintain uncluttered environment
  — use paper tape only
- Monitor laboratory findings—CBC, platelet count, culture reports.
- Administer antiemetics as ordered.
- Daily weights.
- Encourage small, frequent feedings.
- Administer analgesics to relieve the pain of mucositis.
- Encourage the client to balance rest with exercise.
- Provide emotional support and referrals to assist the client/family.

Surgical

- See "Bone Marrow Transplantation," p. 92.

COMMUNITY AND SELF-CARE

- Instruct client regarding:
  — disease process and treatment regime
  — signs/symptoms to report to physician
  — measures to prevent infection:
    - avoid large crowds and wear a mask in public
    - good personal hygiene
    - maintain a balance between exercise and rest
    - maintain a well-balanced diet
    - avoid raw fruits and vegetables and raw meat
    - avoid anyone with an infectious disease
    - change air conditioner and furnace filters weekly
    - remove additional sources of bacteria found in standing water: fish tanks, flower vases, humidifiers

— measures to reduce risk of bleeding:
  - soft toothbrush
  - electric razor
  - avoid blowing nose or straining with stool
  - safety precautions
— see "Chemotherapy," p. 149.
— see "Radiation Therapy," p. 605.
— see "Bone Marrow Transplantation," p. 92.
— importance of follow-up clinic and laboratory visits

- Refer to available community resources.

(For more information, see pp. 1487–1495 of Black and Matassarin-Jacobs: *Medical-Surgical Nursing: Clinical Management for Continuity of Care,* 5th ed.)

Leukoplakia

- Leukoplakia is a potentially precancerous yellow-white or gray-white lesion occurring in the oral mucous membranes. It results from chronic irritation of the mucosa by physical, thermal, or chemical factors. Men are twice as affected as women.
- Treatment is aimed at elimination of the cause.

(For more information, see pp. 1726–1727 of Black and Matassarin-Jacobs: *Medical-Surgical Nursing: Clinical Management for Continuity of Care,* 5th ed.)

Liver Abscess

OVERVIEW

- A liver abscess is a localized collection of pus and organisms within the parenchyma of the liver.
- A liver abscess usually develops after one of the following: bacterial cholangitis, portal vein bacteremia, or amebiasis (infestation with amebae from tropical or subtropical areas).

- Other predisposing factors are diabetes mellitus, infected hepatic cysts, metastatic liver tumors with secondary infection, and diverticulitis.

CLINICAL MANIFESTATIONS

- right upper quadrant pain
- right shoulder pain
- liver enlargement and tenderness
- nausea/vomiting
- weight loss, anorexia
- fever and diaphoresis

ACUTE AND SUBACUTE CARE

Medical Management

- percutaneous drainage of abscess
- antibiotic therapy
- Flagyl or chloroquine phosphate if due to amebic infestation

Surgical Management

- surgical drainage of abscess

Nursing Management

- Monitor vital signs—high temperature and rapid pulse may indicate general sepsis.
- Encourage movement, coughing, and deep-breathing to prevent pulmonary complications.
- Encourage fluid intake.
- Administer antibiotics as ordered.

COMMUNITY AND SELF-CARE

Instruct the client regarding:
- Disease process and treatment regime.
- Importance of completing antibiotic or Flagyl regime.
- Signs/symptoms to report.
- Importance of follow-up care.

(For more information, see p. 1902 of Black and Matassarin-Jacobs: *Medical-Surgical Nursing: Clinical Management for Continuity of Care,* 5th ed.)

Liver Tumors (Primary)

- Primary liver neoplasms may be adenomas or hepatocellular carcinoma.
- Adenomas are benign hepatic cell tumors. They may be related to oral contraceptive use by women. They may be dangerous due to their vascularity, and the possibility of rupture. Treatment may be discontinuation of the hormone if the tumor is hormone dependent. Surgical excision may be necessary in some cases.
- Primary hepatocellular carcinoma (malignant hepatoma) is one of the most common tumors worldwide. It is four times more common in men than women. It may be caused by hepatitis B, hepatitis C, chronic liver disease, cirrhosis, anabolic steroid use, or long-term androgen therapy. Surgical resection of the tumor is the only method of cure and may be attempted if the tumor is confined to one lobe. If interventions fail to terminate the tumor process, the client usually dies of hepatic failure within 3–6 months.
- See "Chemotherapy," p. 149, and "Radiation Therapy," p. 605.

(For more information, see pp. 1895–1896 of Black and Matassarin-Jacobs: *Medical-Surgical Nursing: Clinical Management for Continuity of Care,* 5th ed.)

Liver Transplant

OVERVIEW

- Liver transplant is now considered a feasible form of intervention for a variety of endstage liver diseases.
- Liver transplantation is indicated for clients whose chronic or acute liver disease is progressive, life-threatening, and unresponsive to medical therapy.

- The number of transplants has continued to grow each year. In 1990, over 2500 people in the United States received transplants.
- Common conditions for which transplants are performed are:
  — primary biliary cirrhosis (adult)
  — hepatitis—chronic or fulminant (usually adult)
  — sclerosing cholangitis (adult)
  — biliary atresia (pediatric)
  — Alpha$_1$-antitrypsin deficiency (usually pediatric)
  — confined hepatic malignancy (adult or pediatric)
  — Wilson's disease
  — Budd-Chiari syndrome (hepatic vein obstruction)
- The transplant may be orthotopic (the diseased liver is removed and the new liver implanted in the same location) or heterotopic (the diseased liver is not removed during transplant). Orthotopic is by far the more common of the two.
- The criteria for matching donors and recipients for liver transplantation include compatible blood type and liver size. There is a crucial lack of suitable donor organs for transplantation, and a number of clients will die awaiting the operation.
- The major postoperative complications specific to liver transplantation include infection, occlusion of vessels, and rejection. Symptoms of acute rejection include: fever, tachycardia, right upper quadrant pain or flank pain, and increasing jaundice. Rejection most commonly occurs between the fourth and tenth postoperative days.

ACUTE AND SUBACUTE CARE

Nursing Management

Postoperative Care

In addition to routine postoperative care:

- Observe for signs/symptoms of respiratory compromise.
- Monitor for signs/symptoms of infection.
- Monitor fluid and electrolyte status.
- Monitor lab tests—liver function tests, coagulation studies, WBC, etc.

- Monitor for signs/symptoms of bleeding.
- Monitor blood pressure, pulse, central venous pressure, and pulmonary artery pressures.
- Follow immunosuppressive protocols.
- Monitor wound drains and bile drains for patency.
- Administer immunosuppressive drugs as ordered.
- Monitor for signs of rejection: fever, tachycardia, right upper quadrant pain, increasing jaundice.

COMMUNITY AND SELF-CARE

- Instruct client/significant other regarding:
  — signs/symptoms of rejection
  — prevention of and signs/symptoms of infection
  — immunosuppressive therapy and possible side effects
  — avoidance of over-the-counter medications unless physician approves
  — diet, exercise, and activity
  — care of lines, wound or T-tube
  — follow-up laboratory studies
  — when to call the local physician and/or the transplant team
  — need for Medic-Alert bracelet
  — importance of follow-up visits (liver biopsies are usually performed at months 3 and 6, and then yearly)
- Refer to home health care agency/support groups as needed.

(For more information, see pp. 1898–1901 of Black and Matassarin-Jacobs: *Medical-Surgical Nursing: Clinical Management for Continuity of Care,* 5th ed.)

Liver Tumors (Metastatic)

OVERVIEW

- Metastatic tumors of the liver are tumors that began elsewhere in the body and have spread to the liver.
- The liver is one of the most common sites of metastasis due to the liver's high rate of blood

flow, size, and portal drainage from the major abdominal organs.
- Metastatic liver tumors arise from melanomas and tumors of the gastrointestinal tract, lung, and breast.
- Metastatic tumors spread to the liver by:
  — direct extension from adjacent organs
  — the hepatic arterial system
  — the portal venous system
- Unfortunately, these tumors may be far advanced before clinical manifestations are present, and this condition usually carries a poor prognosis.

CLINICAL MANIFESTATIONS

Manifestations may be vague until the tumor is advanced.

- minor temperature elevation
- gastrointestinal symptoms
- back pain
- right upper quadrant distress
- tenderness
- abdominal distention
- weight loss
- anorexia
- diarrhea or constipation
- nausea
- ascites
- hepatomegaly
- jaundice

Some clients also may develop polycythemia, blood sugar disorders, and hypercalcemia.

ACUTE AND SUBACUTE CARE

Medical Management

- irradiation
- percutaneous biliary drainage or internal placement of a biliary drain to help pass bile into the duodenum and decrease jaundice and discomfort
- regional chemotherapy perfusion of the liver via the hepatic artery to relieve pain and slow tumor growth
- chemotherapy—systemic

Surgical Management

- resection may be an option if the tumor is small and confined to one segment or lobe and if the client can withstand the surgery

Nursing Management

Varies according to the procedures performed and the amount of liver dysfunction.

- Assess for metabolic dysfunctions, bleeding problems, ascites, edema, inability to metabolize drugs, hypoproteinemia, jaundice, and endocrine complications.
- Prepare the client for all procedures and assess for post procedure complications.
- Provide emotional support to the family and client.
- See also "Chemotherapy," p. 149.
- See also "Radiation Therapy," p. 605.

COMMUNITY AND SELF-CARE

- Instruct client/significant other regarding:
  — side effects of chemotherapy
  — skin care of irradiated areas
  — pain management
  — signs/symptoms to report to physician
  — importance of follow-up care
- Refer to home health care agency, hospice, and cancer support groups as needed.

(For more information, see pp. 1896–1898 of Black and Matassarin-Jacobs: *Medical-Surgical Nursing: Clinical Management for Continuity of Care,* 5th ed.)

Lung Abscess

OVERVIEW

- Lung abscess is a collection of pus within the lung tissue that if untreated can cause tissue necrosis.

- Risk factors include: aspirated foreign material; tumors; thick mucous due to accumulation, oversedation, alcohol, and seizure; pneumonia; immunosuppression.

CLINICAL MANIFESTATIONS

- chills, fever, cough
- pleuritic pain, purulent, foul-smelling sputum, hemoptysis
- decreased breath sounds and dullness to percussion, crackles

ACUTE AND SUBACUTE CARE

Medical Management

- antibiotics
- bronchoscopy

Surgical Management

- wedge resection—removal of a portion of the lung
- lobectomy—removal of a lobe of the lung
- pneumonectomy—removal of one lung

Nursing Management

- Maintain hydration.
- Provide postural drainage to facilitate expectoration.
- Note color, quantity, quality, and smell of sputum
- Provide frequent oral cares.
- Observe oral mucosa for overgrowth with Candida Albicans due to long term antibiotic use.

COMMUNITY AND SELF-CARE

Instruct client regarding:

- the length of the antibiotic therapy may last 6 weeks
- the importance of following the medical regime
- the side effects of the antibiotics
- follow-up care

(For more information, see pp. 1138–1139 of Black and Matassarin-Jacobs: *Medical-Surgical Nursing: Clinical Management for Continuity of Care,* 5th ed.)

Lung Cancer

OVERVIEW

- Lung cancer is malignancy in the epithelium of the respiratory tract. There are four major types of lung cancer:
  (1) small cell carcinoma (oat cell)—usually presents as a hilar or central mass; rapid growth with early metastasis to mediastinum, thoracic and extrathoracic structures
  (2) squamous cell cancer—arises from bronchial epithelium; slow growth, metastasis not common. If metastasis occurs, it is usually to the lymphatic system, adrenals, and liver.
  (3) adenocarcinoma—arises from the bronchial mucus gland; grows slowly; metastasizes to lung or other organs
  (4) large cell carcinoma—arises peripherally in the lung as single or multiple masses; grows slowly with metastasis to the kidney, liver, and adrenals
- Survival from lung cancer remains low, especially for clients with small cell carcinomas.
- Lung cancer is the leading cause of death from cancer in the United States.
- Risk factors include: genetic predisposition; cigarette smoking; passive smoke (inhaling smoke from the environment surrounding an active smoker); exposure to radioactive isotopes, polycyclic hydrocarbons, vinyl chloride, mustard gas, metallurgical ores, asbestos fibers, and air pollution.

CLINICAL MANIFESTATIONS

Symptoms vary according to tumor type, location and extent, and previous pulmonary health.

- Centrally located pulmonary tumors
  — coughing, wheezing, stridor, dyspnea
  — chest, shoulder, back pain
  — hemoptysis
  — pericardial effusion, cardiac tamponade, and rhythm disturbances, if extends to pericardium
- Peripheral pulmonary tumors

— sharp, severe pleural pain that worsens on inspiration
— signs/symptoms of pleural effusion

- Apical pulmonary tumors (Pancoast's tumors)
  — no symptoms until tumor extends into surrounding structures
  — arm and shoulder pain from tumor involvement of the first thoracic and eighth cervical nerves of the brachial plexus
  — rib pain
  — Horner's syndrome (due to sympathetic nerve ganglia involvement)
    - pupil contraction on affected side of face
    - partial eyelid ptosis on affected side of face
    - absence of sweating on affected side of the face
- Pleural tumors (malignant mesotheliomas)
  — chest pain
  — dyspnea, cough
  — weight loss, fever
- warning signs of lung cancer:
  — any change in respiratory pattern
  — persistent cough
  — sputum streaked with blood
  — hemoptysis
  — rust-colored or purulent sputum
  — chest, shoulder, or arm pain
  — dyspnea
  — recurrent episodes of pleural effusion, pneumonia, or bronchitis

ACUTE AND SUBACUTE CARE

Medical Management

Treatment depends upon tumor type, stage, and underlying health status.

- radiation therapy—used alone or in combination with chemotherapy or surgery; may also be used for palliation of symptoms
- chemotherapy—small cell lung cancer responds well; use of chemotherapy for non-small cell lung cancer is controversial

Surgical Management

- pulmonary resection is the treatment of choice for early stage non-small cell lung cancer:
  - — wedge resection—removal of a small, localized area of diseased tissue. Pulmonary structure and function are relatively unchanged.
  - — segmental resection—removal of one or more lung segments (a bronchiole and its alveoli)
  - — lobectomy—removal of an entire lobe of the lung. The remaining lung overexpands to fill in the thoracic space previously occupied by the resected tissue.
  - — pneumonectomy—removal of an entire lung. Once the lung is removed, the involved side is an empty space. The phrenic nerve is severed on the affected side to paralyze the diaphragm in an elevated position to reduce the size of this cavity.
- laser therapy—palliative for the relief of endobronchial obstructions caused by nonresectable lung tumors

Nursing Management

Medical

- See "Chemotherapy," p. 149, and "Radiation Therapy," p. 605.

Surgical

Preoperative Care

In addition to routine preoperative care:

- Provide emotional support and facilitate discussion of fears and concerns of client and significant other.
- Instruct client and significant other regarding:
  - — anticipated surgical procedure
  - — early postoperative period and presence of chest tubes (except with pneumonectomy), drainage tubes, intubation, mechanical ventilation, and oxygen therapy
  - — postoperative exercises
    - respiratory exercises and splinting
    - leg exercises
    - arm/shoulder exercises

Postoperative Care

In addition to routine postoperative care:

- Monitor for potential postoperative complications and report to physician immediately.
  - — respiratory failure
  - — tension pneumothorax
  - — pulmonary embolus
  - — pulmonary edema
  - — cardiac dysrhythmias
  - — hemorrhage, hemothorax, hypovolemic shock
  - — thrombophlebitis
  - — subcutaneous emphysema around incision and in the chest and neck
- Monitor breath sounds.
- Monitor dressing and incisional area for bleeding.
- Position client in side-lying position on nonoperative side in immediate postoperative period, until consciousness regained.
- Place client in semi-Fowler's position once vital signs are stable and turn every 1–2 hours as appropriate (head of bed up 30 to 45 degrees).
- Avoid positioning on operative side if wedge resection or segmentectomy performed (hinders expansion of remaining lung tissue).
- Avoid complete lateral positioning after pneumonectomy (may cause mediastinal shift and compression of remaining lung).
- Assist with coughing and deep breathing every 1–2 hours during the first 24–48 hours.
- Evaluate need for suctioning.
- Administer analgesics, assess effectiveness, and schedule pulmonary and leg exercises when medication is at maximal effectiveness.
- Maintain closed chest tube drainage (usually not used after pneumonectomy).
- Monitor amount and type of chest tube drainage.
- Begin passive range of motion exercises of arm and affected shoulder on affected side 4 hours after recovery following anesthesia. Perform twice every 4–6 hours for the first 24 hours. Progress to 10–20 times every 2 hours, eventually progress to active range of motion.
- Encourage ambulation when condition permits.
- Assess client's tolerance of activity.

- Provide emotional support and facilitate discussion of fears and concerns.
- Encourage use of previously successful coping strategies.

COMMUNITY AND SELF-CARE

- Instruct client regarding:
  — wound care
  — continuation of exercise program
  — avoidance of environmental irritants
  — activity limitations and avoidance of heavy lifting
  — signs/symptoms to report to physician (e.g., infection, deteriorating respiratory status)
  — importance of follow-up to detect complications, recurrence of malignancy or metastasis
- Refer to cancer support groups as appropriate.
- Refer to home health care agency as appropriate.

(For more information, see pp. 1151–1166 of Black and Matassarin-Jacobs: *Medical-Surgical Nursing: Clinical Management for Continuity of Care,* 5th ed.)

Lymphadenitis

- Lymph nodes act as defense barriers and are secondarily involved in virtually all systemic infections and in many neoplastic disorders.
- Generalized lymphadenopathy (enlargement of two or three regionally separated lymph node groups) is usually due to inflammation, neoplasm, or immunologic reaction.
- The specific nodes affected in an infectious disease depend upon the location of the infection, the nature of the organism and the severity of the disease.
- In acute lymphadenitis, the inflamed nodes are most commonly located in the cervical region in association with infections of the teeth or tonsils or in the axillary or inguinal regions secondary to infections in the extremities. Generalized lymphadenopathy is characteristic of the secondary stage

of syphilis, viral infection, and bacteremia. The lymph nodes are enlarged, tender, warm, and reddened.

- Chronic lymphadenitis occurs in the course of a longstanding infection. The lymph nodes become scarred with fibrous tissue. Clinically, the nodes are enlarged, firm to palpation, and not tender or warm.
- The management of lymphadenitis is treatment of the underlying cause.

(For more information, see p. 1441 of Black and Matassarin-Jacobs: *Medical-Surgical Nursing: Clinical Management for Continuity of Care,* 5th ed.)

Lymphedema

OVERVIEW

- Lymphedema is swelling due to impaired transcapillary fluid transport and transportation of lymph.
- Failure of lymph transport allows plasma proteins in the interstitial fluid to accumulate, increasing osmotic pressure. The osmotic pressure is reduced by drawing water into interstitial areas. The fluid seeks pathways through the tissues, which causes inflammation, lymphatic thrombosis, and eventually fibrosis.
- Primary lymphedema is an inherited trait that results in abnormal development of lymph vessels.
- Secondary lymphedema occurs because of damage or obstruction of the lymph system by another disease process or procedure. Examples include:
  - neoplasms
  - trauma
  - surgical excision of axillary, inguinal, or iliac nodes
  - irradiation

CLINICAL MANIFESTATIONS

Primary Lymphedema

- bilateral mild edema of ankles and legs in women at puberty
- unilateral edema of the entire leg (men and women)
- bilateral edema present at birth or an early age
- skin vesicles filled with lymph

Secondary Lymphedema

- dull, heavy sensation in affected limb(s)
- nonpitting edema
- reduction but not disappearance of swelling when legs are elevated
- rough skin
- enlargement of affected limb(s)

ACUTE AND SUBACUTE CARE

Medical Management

There is no cure once swelling occurs.

- physical therapy—manual squeezing of the tissue to press stagnant lymphatic fluid to the proximal part of the limb, followed by active and passive exercises to transport the lymph further into the lymphatic system and bloodstream
- pneumatic pumping device
- diuretics
- elastic stockings or arm sleeves

Surgical Management

Surgery is used only if medical management is not beneficial. Though not curable, the final appearance may be more acceptable.

- all skin, subcutaneous tissue, and deep fascia are removed and the extremity is covered with a skin graft
- removal of the bulk of edematous tissue

Nursing Management

- Monitor extremity for signs of infection.
- Provide meticulous skin care.
- Keep extremity elevated above right atrium.

- Apply elastic stockings or sleeves as prescribed.
- Apply and monitor pneumatic compression device.
- Encourage activity and exercises.

COMMUNITY AND SELF-CARE

Instruct client regarding:

- operation of pneumatic compression device
- application of elastic stocking or arm sleeve
- measures to prevent infection
- signs/symptoms of infection to report
- prescribed exercises
- importance of elevating limb above the heart whenever possible

(For more information, see pp. 1439–1441 of Black and Matassarin-Jacobs: *Medical-Surgical Nursing: Clinical Management for Continuity of Care*, 5th ed.)

M

Mechanical Ventilation

OVERVIEW

- Mechanical ventilation is the use of a positive-pressure ventilator with an artificial airway (either tracheostomy or endotracheal tube).
- Indications for mechanical ventilation include inadequate ventilation and hypoxemia.
- Common disorders that may require mechanical ventilation include: pneumonia, adult respiratory distress syndrome (ARDS), rib fractures, cardiogenic shock, Guillain-Barré syndrome, myasthenia gravis, head injury, and airway obstruction.
- Positive-pressure ventilators may be categorized as: (1) those for short-term use (intermittent positive-pressure breathing [IPPB]) and (2) those for continuous use (continuous mechanical ventilation).
  (1) IPPB is use of a pressure-cycled ventilator to deliver pressurized breaths to a spontaneously breathing client in 10–20 minute treatments. It is infrequently prescribed.
  (2) Continuous mechanical ventilation (CMV) is used to: maintain adequate ventilation; deliver precise concentrations of FIO_2; deliver adequate tidal volumes; and to decrease the work of breathing in clients who cannot sustain adequate ventilation on their own.
- Continuous mechanical ventilators may be pressure-cycled (delivers a volume of gas using positive pressure during inspiration until a preselected pressure has been reached) or volume-cycled (delivers a pre-set tidal volume of inspired gas regardless of the pressure required to deliver this volume). A pressure limit can be set to prevent dangerously high pressures from occurring.
- Adverse physiologic effects of positive pressure delivered via a mechanical ventilator include:

— decreased cardiac output
— possible ischemia of the gastric mucosa, leading to bleeding and stress ulceration (due to decreased blood flow to the splanchic area resulting from descent of the diaphragm into the abdomen during the inspiratory phase)
— water retention (due to an increase in antidiuretic hormone)
— possible cerebral edema if severe alkalosis occurs.

- Ventilation may be assisted or controlled.
  — Assisted ventilation is person-cycled. The client's own inspiratory effort turns on ("trips") the ventilator, initiating the mechanical inspiratory phase.
  — Controlled ventilation governs a client's rate of ventilation by automatically cycling the ventilator at a predetermined number of cycles per minute; the ventilator does all of the work of breathing, the client does none.
- Clients who are on controlled ventilation and have spontaneous respirations may "fight" or "buck" the ventilator because they cannot synchronize their own respirations with the machine's cycle. If the nurse is unable to help them relax and breathe with the ventilator, sedatives, and possibly neuromuscular blocking agents may be indicated, such as pancuronium bromide (Pavulon), curare, or verçuronium bromide (Norcuron). Neuromuscular blocking agents block the transmission of nerve impulses and result in muscle paralysis. They do not affect sensorium or perception of pain and always should be used in conjunction with sedation or analgesics.
- Positive end-expiratory pressure (PEEP) and continuous positive airway pressure (CPAP) are ventilator techniques applied during expiration, whereby intrathoracic pressures are not allowed to return to ambient pressure. This helps keep the alveoli open, increases functional residual capacity (FRC), and enhances oxygenation as a result of the enlarged surface area that is available for diffusion.
- CPAP usually is applied to a client with spontaneous respirations.

- PEEP usually is applied during mechanical ventilation with controlled, assist/controlled, or intermittent mandatory ventilation.
- The adverse physiologic effects of positive airway pressure (i.e., CPAP and PEEP) are basically the same as those discussed for mechanical ventilation. There are also the following risks:
  — rupture of the lungs (barotrauma)
  — pneumothorax
  — subcutaneous emphysema
  — pneumomediastinum
  — cardiovascular embarrassment (decreased cardiac output)
  — increased intracranial pressure
- Intermittent mandatory ventilation (IMV) is the setting of a ventilator to deliver a specific respiratory rate. If the client breathes at a rate higher than the machine rate, these breaths will not be positive-pressure ventilations.
- Synchronized intermittent mandatory ventilation (SIMV) is the same as IMV but the preset breaths are activated by the client's inspiratory efforts and are sychronized with the client's breathing.
- Pressure support ventilation (PSV) is a recent ventilation method that augments spontaneous inspiratory effort with a preset level of positive airway pressure. When the client on PSV initiates a breath, the machine is triggered and delivers a flow of gas at the preset pressure. This may be used as a "stand alone" or "mixed" method. Usually IMV and PSV are used together.

ACUTE AND SUBACUTE CARE

Nursing Management

Promote respiratory function.

- Auscultate lungs frequently to assess for adventitious sounds, to validate endotracheal tube placement, and to ensure bilateral ventilation of the lungs.
- Suction as needed, providing pre- and post-hyperinflation and hyperoxygenation.
- Instill normal saline into airway PRN prior to suctioning to loosen secretions and promote coughing.

- Turn and reposition every 2 hours.
- Position on unaffected side.
- Secure endotracheal tube (ETT) properly.
- Use a bite block or oral airway, if needed.
- Monitor arterial blood gas values and pulse oximetry.
- Check the machine and alarms frequently to ensure proper functioning.
- Always have a self-inflating resuscitation bag readily available.
- Use a manual resuscitation bag if the alarm sounds and you cannot quickly correct the problem.
- Monitor peak inspiratory pressures and ventilatory parameters hourly.
- Assess if the client's breathing rate is greater than the mechanical ventilatory rate.
- Maintain patency of endotracheal tube or tracheostomy.
- Prevent loose connections or kinks in the tubing.

Provide a communication method and assist to decrease anxiety.

- Explain all procedures.
- Explain purpose of ventilator to client and family; discuss how it helps breathing, how it feels, how to cooperate with the machine and different types of alarms.
- Develop a means of communication, via writing or picture board.
- Place call light within reach and be sure all staff know that client cannot speak.
- Encourage significant others to talk to client.
- Provide distractions (e.g., TV and radio).
- Medicate with antianxiety medication and sedatives as ordered.
- If client is on neuromuscular blocking agents:
  - — Be sure other staff know the client is on a neuromuscular blocking agent and can still feel pain and hear.
  - — Be sure that client receives sedation in conjunction with neuromuscular blocking agents.
  - — Explain to the client the cause of paralysis and provide reassurance.

Monitor for complications.

- Assess for possible early complications due to mechanical ventilation:

— rapid electrolyte changes
— severe alkalosis
— hypotension secondary to changes in cardiac output.

- Monitor for signs of respiratory distress: restlessness, apprehension, irritability, use of accessory muscles, and increased heart rate.
- Assess for signs/symptoms of barotrauma: increasing dyspnea; agitation; decreased or absent breath sounds; tracheal deviation away from the affected side; subcutaneous emphysema; and decreasing PaO_2 levels.
- Assess for cardiovascular depression: hypotension, tachycardia, bradycardia, dysrhythmias, weak peripheral pulses, increases in pulmonary wedge pressure, or signs of increased heart failure.
- Monitor for signs of inadvertent extubation: vocalization, low-pressure alarm, bilateral decrease in upper lobe airway sounds, gastric distention, and clinical manifestations of inadequate ventilation.
- If inadvertent extubation occurs, manually ventilate with a self-inflating resuscitation bag and notify physician for reintubation.
- Prevent endotracheal tube pressure on nares or oral mucosa.
- Provide good oral care.
- If client is on PEEP or CPAP, assess:
  — blood pressure and heart rate
  — breath sounds
  — signs of increased heart failure
  — subcutaneous emphysema.

Prevent infection.

- Maintain sterile technique when suctioning.
- Monitor color, amount, and consistency of sputum.
- Drain water from tubing; do not drain it back into the humidifier.

Provide adequate nutrition.

- Begin tube feeding as ordered when it is evident the client will remain on the ventilator for a long time.
- Weigh daily.
- Monitor intake and output.

Monitor for gastrointestinal bleeding.

- Monitor bowel sounds.

- Monitor gastric pH and hematest gastric secretions every shift.

Maintain muscle strength.

- Perform range of motion exercises and ambulate to chair when able.
- Encourage client to perform exercises in bed, if able.

(For more information, see pp. 1173–1184 of Black and Matassarin-Jacobs: *Medical-Surgical Nursing: Clinical Management for Continuity of Care,* 5th ed.)

Meningitis (Bacterial)

OVERVIEW

- Bacterial meningitis is an inflammation of the arachnoid or pia mater membranes. The infection spreads throughout the subarachnoid space around the brain and spinal cord and usually involves the ventricles.
- The most common bacteria causing meningitis are *Neisseria meningitidis*, *Streptococcus pneumoniae*, and *Haemophilus influenzae*. These organisms are often present in the nasopharynx. It is not known how they enter the bloodstream and the subarachnoid space.
- Twenty to twenty-five thousand cases occur yearly in the United States.
- The mortality rate is less than 5 per cent, if treated. Residual neurologic deficits are rare.
- Factors predisposing to meningitis include:
  - — head trauma
  - — systemic infection
  - — postsurgical infection
  - — meningeal infection
  - — anatomic defects

CLINICAL MANIFESTATIONS

- headache
- prostration
- chills

- fever
- nausea
- vomiting
- back pain
- stiff neck
- generalized seizures
- irritability
- coma
- signs of meningeal irritation also occur:
  — nuchal (neck) rigidity
  — positive Brudzinski's sign (forward neck flexion with the client supine, produces flexion of both thighs at the hips and flexion movements of the ankles and knees)
  — positive Kernig's sign (pain, hamstring muscle spasm, and resistance to further leg extension at the knee occurs when the thigh is flexed at a right angle to the abdomen, the knee is flexed 90 degrees to the thigh and then the lower leg is extended)

ACUTE AND SUBACUTE CARE

MEDICAL MANAGEMENT

Bacterial meningitis is a medical emergency. Treatment must be instituted immediately, or death can result in hours or days.

- large doses of the appropriate antibiotic intravenously four to six times daily for 10 days (high doses are required to reach the cerebrospinal fluid)
- analgesics for pain (used with caution so as not to mask signs of neurologic deterioration)

NURSING MANAGEMENT

- Monitor fluid and electrolyte imbalance.
- Perform hourly neurologic checks to detect early signs of increasing intracranial pressure or seizures.
- Administer antibiotic therapy as ordered.
- Maintain isolation precautions as ordered.
- Maintain safety precautions.

COMMUNITY AND SELF-CARE

Instruct client/significant other regarding:

- antibiotic therapy
- use of analgesics
- follow-up care

(For more information, see pp. 856–857 of Black and Matassarin-Jacobs: *Medical-Surgical Nursing: Clinical Management for Continuity of Care,* 5th ed.)

Meningitis (Viral)

- Acute viral meningitis (aseptic meningitis) is usually due to mumps virus or one of the picornaviruses.
- Aseptic meningitis involving the subarachnoid space usually resolves within 2 weeks.
- Clinical manifestations include: drowsiness; photophobia; headache; pain when moving the eyes; neck and spine stiffness with flexion; weakness; rash; fever; and positive Brudzinski's and Kernig's signs (for definitions, see "Meningitis (Bacterial)," p. 472).
- Treatment is symptomatic and involves bedrest and control of fever, headache, pain, and seizures.

(For more information, see p. 859 of Black and Matassarin-Jacobs: *Medical-Surgical Nursing: Clinical Management for Continuity of Care,* 5th ed.)

Menorrhagia

OVERVIEW

- Menorrhagia is characterized by excessive vaginal bleeding at normal intervals.
- The risk factors include: uterine fibroids, adenomyosis, anatomic lesions, spontaneous abortion, inflammatory processes (endometriosis, salpingitis), blood dyscrasias, hypothyroidism,

intrauterine device (IUD), endometrial carcinoma, and medications (anticoagulants).

CLINICAL MANIFESTATIONS

- blood loss is variable
- anemia

ACUTE AND SUBACUTE CARE

Medical Management

- estrogens, progestins, and oral contraceptives
- antifibrinolytic agents

Surgical Management

- Dilatation and curettage (D&C)—unnecessary in most cases.
- Endometrial ablation—laser fiber used to destroy the endometrium.

Nursing Management

In addition to routine preoperative and postoperative care:

- Use sterile perineal pads.
- Check and change pad. May have vaginal packing, which is removed in 24 hours
- Monitor closely for excessive bleeding during the first few hours.
- Make sure the client can urinate before going home.
- Report excess bleeding, inability to urinate, and excessive pain to the physician. Minimal uterine cramping may occur.
- Administer mild analgesics for pain.
- Avoid aspirin for the first 24-48 hours.
- Provide reassurance and support.

COMMUNITY AND SELF-CARE

Instruct client/significant other regarding:

- avoidance of strenuous activity for 1 week
- avoidance of douching, vaginal or rectal intercourse for about 1 week

- that vaginal discharge may be pink followed by dark-red or dark-brown
- report any complications of excessive bleeding, pain, or fever to the physician
- follow-up care

(For more information, see p. 2391 of Black and Matassarin-Jacobs: *Medical-Surgical Nursing: Clinical Management for Continuity of Care,* 5th ed.)

Multiple Myeloma

OVERVIEW

- Multiple myeloma is an abnormal proliferation of plasma cells.
- With this overproduction, bone destruction also occurs. In addition, multiple myeloma is characterized by disruption of red blood cell, leukocyte, and platelet production, secondary to crowding of the bone marrow by plasma cells.
- Complications of multiple myeloma include hypercalcemia (from release of calcium with bone destruction), renal failure (from particles of coagulated protein that block the tubules) and neurologic disorders (secondary to spinal cord compression).
- This condition commonly occurs in clients over 40 years of age. It is more common in males and blacks.

CLINICAL MANIFESTATIONS

Onset is insidious and gradual. Most clients pass through a long presymptomatic period that lasts from 5–20 years. Diagnosis at this stage is usually made by chance as a result of an elevated serum protein during a screening examination.

- backache or bone pain that worsens with movement
- presence of pathologic fractures
- hypercalcemia—anorexia, nausea, vomiting, constipation, confusion, abdominal pain

- renal failure
- paresthesia, paralysis

ACUTE AND SUBACUTE CARE

Medical Management

- chemotherapy—melphalan and prednisone or a combination of alkylating agents—cyclophosphamide, carmustine, vincristine
- radiation therapy
- hypercalcemia management—mithramycin C, furosemide, corticosteroids, IV hydration or etidronate disodium or gallium nitrate with IV hydration
- bone marrow transplantation

Surgical Management

- laminectomy (the excision of a vertebral posterior arch to relieve spinal cord compression)

Nursing Management

Medical

- Administer ordered chemotherapy. See "Chemotherapy," p. 149.
- Assess for signs of hypercalcemia and administer ordered therapy.
- Encourage fluids to maintain an output of 1.5–2.0 liters/day.
- Monitor intake and output.
- Daily weights.
- Monitor laboratory findings—CBC, BUN, creatinine, serum calcium.
- Administer antiemetics.
- Administer analgesics.
- Institute appropriate safety measures.
- See "Bone Marrow Transplantation," p. 92.

Surgical

- See "Herniated Intervertebral Disc," p. 346, for care of the laminectomy client.

COMMUNITY AND SELF-CARE

- Instruct client regarding:

— disease process and treatment regime
— potential chemotherapy side effects and interventions—see "Chemotherapy," p. 149.
— see "Bone Marrow Transplantation," p. 92.
— signs/symptoms of hypercalcemia
— importance of adequate fluids, low-calcium diet
— household safety measures
— importance of follow-up visits
- Refer to available community resources.

(For more information, see pp. 1498–1500 of Black and Matassarin-Jacobs: *Medical-Surgical Nursing: Clinical Management for Continuity of Care,* 5th ed.)

Multiple Sclerosis

OVERVIEW

- Multiple sclerosis (MS) is a progressive degenerative disease that affects the myelin sheath of neurons in the central nervous system (CNS).
- The myelin sheath is essential for normal conduction of nerve impulses to and from the brain and spinal cord. In MS, patches of myelin deteriorate at irregular intervals along the nerve axon, causing slowing of nerve conduction. Although this may occur anywhere in the CNS, the areas most commonly involved are the optic nerves, cerebrum, and cervical spinal cord. The exact cause of MS is unknown.
- Precipitating factors that can precede the onset or an exacerbation of MS include: infection, physical injury, emotional stress, pregnancy, and fatigue.
- MS has two major courses: (1) exacerbating remitting—client has episodes of neurologic dysfunction (exacerbations) from which he or she recovers and is able to function normally (remission), and (2) chronic progressive—client experiences a steady decline in neurologic function that can occur over several years.
- The onset of MS usually occurs between the ages of 20 and 40 years old, and it affects women twice as often as men.

- Life expectancy is about 85 per cent of the general population. The usual cause of death is bacterial infection of the lungs, bladder, or pressure ulcers.

CLINICAL MANIFESTATIONS

- weakness or tingling sensations (paresthesias) of one or more extremities
- vision loss
- loss of coordination
- bowel and bladder dysfunction
- seizures
- fatigue that worsens as the day progresses
- muscle spasticity
- depression

ACUTE AND SUBACUTE CARE

Medical Management

- corticosteroid therapy—adrenocorticotropic hormone, prednisone, azathioprine (Imuran)
- interferon beta 1b (Betaseron)—genetically engineered complex protein with antiviral and immunoregulatory properties has recently been approved and has shown to reduce the number of MS exacerbations
- seizure control—Dilantin
- antidepressant therapy—Elavil
- antispasmodic therapy—Lioresal, Valium, Dantrium

Nursing Management

- Institute measures for neurogenic bladder:
  - — maintain fluid intake at 2000 ml/24 hours
  - — avoid fluid intake after the evening meal
  - — encourage to attempt voiding every 3 hours
  - — intermittent catheterization if indicated.
- Encourage high-fiber diet.
- Administer stool softeners as ordered.
- Institute a bowel training program.
- Assess ability to perform activities of daily living.
- Provide adequate rest periods.
- Plan activities at client's peak energy level (usually in morning).

- Collaborate with Physical and Occupational Therapy for methods to reduce energy consumption and adaptive devices for ambulation and self-care.
- Encourage and promote range of motion and muscle strengthening exercises.
- Determine areas of numbness and intervene to prevent injury and development of pressure ulcers.
- Provide emotional support to client and family.

COMMUNITY AND SELF-CARE

- Instruct client/family regarding:
  - — disease process and prognosis
  - — avoidance of physical and emotional stressors that may precipitate an exacerbation
  - — skin care measures
  - — bowel/bladder training regime
  - — intermittent catheterization technique
  - — importance of adequate rest
  - — exercise regime
  - — use of adaptive devices
  - — importance of follow-up appointments
- Refer to community resources—support groups, respite care, Visiting Nurse Association.

(For more information, see pp. 873–877 of Black and Matassarin-Jacobs: *Medical-Surgical Nursing: Clinical Management for Continuity of Care,* 5th ed.)

Muscular Dystrophy

OVERVIEW

- Muscular dystrophy (MD) is a hereditary, progressive, degenerative disease of skeletal muscle.
- Types of MD include:

Duchenne MD

- — most common
- — onset before age 3
- — symmetric weakness of pelvis and shoulder girdle muscles (early involvement), becomes generalized in later stages

- — heart involvement
- — contractural deformities—common
- — scoliosis—common
- — IQ—decreased
- — course—steadily progressive

Becker MD

- — onset between ages of 5 and 15 years
- — weakness of pelvis and shoulder muscles and in later stage becomes generalized (facial muscles are spared)
- — contractural deformities—less common
- — scoliosis—not severe
- — heart involvement—late, uncommon
- — IQ—normal
- — course—slowly progressive

Limb Girdle MD

- — not common
- — onset —by second decade
- — muscle involvement—shoulders and pelvic girdle, (early)—periphery (late)
- — contractural deformities—late, mild
- — scoliosis—mild, late
- — heart involvement—rare
- — IQ—normal
- — course—slowly progressive

CLINICAL MANIFESTATIONS

- see above
- elevated CPK, abnormal muscle biopsy results, and abnormal electromyogram (EMG)

ACUTE AND SUBACUTE CARE

Medical Management

- supportive, depends on the type and severity of the disease
- long-leg braces
- spinal braces
- exercise programs

Nursing Management

- supportive, based on the type and severity of the disease

COMMUNITY AND SELF-CARE

- based on the type and severity of the disease

(For more information, see pp. 2125–2126 of Black and Matassarin-Jacobs: *Medical-Surgical Nursing: Clinical Management for Continuity of Care,* 5th ed.)

Myasthenia Gravis

OVERVIEW

- Myasthenia gravis (MG) is an autoimmune disease that presents as muscular weakness and fatigue that worsens with exercise and improves with rest.
- Myasthenia gravis is caused by loss of acetylcholine receptors in the postsynaptic neurons of the neuromuscular junction. The cause of myasthenia gravis is unknown.
- Myasthenia gravis may occur at any age, although there are two peaks of onset. In early-onset myasthenia gravis, at age 20–30 years, women are more often affected than men. In late-onset, after age 50, men are more often affected.
- The course of MG varies, with remissions and exacerbations. Signs and symptoms may progress quickly or slowly and fluctuate from day to day. The severity of the disease varies greatly from person to person.

CLINICAL MANIFESTATIONS

- increasing weakness with sustained muscle contraction. (If client is asked to hold arms up, the power of muscle contraction diminishes, and arms drift downward. After a period of rest, the muscles regain their strength.)
- muscle weakness increased at end of day
- ptosis (drooping of upper eyelid)
- diplopia (double vision)
- expressionless face and tendency for mouth to hang open due to weakness of the facial muscles
- dysphagia (muscles of chewing and swallowing involved)

- nasal quality to speech
- respiratory distress (respiratory muscle involvement)

ACUTE AND SUBACUTE CARE

MEDICAL MANAGEMENT

- short-acting anticholinesterase compounds—pyridostigmine (Mestinon), neostigmine (Prostigmin)
- corticosteroids—prednisone (reduces level of serum acetylcholine receptor antibodies)
- plasmapheresis—to remove plasma proteins containing antibodies believed to cause MG

SURGICAL MANAGEMENT

- thymectomy—removal of thymus gland that may alter some immunologic control mechanism that affects the production of antibodies to the anticholinesterase receptor

NURSING MANAGEMENT

Medical

- Administer anticholinesterase drugs precisely on time to maintain blood levels.
- Ensure suctioning equipment is maintained at bedside and instruct client on self-suctioning.
- Initiate aspiration precautions.
- Plan activities at time of client's highest energy level and allow for rest periods.
- Assess muscle strength before and after activity.
- Observe for myasthenia crisis (an exacerbation of myasthenic symptoms caused by under-medication with anticholinesterase drugs):
  — increased pulse and respirations
  — increased blood pressure
  — severe respiratory distress, cyanosis
  — bowel and bladder incontinence
  — absence of cough and swallow reflex
  — increased secretions, increased lacrimation
  — restlessness.
- Intervene in myasthenia crisis:

- support respiratory function—suction excess secretions, administer supplemental oxygen and assisted ventilation
- administer additional anticholinesterase (cholinergic) medication.

- Observe for cholinergic crisis (an acute exacerbation of muscle weakness caused by over-medication with anticholinesterase [cholinergic] drugs):
  - nausea, vomiting, diarrhea
  - abdominal cramps
  - blurred vision
  - excessive pulmonary secretions
  - weakness with difficulty swallowing, chewing, speaking, and breathing
  - apprehension.
- Intervene in cholinergic crisis:
  - support respiratory function—suction, administer supplemental oxygen and assisted ventilation
  - hold cholinergic drugs until cholinergic effects decrease
- Collaborate with Physical and Occupational Therapy for exercises and adaptive devices.

Surgical

Nursing management is similar to care following thoracic surgery.

COMMUNITY AND SELF-CARE

- Instruct the client regarding:
  - disease process and prognosis
  - importance of medication regime
    - timing of doses
    - no omission of doses.
  - importance of available suctioning equipment in the home
  - self-suctioning technique or teaching household members suctioning technique
  - symptoms of myasthenia crisis and cholinergic crisis and crisis intervention
  - factors that may predispose client to an exacerbation—infection, emotional stress, surgery, physical stress
  - need for adequate rest periods

— use of adaptive devices and exercises
— importance of wearing medical alert identification
— importance of follow-up appointments

- Refer to available community resources.

(For more information, see pp. 883–886 of Black and Matassarin-Jacobs: *Medical-Surgical Nursing: Clinical Management for Continuity of Care,* 5th ed.)

Myocarditis

OVERVIEW

- Myocarditis is an inflammation of the myocardial wall.
- It can be caused by almost any bacterial, viral, or parasitic organism, as well as radiation, toxic agents such as lead, and drugs such as lithium and cocaine.
- Myocardial damage is usually the result of direct invasion or the toxic effects of the microorganism in cardiac myocytes. Usually myocarditis involves both ventricles. The disease process may cause impairment of contractility and dysrhythmias.
- Myocarditis affects clients of all ages and may be acute or chronic.
- In the United States, most cases of myocarditis are due to viral infections. The most common viruses are coxsackieviruses A and B, mumps, influenza virus A and B, rubella virus, measles virus, cytomegalovirus, and Epstein-Barr virus.

CLINICAL MANIFESTATIONS

- fatigue, dyspnea, palpitations
- chest pain experienced as a mild continuous pressure distinguishable from effort-induced angina
- fever
- tachycardia
- dysrhythmias

ACUTE AND SUBACUTE CARE

MEDICAL MANAGEMENT

In most cases, myocarditis is self-limiting and uncomplicated. If myocardial involvement becomes extensive, myofibril degeneration can lead to heart failure, cardiomegaly, and cardiomyopathy.

- specific therapy for underlying infection
- bedrest to decrease cardiac workload
- supplemental oxygen
- antipyretics

NURSING MANAGEMENT

- Assess for changes in cardiac or respiratory status.
- Treat fever with rest, cooling measures, forced fluids, and antipyretics.
- Administer antimicrobial therapy as ordered.
- Encourage fluids and a well-balanced diet.
- Administer PRN analgesics.
- Provide adequate rest periods.
- Implement progressive activity schedule.

COMMUNITY AND SELF-CARE

Instruct client regarding:

- disease process and treatment regime
- need to monitor pulse rate and rhythm and report any sudden changes
- importance of completing prescribed antibiotics
- need for follow-up visits

(For more information, see pp. 1334–1335 of Black and Matassarin-Jacobs: *Medical-Surgical Nursing: Clinical Management for Continuity of Care,* 5th ed.)

N

Narcolepsy

- Narcolepsy is a sleep disorder characterized by excessive daytime sleepiness. The client experiences repeated episodes of drowsiness followed by brief naps, especially when engaged in monotonous activities. Clients report having fallen asleep at work or while driving.
- Prevalence is one in 1,000 clients in the United States.
- Narcoleptic clients may experience other associated symptoms, which, when combined with excessive sleepiness, constitute a narcolepsy tetrad:
  (1) cataplexy—sudden loss of muscle tone at times of unexpected emotion (e.g., fright)
  (2) sleep paralysis—inability to move for one to several minutes after awakening
  (3) hypnagogic hallucinations—hallucinatory experiences that occur at sleep onset or awakening
- Impaired release of dopamine may be a factor in narcolepsy.
- Treatment consists of low doses of stimulants to improve alertness and tricyclic antidepressants to control cataplexy.

(For more information, see pp. 400–401 of Black and Matassarin-Jacobs: *Medical-Surgical Nursing: Clinical Management for Continuity of Care,* 5th ed.)

Nasal Fracture

OVERVIEW

- Simple nasal fractures may be reduced in an emergency facility. For more extensive fractures, surgery may be performed under local anesthesia with mild sedation.

- Intranasal packing, internal or external splints, and an external dressing may be applied.

ACUTE AND SUBACUTE CARE

Nursing Management

- See "Nasal Septoplasty," p. 489.

(For more information, see p. 1102 of Black and Matassarin-Jacobs: *Medical-Surgical Nursing: Clinical Management for Continuity of Care,* 5th ed.)

Nasal Polypectomy

OVERVIEW

- Nasal polypectomy is the removal of nasal polyps with a snarelike instrument. The bleeding sites are cauterized, and intranasal packing is inserted. Local anesthesia generally is used.

ACUTE AND SUBACUTE CARE

Nursing Management

Postoperative Care

In addition to routine postoperative care:

- Maintain nasal packing, ice packs, and a semi-to-high-Fowler's position to minimize bleeding and edema.
- Assess for changes in vital signs.
- Assess for signs of posterior nasal bleeding:
  - — frequent swallowing
  - — blood in the throat or oropharynx.

COMMUNITY AND SELF-CARE

Instruct client regarding:

- the use of humidification, frequent mouth care, and increasing oral fluids to minimize oropharyngeal discomfort and dryness from mouth breathing
- avoidance of cleaning the nose

- avoidance of aspirin or aspirin-containing products
- sneezing through an open mouth
- maintaining ice compresses for the first 48 hours

(For more information, see p. 1102 of Black and Matassarin-Jacobs: *Medical-Surgical Nursing: Clinical Management for Continuity of Care,* 5th ed.)

Nasal Septoplasty

OVERVIEW

- Nasal septoplasty is performed for a deviated nasal septum when the deviation is causing obstruction to nasal breathing, dryness of the nasal mucosa causing bleeding, or a cosmetic deformity. An incision is made on either side of the septum; the mucous membrane is elevated, and the offending portion of cartilage is straightened or removed. A local anesthetic with mild sedation commonly is used.
- Intranasal packing and internal splints may be used to control bleeding and prevent hematoma formation.

ACUTE AND SUBACUTE CARE

Nursing Management

In addition to routine postoperative care:

- Maintain patent airway.
- Assess for edema and hemorrhage.
- Provide analgesics as ordered and assess for adequate pain relief.
- See "Nasal Polypectomy," p. 488 for other nursing management.

(For more information, see p. 1102 of Black and Matassarin-Jacobs: *Medical-Surgical Nursing: Clinical Management for Continuity of Care,* 5th ed.)

Near Drowning Accidents

OVERVIEW

- Near-drowning is a diagnosis given to clients who initially survive suffocation after submersion in water or a fluid medium. "Immersion syndrome" is another term for this diagnosis.
- Fresh water drowning is more common than salt water drowning.
- Common risk factors for near drowning include alcohol or drug ingestion, overestimation of swimming skills, hypothermia, hyperventilation, and hypoglycemia.
- Fresh water and salt water wash out alveolar surfactant. Fresh water also changes the surface tension of surfactant. The loss of surfactant leads to alveolar collapse, intrapulmonary shunting, and hypoxemia. Poor perfusion and hypoxemia result in acidosis and eventual pulmonary edema. Alterations in fluid-electrolyte balance often are seen.

ACUTE AND SUBACUTE CARE

Nursing Management

- Obtain a history of the submersion. Include the length of submersion, temperature of the water, type of water, and any associated injuries (such as spinal cord injuries).
- Maintain airway, breathing, and circulation (ABCs).
- Assess for any signs of hypoxia (confusion, irritability, lethargy, or unconsciousness).
- Assist with intubation and ventilate with 100 per cent oxygen and 5–10 cm of positive end-expiratory pressure (PEEP) to prevent the alveoli from collapsing.
- Remove wet clothing and wrap in a warm blanket.
- Rewarm the client slowly.
- Correct acid-base or electrolyte abnormalities as ordered.
- Monitor diagnostic studies.
- Observe client for at least 24 hours for any complications, especially pulmonary edema.

(For more information, see p. 2522 of Black and Matassarin-Jacobs: *Medical-Surgical Nursing: Clinical Management for Continuity of Care,* 5th ed.)

Nephrotic Syndrome

OVERVIEW

- Nephrotic syndrome is a set of clinical symptoms arising from protein-wasting secondary to diffuse glomerular damage. The glomerular basement membrane becomes abnormally permeable to protein molecules, particularly albumin. Proteins are excessively filtered into the tubules and excreted into the urine.
- Common causes are glomerulonephritis or systemic disorders, such as diabetes mellitus, lupus erythematosus, amyloidosis, hepatitis B, carcinoma, leukemia, infectious disease, and pre-eclampsia. Other predisposing factors include allergic reactions and medications.

CLINICAL MANIFESTATIONS

- proteinuria, hypoalbuminemia, and edema
- hyperlipidemia and normocytic anemia
- waxy pallor of the skin
- anorexia, malaise, irritability, amenorrhea

ACUTE AND SUBACUTE CARE

Medical Management

- steroids, loop diuretics, and plasma volume expanders
- cytotoxic agents, indomethacin, and antiplatelet agents
- long-term anticoagulant therapy to prevent renal vein thrombosis.
- diet of normal or high levels of protein, adequate carbohydrate, and adequate calories with a mild sodium restriction
- fluid restriction if client is hyponatremic

Nursing Management

- Assess for signs/symptoms of complications:
  - — renal failure
  - — hypovolemia
  - — thromboembolism
  - — abnormal thyroid function
  - — increased susceptibility to infections
- Discuss ways to reduce edema and prevent skin breakdown.
- Assess for signs/symptoms of electrolyte imbalance from diuresis.
- Strict intake and output.
- Daily weights.
- Measure edematous areas daily.

COMMUNITY AND SELF-CARE

- Instruct the client regarding:
  - — long-term anticoagulant therapy and safety precautions
  - — need for meticulous skin care
  - — dietary restrictions
  - — activity restrictions
- Discuss with the client/significant other coping with long-term illness; make referrals as needed.

(For more information, see pp. 1634–1635 of Black and Matassarin-Jacobs: *Medical-Surgical Nursing: Clinical Management for Continuity of Care,* 5th ed.)

Neurogenic Bladder Dysfunction

OVERVIEW

- There are five major types of neurogenic bladder dysfunction:
  - — Uninhibited—the urge to void causes urine excretion.
  - — Sensory Paralytic—the client cannot perceive bladder fullness, which leads to retention with overflow incontinence.
  - — Motor Paralytic—the client perceives the bladder filling but is unable to initiate micturition.

— Autonomous—the client cannot perceive bladder fullness nor initiate or maintain urination without "assistance."
— Reflex—the client has no sensation and the bladder contracts reflexively but does not empty completely.

- All types are caused by central or peripheral nervous system lesions.

CLINICAL MANIFESTATIONS

- urine retention or incontinence depending upon the type of dysfunction

ACUTE AND SUBACUTE CARE

Medical Management

- bladder training is attempted with or without intermittent catheterization or pharmacologic therapy
- medications may include anti-spasmodics and anticholinergics

Surgical Management

- external sphincterotomy (incision of the bladder neck) to restore normal emptying
- for uninhibited bladder dysfunction, injection of alcohol into the subarachnoid space or cutting of the sacral nerves may inhibit reflex bladder contractions. Electrodes implanted in the epidural space also serve this purpose.

Nursing Management

- Instruct the client/significant other regarding:
  — methods to apply external pressure on the abdomen to help control the detrusor muscle
  — the Credé maneuver
  — methods to stimulate trigger points on lower abdomen, inner thighs, and pubic area to initiate micturition (i.e., stroking, pinching, applying ice)
  — intermittent self catheterization
  — amount of fluid to drink.

- Monitor and instruct patient/significant other on signs and symptoms of autonomic dysreflexia, which can occur from bladder distention. This is a medical emergency and must be treated immediately. (See "Spinal Cord Injury," p. 662.)

COMMUNITY AND SELF-CARE

- Determine client's ability to function in the home setting and significant others available for assistance.
- Include significant others in all teaching.
- Assess need for home health care follow-up.
- Instruct the client/significant other regarding:
  - — signs/symptoms of urinary tract infection and to report to physician
  - — self-catheterization technique
  - — bladder training program
- Monitor urinary function regularly with renal function lab tests and yearly renal ultrasounds.

(For more information, see pp. 1612–1619 of Black and Matassarin-Jacobs: *Medical-Surgical Nursing: Clinical Management for Continuity of Care,* 5th ed.)

Neurologic Fungal Infections (Coccidioidomycosis, Cryptococcosis)

- Central nervous system (CNS) fungal infections are rare, and if present, usually are complications from another disease (e.g., leukemia, organ transplantation, acquired immunodeficiency syndrome [AIDS]) that has altered the immune system.
- Cryptococcosis is the most frequent CNS fungal infection. The cryptococcus is a common soil fungus. Diagnosis is confirmed by finding *Cryptococcus neoformans* in the cerebrospinal fluid. This infection is fatal, unless treated within a few weeks.
- The incidence of cryptococcosis has risen with the AIDS epidemic.
- Coccidioidomycosis mainly involves the lungs but may spread to the meninges.

- The most common opportunistic infection to attack the CNS of the AIDS patient is toxoplasmosis. It is usually manifested as single or multiple brain abscesses.
- Clinical manifestations are similar to those seen with bacterial infections of the CNS (see "Meningitis (Bacterial)," p. 472).
- Treatment for both of these infections is intravenous amphotericin B combined with flucytosine for 4–6 weeks. Recovery is usually certain except for clients with advanced infections or other overwhelming, fatal disease. There is, however, a 50–60 per cent relapse rate in clients with AIDS. Treatment for toxoplasmosis is comprised of pyrimethamine (Daraprim), sulfadiazine, or clindamycin (Cleocin), and leucovorin (folinic acid).

(For more information, see p. 860 of Black and Matassarin-Jacobs: *Medical-Surgical Nursing: Clinical Management for Continuity of Care,* 5th ed.)

Non-Hodgkin's Lymphoma

OVERVIEW

- Non-Hodgkin's disease is a lymphoma that results in uncontrolled proliferation of lymphocytes.
- Involvement of the disease starts in the lymph nodes, although a significant number arise outside the lymphoid system.
- Lymphomas are classified as either (1) Hodgkin's—contains Reed-Sternberg cell or (2) non-Hodgkin's—without the Reed-Sternberg cell.
- There are many classification systems used to differentiate non-Hodgkin's lymphoma based on histology and cytologic characteristics.
- Overall, the prognosis of non-Hodgkin's lymphoma is poorer than that of Hodgkin's disease.
- Non-Hodgkin's lymphoma is more common in adults in their middle and older years, and is more common in males than females.

CLINICAL MANIFESTATIONS

- painless, enlarged lymph nodes
- fevers and night sweats
- weight loss
- hepatosplenomegaly
- nonproductive cough, dyspnea (mediastinal involvement)
- progressive anemia with fatigue and malaise

ACUTE AND SUBACUTE CARE

Medical Management

- chemotherapy
- radiation therapy

Surgical Management

- tumor debulking prior to radiation or chemotherapy

Nursing Management

- Administer ordered chemotherapy.
- See "Chemotherapy," p. 149.
- See "Radiation Therapy," p. 605.
- Monitor laboratory findings—CBC, platelet count, renal profile.
- Encourage balanced diet.
- Encourage rest.

COMMUNITY AND SELF-CARE

- Instruct client regarding:
  — disease process and treatment regime
  — see "Chemotherapy," p. 149.
  — see "Radiation Therapy," p. 605.
  — signs/symptoms to report to physician
  — importance of follow-up visits
- Refer to available community resources (cancer support groups).

(For more information, see p. 1503 of Black and Matassarin-Jacobs: *Medical-Surgical Nursing: Clinical Management for Continuity of Care,* 5th ed.)

O

Obesity

OVERVIEW

- Obesity is weight 20 per cent or greater than the desirable weight for adults of a given sex and height.
- It is caused by a caloric intake that exceeds energy expenditure.
- Complications include: atherosclerosis, ischemic heart disease, hypertension, and diabetes mellitus.
- Some studies show a link between obesity with breast, endometrial, and ovarian cancer.

CLINICAL MANIFESTATIONS

- weight as defined above

ACUTE AND SUBACUTE CARE

Medical Management

- caloric restriction with an exercise program
- use of support groups (TOPS, Overeaters Anonymous, Weight Watchers) for appetite re-education in which the client learns to eat and be satisfied with nutritious, well-balanced foods that are low in calories

Surgical Management

- jaw wiring to reduce food intake
- gastric stapling (gastroplasty)—involves stapling the top part of the stomach with creation of a small pouch to receive digested food. The client can eat only about 30 ml of food every 5 minutes.

Nursing Management

Medical

- Instruct on healthy diet with correct portion size.
- Assist to develop a regular exercise program.
- Assist to develop other ways to deal with stress, boredom, and anxiety.
- Obtain weights at regular intervals.
- Assist to develop improved self esteem.
- Assist to find areas of self regard.

COMMUNITY AND SELF-CARE

- Instruct client regarding:
  — reinforcement of nutritional plan and exercise program
- Refer to support groups (TOPS, Overeaters Anonymous, Weight Watchers).

(For more information, see pp. 1760–1761 of Black and Matassarin-Jacobs: *Medical-Surgical Nursing: Clinical Management for Continuity of Care,* 5th ed.)

Ocular Tumors, Malignant

OVERVIEW

- Retinoblastoma is a highly malignant intraocular tumor. It is a relatively rare form of cancer, occurring most often in children. Retinoblastomas grow rapidly along the optic nerve and invade the brain.
- Choroidal melanomas are often detected during a routine ocular examination because there is no pain associated with the development of the tumor. By the time the tumor has grown large enough to obstruct vision, there may be involvement of the macula and metastasis.

CLINICAL MANIFESTATIONS

- visual changes

ACUTE AND SUBACUTE CARE

Medical Management

- radiation therapy using seed placement
- cycloplegic eye drops (decrease ciliary muscle spasm)
- antibiotic/steroid eye drops

Surgical Management

- photocoagulation and/or cryotherapy
- enucleation (removal of the eyeball)

Nursing Management

Medical

- Administer eye drops as ordered.
- Maintain radiation precautions while seeds in place.

Surgical-Enucleation

Postoperative Care

In addition to routine postoperative care:
- Maintain pressure dressing over the eye.
- Prepare the client for dressing removal the next day by explaining what the eye will look like. The socket and lid will be swollen and the plastic conformer (placed to maintain socket shape) will be visible.
- Perform eye care.
- Apply antibiotic ophthalmic ointment.
- Implement safety measures (client will need to adjust to monocular vision).

COMMUNITY AND SELF-CARE

Postoperative

Instruct client regarding:
- technique for instilling eye drops
- eye care
- measures for a safe home environment
- need for extra precaution with remaining eye (i.e., wear eye protection when engaging in any activity that may result in injury)
- importance of follow-up visits. Prosthesis will be fitted in 4–6 weeks.

(For more information, see pp. 970–971 of Black and Matassarin-Jacobs: *Medical-Surgical Nursing: Clinical Management for Continuity of Care,* 5th ed.)

Osteoarthritis

OVERVIEW

- Osteoarthritis (OA) is a noninflammatory joint disease, characterized by degeneration and loss of articular cartilage in synovial joints. It was previously called degenerative joint disease (DJD).
- Osteoarthritis is classified as:
  (1) primary (idiopathic)—is associated with aging. This is the most common type, existing in about 60 million people in the United States. It occurs in about 50 per cent of all people by the age of 16 years. Weight-bearing joints are the most commonly affected.
  (2) secondary—due to conditions that lead to damage of joint surfaces: repetitive strain and sprains, joint dislocation, fractures, medications (steroids, cholchicine, etc.)
- With OA there is a loss of articular cartilage due to enzymatic destruction. Layers of the cartilage loosen and eventually the subchondral bones become unprotected, then dense.

CLINICAL MANIFESTATIONS

- aching pain
- crepitus and stiffness in involved large weight-bearing joints
- enlarged joints
- contractures
- muscle spasms

ACUTE AND SUBACUTE CARE

Medical Management

- pain management
- nonsteroidal anti-inflammatory drugs
- local steroid injections

- splints
- traction
- heat treatments
- weight loss and exercise regime

Surgical Management

- osteotomy—removal of a section of bone to realign a joint, and decrease joint strain
- arthrodesis—fusion of a joint
- total hip replacement (arthroplasty)—placement of a prosthetic implant to restore motion to the joint and function to the muscles, ligaments, and other soft tissue structures
- total knee replacement—like total hip, a metal and polyethylene implant is used

Nursing Management

Medical

- Administer analgesics and anti-inflammatory drugs.
- Apply heat treatments.
- Consult Physical Therapy for braces, splints, or assistive devices.
- Encourage to establish an exercise regime.
- Implement appropriate safety measures.

Surgical

Total Hip/Total Knee

In addition to routine preoperative care:
- Teach the client how to use crutches and/or walker.
- Assist to practice transfer technique from bed to chair.
- Instruct and assist to practice postoperative exercises.

Total Hip Replacement

In addition to routine postoperative care:
- Monitor dressing and Hemovac drains for excessive drainage.
- Maintain affected leg in abducted position and straight alignment.
- Assess nerve function and circulation in affected leg every 1–2 hours.
- Encourage and supervise ordered exercises.

- Prevent flexion of the hip of more than 90 degrees when positioning or transferring.
- Initiate weight bearing and ambulation as ordered.
- Administer prophylactic antibiotics (steroid therapy, cytotoxic therapy, and implantation of a foreign object put the client at risk for infection).
- Monitor white blood count, temperature, and incision site for signs of infection.
- Monitor for signs of adrenocortical insufficiency (clients on steroids prior to surgery may exhibit signs of insufficiency secondary to the stress of surgery):
  — tachycardia
  — hypotension
  — diaphoresis
  — decreasing level of consciousness
- Institute measures to prevent thrombophlebitis:
  — support stockings
  — in bed exercises
  — low dose heparin
- Monitor for signs/symptoms of pulmonary embolism:
  — respiratory distress
  — tachycardia
  — hypertension
  — tachypnea
  — fever

Total Knee Replacement

- Maintain knee in maximum extension.
- Monitor use of continuous passive motion machine (CPM). The CPM should be used at all times except when not lying supine. The initial CPM setting is at 30 degrees of flexion and full extension. The degrees of flexion are slowly increased each day, until 90 degrees of flexion is reached.
- Encourage and supervise ordered exercises.
- Insitute weight bearing and ambulation as ordered.
- Monitor for possible complications: thrombophlebitis, pulmonary embolism, infection, and adrenal insufficiency.

COMMUNITY AND SELF-CARE

Medical

Instruct the client regarding:
- techniques to reduce stress on the joints
- how to use assistive devices
- use of PRN analgesics
- prescribed exercises
- application of heat compresses
- weight loss diet and exercise regime.

Surgical (total hip/total knee)

Instruct the client regarding:
- importance of not flexing the hip greater than 90 degrees and avoiding extremes of internal rotation for 6 months to 1 year
- importance of not crossing one leg over the other
- importance of prescribed exercises
- avoidance of sitting continuously for longer than 1 hour
- avoidance of actions that place a strain on the hip joint—excessive bending, heavy lifting, jogging, and jumping
- avoidance of sitting in low-reclining or rocking chairs
- use of assistive devices (crutches/walker) until full weight bearing is allowed
- driving restrictions
- incision care

(For more information, see pp. 2108–2120 of Black and Matassarin-Jacobs: *Medical-Surgical Nursing: Clinical Management for Continuity of Care,* 5th ed.)

Osteomalacia

OVERVIEW

- Osteomalacia is a disease in which the bone becomes abnormally soft because of a disturbed calcium and phosphorus balance secondary to a vitamin D deficiency, which results in marked deformities of the weight-bearing bones and pathologic fractures.

- Osteomalacia is always due to inadequate concentration of calcium or phosphorus. Inadequate calcium or vitamin D in the diet may cause a decrease in the absorption of calcium from the intestine. Increased urinary excretion of calcium or loss of calcium or phosphorus during pregnancy and lactation may cause osteomalacia.
- Osteomalacia occurs mainly in the spine, pelvis, and lower extremities.
- Osteomalacia is similar to rickets, which occurs in children; therefore, the condition is called adult rickets.
- Osteomalacia mainly affects women.
- Risk factors include:
  - — hypoparathyroidism
  - — renal tubular disorders
  - — hepatobiliary disease
  - — small intestine disease
  - — use of long-term anticonvulsants, tranquilizers, sedatives, and muscle relaxants

CLINICAL MANIFESTATIONS

- scoliotic or kyphotic deformities of the spine
- bone pain
- bowing and bending deformities of the long bones
- decreased serum calcium and phosphorus

ACUTE AND SUBACUTE CARE

Medical Management

- vitamin D replacement
- supplemental calcium
- pain management
- dietary modifications—high calcium, high phosphorus
- management of fractures, if present

Surgical Management

- repair of fractures

Nursing Management

- Administer vitamin and mineral supplements as ordered.
- Administer analgesics.
- Consult Physical Therapy for adaptive devices for ambulation or activities of daily living and strengthening exercises.
- Monitor laboratory findings—calcium and phosphorus levels.
- Encourage diet high in calcium and phosphorus.

COMMUNITY AND SELF-CARE

Instruct client regarding:
- disease process and treatment regime
- use of adaptive devices
- use of PRN analgesics
- dietary modifications—high calcium, high phosphorus

(For more information, see pp. 2106–2107 of Black and Matassarin-Jacobs: *Medical-Surgical Nursing: Clinical Management for Continuity of Care,* 5th ed.)

Osteomyelitis

OVERVIEW

- *Osteomyelitis* is a term used to describe any infection of the bone. Acute osteomyelitis responds to a 4–6 week course of intravenous antibiotics, whereas chronic osteomyelitis persists longer than 4 weeks and involves sequestered (necrotic bone that has separated from living tissue) areas of infection.
- Osteomyelitis is generally bacterial in origin, but may also be caused by viral or fungal infections. Staphylococcus aureus is the most common organism, but Escherichia coli, Klebsiella, Proteus, Pseudomonas, and Salmonella may also cause osteomyelitis. These organisms may be directly introduced into the bone, may be spread from adjacent soft tissue infection or travel through the

blood to the site. The bacteria are able to multiply readily in bone because bone has a slow circulatory system.

CLINICAL MANIFESTATIONS

- fever (usually above 101° F. [38° C.])
- localized pain or tenderness
- erythema (redness)
- heat and swelling around the infected bone
- elevated WBC and ESR (erythrocyte sedimentation rate)
- positive blood cultures

ACUTE AND SUBACUTE CARE

Medical Management

- needle aspiration (to relieve pressure within the bone)
- antibiotic therapy for 4–6 weeks

Surgical Management

Chronic Osteomyelitis

- sequestrectomy (removal of the dead bone) and saucerization (removal of scar tissue, infected tissue, sequestra and necrotic bone, leaving a saucer-like depression)
  — surgery is followed by a 4–6 week course of IV antibiotics, followed by a course of oral antibiotics

Nursing Management

Medical

- Administer antibiotics as prescribed.
- Monitor temperature and administer PRN antipyretics.
- Administer PRN analgesics and anti-inflammatory agents and assess effectiveness.
- Provide wound care as indicated.
- Encourage progressive exercise/ambulation program.
- Monitor laboratory findings—WBC, ESR, blood culture reports.

Surgical

Postoperative Care

In addition to routine postoperative care:
- Administer antibiotics as prescribed.

COMMUNITY AND SELF-CARE

Because of the extended IV antibiotic regime for both acute and chronic osteomyelitis, the client is often sent home with IV access in place and a referral made to a home health care agency to complete antibiotic therapy.

Instruct client regarding:
- disease process and need for long-term antibiotic therapy
- care of IV access catheter and site
- wound/incision care
- signs/symptoms to report (fever, increased wound drainage, increased pain)
- use of PRN analgesics
- importance of follow-up appointments

(For more information, see pp. 2121–2122 of Black and Matassarin-Jacobs: *Medical-Surgical Nursing: Clinical Management for Continuity of Care,* 5th ed.)

Osteoporosis

OVERVIEW

- Osteoporosis is a common age-related metabolic bone disease in which there is a severe general reduction in the skeletal bone mass and an increased susceptibility to fractures, especially in the wrist, hip, and vertebral column. Bone resorption occurs faster than bone formation.
- Bone is a dynamic tissue that undergoes continuous remodeling, the process by which old bone is replaced by new, with little or no net change in the mass or shape of the bone. Although there is disagreement about exactly when bone loss naturally begins, it is well established that at the time of menopause, women experience a marked accel-

eration in bone loss. Peak bone mass and the subsequent rate and duration of bone loss are important determinants of whether skeletal integrity will be compromised to the degree that it eventually results in a low-trauma (fragility) fracture.

- Osteoporosis can be classified as:
  - primary—refers to the occurrence of the condition among older persons in whom no secondary predisposing condition exists. This includes both postmenopausal osteoporosis and the osteoporosis of aging.
  - secondary—results from an associated condition such as hyperparathyroidism, long-term corticosteroid or heparin administration
- In the United States alone, osteoporosis affects 25 million individuals and is responsible for 1.3 million fractures each year. One-third of American women over age 50 will eventually have a vertebral fracture.
- Risk factors include:
  - female gender—bone loss related to menopause is considered to be the most important reason for this difference. In postmenopausal women, estrogen production and bone calcium storage decrease. Estrogen appears to protect against bone loss.
  - advanced age
  - family history
  - sedentary lifestyle
  - small-framed body build
  - inadequate dietary intake of calcium
  - excessive alcohol consumption
  - long-term use of corticosteroids, anticonvulsants, furosomide
  - heavy cigarette smoking

CLINICAL MANIFESTATIONS

Osteoporosis often is not diagnosed until the client presents with a fracture.

- shortened stature
- marked kyphosis of the thoracic spine (dowager hump)
- impaired breathing (due to deformities of the spine and rib cage)

- pain at the site of fracture

ACUTE AND SUBACUTE CARE

Medical Management

- management of fractures, if present
- Physical therapy
- calcitonin therapy—inhibits bone loss
- estrogen preparations
- flexible corset to relieve back pain
- pain management
- dietary modification—high calcium

Surgical Management

- repair of fractures

Nursing Management

- Administer analgesics as ordered.
- Administer calcitonin and estrogen therapy as ordered.
- Consult with physical therapy for muscle strengthening exercises and adaptive devices for ambulation and activities of daily living.
- Encourage high-calcium diet.
- Institute appropriate safety measures.
- Monitor laboratory findings—calcium and phosphorus levels.

COMMUNITY AND SELF-CARE

Instruct client regarding:

- disease process and treatment regime
- dietary modifications—high calcium
- importance of weight-bearing exercises (walking, tennis, stair climbing) to increase bone mass
- use of PRN analgesics
- use of adaptive devices and muscle strengthening exercises
- safety measures in the home environment

(For more information, see pp. 2098–2104 of Black and Matassarin-Jacobs: *Medical-Surgical Nursing: Clinical Management for Continuity of Care,* 5th ed.)

Otitis Media

- Otitis media is infection of the middle ear. It may be acute (sudden in onset and short in duration) or chronic (repeated infections usually associated with drainage). Repeated infections can cause perforation and hearing loss. Clinical manifestations include ear pain and immobile, reddened ear drum.
- Serous otitis media is fluid in the middle ear and may be found in conjunction with upper respiratory infections or allergies.
- The treatment for otitis media is antibiotic therapy.
- A surgical procedure called a myringotomy may be performed for recurrent otitis media. An incision is made into the tympanic membrane through which fluid is removed and a transtympanic tube inserted. This tube normally extrudes by itself in 3–12 months.
- The nurse instructs the client to:
  — obtain prompt treatment for allergic or upper respiratory infections
  — avoid getting water in the ear (by using cotton balls)
  — seek medical attention for decreased hearing, pain in the ear, or drainage from the ear.
- Following surgery, the nurse instructs the client to:
  — blow the nose gently, one side at a time
  — sneeze or cough with mouth open for 1 week after surgery
  — avoid physical activity for 1 week and exercises or sports for 3 weeks after surgery
  — avoid heavy lifting
  — keep ear dry for 4–6 weeks after surgery
  — not shampoo for 1 week after surgery
  — protect ear when necessary with two pieces of cotton (outer piece saturated with petroleum jelly)
  — avoid airplane flights for the first week after surgery
  — report any drainage other than slight bleeding

For more information, see pp. 1005–1006 of Black and Matassarin-Jacobs: *Medical-Surgical Nursing: Clinical Management for Continuity of Care,* 5th ed.)

Ovarian Cancer

OVERVIEW

- Ovarian cancer is the leading cause of death from reproductive malignancies.
- The exact etiology is unknown, although there does appear to be a familial association.
- Risk factors include: family history, age over 40 years, nulliparity, infertility, history of heavy menstrual bleeding, dysmenorrhea, North American or European descent, and possibly obesity with a diet high in animal fat.
- Ovarian cancer tends to grow and spread silently without symptoms until pressure is placed on other organs or metastasis occurs. Because it is so difficult to detect, early diagnosis generally is not made and thus, the long-term survival rate is poor.

CLINICAL MANIFESTATIONS

- abdominal distention
- urinary frequency and urgency
- pleural effusion
- malnutrition
- pain from pressure of the growing tumor
- constipation
- ascites
- urinary or bowel obstruction

ACUTE AND SUBACUTE CARE

Medical Management

- irradiation or chemotherapy following surgery for stage I ovarian cancer
- chemotherapy and irradiation (including the pelvis and abdomen) following surgery for stage II ovarian cancer

Surgical Management

- total abdominal hysterectomy with bilateral salpingo-oophorectomy (TAH-BSO), omentectomy, and removal of all visible tumor is the surgery of choice

NURSING MANAGEMENT

- Instruct client to get routine pelvic exams and bimanual rectovaginal exams.

See sections on "Chemotherapy," p. 149, "Radiation Therapy," p. 605, and "Uterine Tumors, Benign," p. 743 (for care following TAH-BSO).

For more information, see pp. 2412–2413 of Black and Matassarin-Jacobs: *Medical-Surgical Nursing: Clinical Management for Continuity of Care,* 5th ed.)

P

Pacemakers

OVERVIEW

- A pacemaker is a device that delivers electrical stimuli to the heart through electrodes that have been implanted in the heart muscle. A pacemaker initiates the heart beat when the heart's intrinsic conduction system fails or is unreliable.
- An artificial pacemaker is indicated when the conduction system fails to: (1) generate an impulse spontaneously, (2) transmit impulses from the SA node and atria through the AV junction to the ventricles, or (3) maintain primary control of the pacing function of the heart.
- Possible indications for pacemaker placement include:
  - — acute MI
  - — electrolyte imbalance
  - — autonomic nervous system failure
  - — drug toxicities (antiarrhythmics)
  - — cardiac surgery
  - — complete heart block
  - — second-degree AV block with symptomatic bradycardia
- Pacemakers consist of a pulse generator (the pacemaker's power source) responsible for sending out appropriately timed signals, and a lead-electrode system (the sensory circuit) responsible for identifying and analyzing intrinsic activity and responding appropriately. The lead delivers the electrical impulse from the pulse generator to the myocardium. The lead is a flexible conductive wire encased by insulating material. The electrode is at the end of the lead and delivers the impulse directly to the myocardium. Not only does this system deliver electrical impulses, but it relays information about spontaneous intracardiac signals back to the sensing circuit in the pulse generator.

- The pulse generator can be external or internal. The external unit is designed for temporary pacing, primarily for support of transient dysrhythmias. If permanent, the pulse generator is placed into a small tunnel burrowed within the subcutaneous tissue below the right or left clavicle or in the abdominal cavity.
- There are three major modes of delivering energy to the myocardial tissue.
  (1) external (transcutaneous)—pacing is stimulated through large gelled electrode pads placed anteriorly and posteriorly and connected to an external pacemaker
    — used in emergency cardiac care and preferred for clients who are anticoagulated or may require thrombolytic therapy
  (2) epicardial (transthoracic)—electrical energy travels from external generator through thoracic musculature directly to epicardial surface of the heart
    — most common during and immediately following cardiac surgery
  (3) endocardial (transvenous)—pacing electrode is inserted via the transvenous route (via the antecubital, femoral, jugular, or subclavian vein) and threaded into the right atrium or ventricle so that it comes in direct contact with the endocardium
- Pacemakers are classified according to a five-letter code: the first letter denotes the cardiac chamber to be paced (the atrium [A], the ventricle [V], or both [dual] chambers [D]); the second letter denotes the chamber to be sensed (the atrium [A], the ventricle [V], dual [D] or none [O]); the third letter, the type of response; that is, sensed intrinsic activity will cause the pacemaker's impulse to be "triggered" [T] (to pace) or "inhibited" [I] (not to pace) or both [D]. For example, a VVI pacemaker paces in the ventricle, senses in the ventricle and will inhibit pacing if the client's intrinsic rhythm is sensed. Letter four, rate adaptiveness and programmability, and letter five, antitachydysrhythmic functions are infrequently seen in practice.
- Pacemaker function—the pacemaker has a sensor that senses if the intrinsic beat has occurred; if

not, the pacer sends out an impulse to begin myocardial depolarization through the pulse generator. The pulse generator captures the myocardium and maintains the heart's rhythm. For a predetermined time after the pacemaker impulse, the pacemaker is incapable of sensing incoming signals. This refractory period prevents the pacemaker from sensing its own generated activity.

- Pacing modes:
  (1) Asynchronous (fixed rate) Pacing (AOO, VOO, DOO)—pace only, do not sense
    - Pacing mode delivers an electrical impulse to the heart at a preset fixed rate regardless of intrinsic cardiac activity.
    - There is no sensory mechanism; the pacing mechanism ignores the client's intrinsic rhythm.
    - Major disadvantages:
      - potential tachycardia when both the pacemaker and SA node fire.
      - atrial and ventricular synchrony do not occur.
      - risk that a ventricular pacemaker stimulus may occur during the vulnerable period producing ventricular tachycardia or ventricular fibrillation.

  (2) Noncompetitive (demand) Pacing (VVI, VVT, AAI, AAT)
    - Pacemaker fires only on demand or when needed to stimulate atrial or ventricular contraction.
    - If intrinsic beats are sensed, the pacemaker is inhibited. If a spontaneous P wave or QRS does not occur, the pacemaker discharges at a preset delay interval to either the atria (atrial demand pacing) or ventricle (ventricular demand pacing).
    - Major disadvantage:
      - atrial and ventricular contractions are not synchronous

  (3) Synchronous Pacing (VAT, VDD)
    - The sensing electrode is placed in the atrium and the pacing electrode in the ventricle. Thus, the pacemaker unit senses atrial activ-

ity and elicits a stimulus to prompt ventricular depolarization.
- Allows the heart rate to vary, and atrial-ventricular synchrony occurs.
- A built-in safety mechanism causes ventricular depolarizations to occur at a fixed rate should atrial rates become too fast.

(4) Atrioventricular Sequential Pacing (DVI)
- The ventricle is sensed and the atrium paced. If the ventricle does not depolarize after a preset interval, it is also paced. If the ventricle depolarizes on its own, ventricular output through the pacemaker is inhibited.
- The atrium is paced regardless of its own intrinsic activity; therefore, competition may occur, leading to atrial fibrillation.

(5) Optimal Sequential Pacemaker (DDD)
- Pacemakers consist of both atrial and ventricular circuits that sense and pace their respective chambers. If spontaneous atrial activity does not occur, the atrium is paced. Any sensed atrial activity inhibits pacing function. If ventricular depolarization does not occur in the preset time interval, the ventricle is paced.
- The advantage of this mode is that it more closely mimics the normal heart. Atrial-ventricular synchrony is maintained, and the heart rate can change to meet metabolic demands.

- Methods of pacing:
  - Temporary pacing:
    - used in short-term pacing
    - the pulse generator is external
    - pacing electrodes are inserted by transcutaneous, transthoracic, or transvenous routes
  - Permanent pacing:
    - indicated in long-term management
    - pacing electrode is inserted either via transvenous route or by direct application to the epicardial surface during thoracotomy
    - the pulse generator is implanted in the subcutaneous tissue below the clavicle

ACUTE AND SUBACUTE CARE

Nursing Management

- Monitor client's cardiac rhythm continuously.
- Assess for signs/symptoms of decreased cardiac output.
- Instruct client to avoid excessive extension or abduction of the arm on the operative side.
- Assess for possible complications: wound infection, phlebitis at the insertion site, pneumothorax, atelectasis, pericardial fluid accumulation, diaphragmatic stimulation (seen as twitching at the pacemaker site or hiccupping) and dysrhythmias.
- Evaluate rhythm strip for possible signs of pacemaker malfunction:
  - — failure to pace properly—intermittent absence of pacing artifact or rapid, inappropriate firing. Possible causes; battery failure, lead dislodgement, fracture of lead wire, disconnection between catheter and generator.
  - — failure to capture—pacing artifact present but not followed by a QRS complex or P wave. The impulse does not generate depolarization. Possible causes: low voltage, battery failure, faulty connection, fractured wire.
  - — failure to sense—inability of the sensor to detect the client's intrinsic beats and the pacemaker sends out impulses too early. Possible causes: improper catheter position, tip or lead dislodgement, battery failure, sensitivity set too low.
  - — oversensing—pacemaker senses electrical activity within the myocardium that should be ignored. Possible causes; sensitivity set too high, electromagnetic interference.
- Monitor for signs and symptoms of pacemaker malfunction—syncope, tachycardia or bradycardia, and palpitations.
- Monitor activity tolerance.

COMMUNITY AND SELF-CARE

Instruct the client regarding:

- wound care—assess wound daily; report signs of inflammation. Avoid constrictive clothing that puts excessive pressure on wound and generator.

- importance of taking pulse daily and to notify physician if pulse slower than set rate
- when to seek medical attention—if experiencing palpitations, vertigo, or syncope
- avoidance of areas with high voltage, magnetic force fields, or radiation:
  - large running motors
  - power plants
  - arc welding machines
- importance of carrying identification card
- avoidance of activity that can cause blunt trauma to the pulse generator
- avoidance of vigorous movement of the arms and shoulders and lifting weights greater than 5–10 pounds for first 6 weeks
- importance of regular physician visits
- need for regular telephone monitoring of the client's electrocardiogram
- indications of battery depletion—pulse rate below set rate, syncope, shortness of breath

(For more information, see pp. 1314–1323 of Black and Matassarin-Jacobs: *Medical-Surgical Nursing: Clinical Management for Continuity of Care,* 5th ed.)

Paget's Disease

OVERVIEW

- Paget's disease is defined as a disorder of bone architecture characterized by an initial phase of increased rate of bone tissue breakdown by osteoclasts, followed by excessive abnormal bone formation by osteoblasts. The diseased bone is structurally weak and prone to fracture. Paget's disease most frequently affects the femur, tibia, lower spine, pelvis, and cranium.
- The exact cause of Paget's disease is unknown.
- In the United States, 2.5 million people over the age of 40 are affected with Paget's disease.

CLINICAL MANIFESTATIONS

- may be asymptomatic
- bone pain
- skeletal deformity (barrel-shaped chest, bowing of the tibia/femur or kyphosis)
- changes in skin temperature (warm and flushed)
- pathologic fractures
- cranial nerve compression (vertigo, hearing loss, blindness)

ACUTE AND SUBACUTE CARE

Medical Management

- pain management—aspirin, indomethacin, ibuprofen
- management of fractures
- calcitonin and etidronate administration—decreases bone resorption
- mithramycin administration—decreases serum calcium

Surgical Management

- repair of fractures

Nursing Management

- Administer ordered medications.
- Administer PRN analgesics.
- Consult Physical Therapy for adaptive devices for ambulation and activities of daily living.
- Institute safety measures.

COMMUNITY AND SELF-CARE

Instruct client regarding:

- disease process and treatment regime
- use of PRN analgesics
- use of adaptive devices
- safety measures

(For more information, see pp. 2104–2106 of Black and Matassarin-Jacobs: *Medical-Surgical Nursing: Clinical Management for Continuity of Care,* 5th ed.)

Pain Assessment and Intervention

OVERVIEW

- Pain is a personal and subjective experience with few or no objective measurements. Pain is defined by each of us from our own personal experiences.
- The International Association for the Study of Pain defines pain as "an unpleasant sensory and emotional experience associated with actual or potential tissue damage, or described in terms of such damage."[1]
- McCaffery defines pain as "whatever the experiencing person says it is and existing whenever the person says it does."[2]
- Pain is a process made up of transduction, transmission, and modulation of pain.

Pain Transduction

- The chain of events that leads to pain begins when pain fibers are excited by multiple types of stimuli. The stimuli consist of mechanical events (such as stretching or pressure), heat or cold, and chemical changes (such as ischemia). Specific fibers react to these stimuli. The fibers are classified as mechanical, thermal, or chemical nociceptors. Nociceptors (nerve receptors for pain) are free nerve endings occurring in almost all types of tissue. The level of pain input into nociceptors is increased by a variety of chemical substances that are released when tissue injury occurs. These substances act as chemical mediators and include bradykinin, serotonin, histamine, substance P, acetylcholine, and others.

Pain Transmission

- Once nociceptors are stimulated, the impulse they discharge travels as electrical activity to the spinal cord and on to the brain. This electric activity becomes the experience of pain when it reaches the brain.

- Modulation of pain may occur via the dorsal horn in the spinal cord, via descending pathways or via endogenous chemicals.
- Once pain has been received and transmitted, it must be perceived or interpreted. The following factors affect a client's *perception* of pain:
  - — pain threshold—the lowest perceivable intensity of stimuli that is transmitted as pain
  - — tolerance for pain—the amount of pain the client is willing to endure. Only the client knows this.
  - — past experiences with pain
- The client's *response* to pain is influenced by many variables:
  - — situational factors (setting in which the pain occurs)
  - — sociocultural factors (race, culture, ethnicity)
  - — age—age may release a client from culturally imposed norms in relation to pain expression
  - — sex (boys may be expected to express less pain than girls)
  - — meaning of pain—if the cause of pain is known, it may help the client respond to it. Pain that is associated with a threat to body image may be much worse than pain that is not.
  - — anxiety—if anxiety is high, pain is felt as greater
  - — fatigue and insomnia
  - — stress
  - — depression and the associated isolation
- Pain may be acute or chronic.
  - — Acute pain is usually of short duration (less than 6 months) and has an identifiable, immediate onset. Acute pain is seen as having a limited and often predictable duration. It also is seen as a useful and limiting pain in that it indicates injury and motivates the individual to get relief from the pain. The physiologic response to acute pain is due to sympathetic nervous system stimulation. The client probably will exhibit: increased or decreased blood pressure, tachycardia, diaphoresis, tachypnea, focusing on the pain, and guarding the affected body part.

— Chronic pain is usually considered to be pain that lasts more than 6 months (or 1 month beyond the normal end of the condition causing the pain) and has no foreseeable end except for very slow healing or death. It is continual or persistent and recurrent. It often has an identifiable cause and is much more difficult to treat than acute pain. Chronic pain is seen as useless because it is not a sign of impending damage. It is often described using affective terms, e.g., hateful or sickening. Chronic pain often is frustrating and difficult to live with. Clients become increasingly engrossed in their illness and eventually may exhibit the following symptoms:
  - depressed mood
  - increased or decreased appetite and weight
  - drastically restricted activity level
  - social withdrawal
  - preoccupation with physical symptoms
  - poor sleep and chronic fatigue.

- Nurses must be aware that:
  - — pain that has a psychological origin (e.g., a tension headache) is just as real as pain of a physiologic origin
  - — pain is individualized. There is no standard pain produced by a particular stimulus. An identical surgical incision in different people produces different amounts of pain.
  - — age is not a determinant of pain, although it may influence expression. Very young and very old clients may experience as much pain as other persons, but have difficulty expressing it.
  - — a person cannot learn to increase tolerance for pain. Prolonged pain actually lowers the client's tolerance of pain.
  - — pain is exhausting. People will sleep, however poorly, in spite of pain.
  - — clients with any unrelieved pain may experience depression or anxiety. If pain continues, these symptoms may increase, but they are caused by the pain, not the reverse.

ASSESSING A CLIENT'S PAIN

- Obtain an accurate history, assessing the following:

— the location of the client's pain (internal or external, one location or multiple areas, unilateral or bilateral)
— the extension or radiation of the client's pain (Is the pain on the surface or deep inside? Does it cover a wide area or can the client point to where it is?)
— the onset and pattern (Does it occur in cycles? What triggers it? Is it sudden or gradual?)
— duration (How long does it last? Is the client ever free of pain?)
— character or quality (Is it dull, sharp, throbbing, shooting?)
— precipitating or alleviating factors
— intensity (Ask: On a scale of 0 to 10, with 0 being no pain and 10 being the worst pain you can imagine, how would you rate your pain?)
— associated symptoms (Ask: Are there any other problems caused by your pain?)
— effect on activities of daily living
— methods of pain relief (Ask about invasive and noninvasive pain relief methods. Ask what has *not* worked to relieve the pain.)

- Ask the client to show where the pain is and describe how it feels.
- Assess for sympathetic responses (associated with low to moderate pain intensity or superficial pain): pallor; increased pulse, blood pressure and respirations; skeletal muscle tension; dilated pupils; and diaphoresis.
- Assess for parasympathetic responses (often associated with pain of severe intensity or with deep pain):
  — decreased blood pressure and pulse
  — nausea and vomiting
  — weakness
  — prostration
  — pallor
  — possible loss of consciousness
- Assess for behavioral responses:
  — moaning, sighing, grimacing, quietness, withdrawal from others
  — crying, restlessness
  — holding or protecting the painful area
  — lying motionless

— assuming a position that minimizes pain (fetal position, drawing up legs)

- Use pain assessment tools, such as the visual analog or visual descriptor scales

ACUTE AND SUBACUTE CARE

Nursing Management

- Alleviate anxiety and assist client to relax.
- Utilize distraction or diversion, such as deep breathing, reading, conversation, listening to the radio or watching TV.
- Combat anticipatory fear of pain by explaining the type of pain the client may feel.
- Eliminate any other sources of discomfort, such as full bladder, improperly positioned drainage tubes, or uncomfortable position.
- Ensure the client receives adequate sleep (over-tiredness decreases pain tolerance).
- Apply heat and cold, depending on effectiveness for the client.
- Administer pain medications as prescribed and assess effectiveness.
- Provide or facilitate consult for noninvasive interventions:
  — meditation
  — cutaneous stimulation—stimulation of the skin to relieve pain. The stimulus can be heat, cold, massage, menthol application, or vibration.
  — progressive relaxation training—the client is taught to gradually tighten, then deeply relax various muscle groups, proceeding systematically from one area of the body to the next.
  — guided imagery—may be combined with other techniques for maximal benefit. The client is asked to visualize a relaxing scene.
  — rhythmic breathing—client is instructed to time breathing to match the rhythm of a clock, music, or metronome
  — biofeedback—wide variety of techniques that provide a client with information about changes in bodily function of which the client is usually

unaware, such as blood pressure. The client learns self-control over physiologic variables that relate to the pain, such as muscle contraction and blood flow.

— hypnosis—induction of a trance-like state, followed by a suggestion to alter the character of the pain or the individual's attitude toward it. Requires a skilled professional.
— acupressure—a noninvasive pain relief method using pressure, massage, or other cutaneous stimulations over acupuncture points
— acupuncture—skillful insertion of very thin metal needles into the body at designated locations to relieve pain
— music therapy

• Provide/assist with invasive interventions as prescribed.
  — nurse-administered (demand) analgesia—administration of pain medication by the nurse on an "as needed" or scheduled basis.
    - advantages include: allows the nurse to assess the pain, and therefore helps the nurse to detect or avoid untoward reactions or side effects. Permits dose adjustment as necessary.
    - disadvantages:
      (1) Pain relief is often delayed or undercontrolled due to overconcern about possible narcotic side effects and fear of inducing narcotic addiction.
      (2) Client may have anxiety due to fear that nurse will not deliver the dose promptly.
      (3) There are wide swings in blood levels of analgesics.
  — Patient controlled analgesia—method involves an intravenous solution pump that contains the analgesic and is controlled by the client. The client can self-administer a dose of analgesic by pressing a button that then releases a preset dose of analgesic. The pumps are programmed to deliver preset demand doses of analgesic until a maximum dose is reached. There is then a minimal interval when no further analgesic can be administered. The client controls the administration of pain medication within the

limits set by the program. There are many advantages to this system:
- the client reports improved pain control
- the client has less anxiety about waiting for the nurse to administer pain medications
- there is near-constant blood concentration of analgesic

— Assist physician with administration of intraspinal analgesia—new advancement in the treatment of postoperative or chronic malignant pain. Narcotics are injected through a small catheter into the epidural or intrathecal space, either by repeated bolus doses given by the anesthesiologist, by a constant infusion via an infusion pump, or via a patient-controlled analgesia pump. The epidural space is outside the dura mater of the spinal cord and brain. The intrathecal space is inside the dura mater and contains the spinal fluid. The dorsal horns of the spinal cord contain receptors for endogenous opioid substances. These receptors bind narcotics and provide excellent pain relief of long duration (8–24 hours) without causing motor nerve blockade. Possible side effects include pruritus, hypotension, respiratory depression, and urinary retention. Nursing care is according to individual hospital protocol.

— Transcutaneous electric nerve stimulation (TENS)—placement of electrodes on the skin to stimulate a superficial nerve close to the pain as a method of pain relief. Positive and negative poles are placed within several inches of each other. Voltage and pulsation are controlled by the client. The overall efficiency of TENS in individuals with chronic pain is about 25 per cent.

- Discharge teaching depends upon the pain treatment modality.

(For more information, see pp. 342–392 of Black and Matassarin-Jacobs: *Medical-Surgical Nursing: Clinical Management for Continuity of Care,* 5th ed.)

REFERENCES:
1. International Association for the Study of Pain (1986). Pain terms: A current list with definitions and notes on usage. Pain, 3:5216-5221.
2. McCaffery, M. (1981). Nursing management of the patient with pain (2nd Ed.). Philadelphia: J. B. Lippincott.

Pancreatic Cancer

OVERVIEW

- Pancreatic cancer is the fifth most common cause of cancer death. Ninety per cent of pancreatic cancer clients die within the first year after diagnosis.
- Pancreatic cancer appears to be linked to diabetes mellitus, alcohol use, history of previous pancreatitis and the ingestion of a high-fat diet.

CLINICAL MANIFESTATIONS

- jaundice
- weight loss
- abdominal pain

ACUTE AND SUBACUTE CARE

MEDICAL MANAGEMENT

- palliative based on symptoms:
  — analgesics
  — nutritional supplements
- chemotherapy—limited success

SURGICAL MANAGEMENT

- pancreatic resection—removal of tumor-involved area of the pancreas
- palliative—to remove obstruction

NURSING MANAGEMENT

Medical

- Administer analgesics and assess effectiveness.

- Encourage a well-balanced diet.
- See "Chemotherapy," p. 149.

Surgical—Pancreatic Resection

Postoperative Care

In addition to routine postoperative care:

- Monitor proper functioning and output of drains.
- Monitor for hyperglycemia.
- Administer pancreatic enzyme replacement therapy (Pancrease) when taking food by mouth.

COMMUNITY AND SELF-CARE

- Instruct client regarding:
  — management of side effects (if chemotherapy prescribed)
  — if postoperative:
    - wound care
    - signs/symptoms of infection
    - pancreatic enzyme replacement therapy
    - insulin therapy
- Refer to available community resources (home health care, hospice).

(For more information, see pp. 1930–1931 of Black and Matassarin-Jacobs: *Medical-Surgical Nursing: Clinical Management for Continuity of Care,* 5th ed.)

Pancreatic Pseudocyst

OVERVIEW

- Pancreatic pseudocysts are localized collections of pancreatic secretions (high concentrations of amylase, lipase, and trypsin) in a cystic structure, usually adjacent to the pancreas rather than within the parenchyma.
- Pseudocysts develop in up to 10 per cent of clients after an attack of acute alcoholic pancreatitis, but they may also be associated with acute pancreatitis of other causes, chronic pancreatitis, trauma, and pancreatic neoplasm.

CLINICAL MANIFESTATIONS

- abdominal pain
- early satiety
- nausea and vomiting

ACUTE AND SUBACUTE CARE

Medical Management

Treatment is based on the presence or absence of symptoms, the client's age, and the size of the cyst. In about 25 per cent of the cases, the pseudocyst resolves spontaneously.

- symptom management:
  — analgesics
  — antiemetics
- frequent ultrasound studies to determine if the cyst is decreasing in size

Surgical Management

- internal drainage — creating an ostomy between the pseudocyst and the stomach (cystogastrostomy), jejunum (cystojejunostomy), or duodenum (cystoduodenostomy)
- external drainage — insertion of a drainage tube to an external collection device
- pancreatic resection, distal pancreatectomy

Nursing Management

Medical

- Administer analgesics and antiemetics as prescribed and assess effectiveness.

Surgical

Postoperative Care

In addition to routine postoperative care:

- Monitor proper function and output of drainage tube.

COMMUNITY AND SELF-CARE

Instruct client regarding:

- wound care, if postoperative

- importance of abstinence from alcohol (if alcohol-related) and available community resources for alcohol cessation

(For more information, see pp. 1929–1930 of Black and Matassarin-Jacobs: *Medical-Surgical Nursing: Clinical Management for Continuity of Care,* 5th ed.)

Pancreatic Transplantation

OVERVIEW

- Advances in pancreatic transplantation techniques continue to be made, and it is hoped that eventually pancreas transplantation will have an impact on the treatment of diabetes mellitus.
- A candidate for a pancreas transplant is most likely to have type II diabetes. Because there is a higher graft success rate in the population that receives a combined pancreas-renal transplant compared with a pancreas transplant alone, both transplants are often performed concurrently.
- Several surgical approaches are used with pancreas transplants. They include transplanting (1) a segmental portion, (2) an entire pancreas with or without all or part of the ampulla of Vater or part of the duodenum, or (3) isolated islet grafts. The major concern when the entire pancreas is transplanted is management of the exocrine secretions from the pancreatic duct. When the entire pancreas is transplanted, it is placed in the lower pelvic cavity and the duct is connected to the urinary bladder to allow for drainage of the pancreatic enzymes. Islet cell grafts are a specific approach to treatment but there are difficulties with isolating and preserving the grafts. They have been transplanted into sites such as the portal vein, renal capsule, and pertioneal cavity, among many other sites.
- Graft rejection is a major complication. Immunosuppressants such as cyclosporine are used to lower the rate of rejection.

ACUTE AND SUBACUTE CARE

Nursing Management

The nursing management is similar to that of a client who has undergone liver transplantation.

In addition to routine postoperative care:

- Monitor hemoglobin and blood glucose results.
- Monitor for signs/symptoms of rejection. (A successful pancreatic transplantation is assessed by analyzing the blood glucose and C-peptide levels. C-peptide levels are elevated and there is a normal blood sugar level 2–3 days postoperatively in a successful transplant).
- Monitor intake and output.
- Monitor for signs/symptoms of infection.
- Advance activity as tolerated.
- Administer immunosuppressants as ordered.

COMMUNITY AND SELF-CARE

Instruct the client regarding:

- disease process and treatment regime
- importance of immunosuppressive therapy
- signs/symptoms of rejection
- activity and lifting restrictions
- blood glucose monitoring
- importance of follow-up care

(For more information, see p. 1931 of Black and Matassarin-Jacobs: *Medical-Surgical Nursing: Clinical Management for Continuity of Care,* 5th ed.)

Pancreatitis, Acute

OVERVIEW

- Acute pancreatitis is an inflammation of the pancreas that may result in autodigestion of the pancreas by its own enzymes.
- The precise mechanism causing pancreatic damage is unclear. The pathologic changes may be due to premature activation of proteolytic and lipolytic pancreatic enzymes (these enzymes are nor-

mally activated in the duodenum). This causes tissue damage in the pancreas. Exactly how the enzymes are activated is unknown, but they may be triggered by reflux of bile from the duodenum into the pancreatic duct or by pancreatic duct obstruction. The net effect is autodigestion of the pancreas.

- In 90 per cent of the cases of acute pancreatitis, the cause is related to excessive alcohol intake or biliary tract disease. The exact mechanism of alcohol-related injury is unknown. For gallstone-related pancreatitis, it is believed that gallstones migrating through the ampulla of Vater cause diversion of bile into the pancreatic duct and subsequent pancreatic parenchyma injury. Other causative factors include: hyperlipidemia, hypercalcemia, pancreatic trauma, and drugs (azathioprine, estrogen).
- Acute pancreatitis is a fairly common, but potentially lethal inflammatory process that results in varying degrees of pancreatic edema, fat necrosis, and hemorrhage. Typically, the manifestations disappear once the causative factors are eliminated. Nine out of 10 clients experience the disease with mild or moderate symptoms and improve with supportive care.

CLINICAL MANIFESTATIONS

- abdominal pain—begins in mid-epigastrium and reaches maximal intensity several hours later and may radiate to the back
  - alcohol-associated pancreatitis—pain begins 12–48 hours after an episode of inebriation
  - gallstone-related pancreatitis—pain begins after a large meal
- nausea and vomiting
- fever
- tachycardia
- epigastric tenderness, abdominal distention
- jaundice (gallstone-related)
- hypotension, hypovolemia, hypoperfusion
- hyperglycemia (as a result of damage to the islets)
- hypocalcemia
- elevated white blood count
- elevated serum amylase and lipase levels

ACUTE AND SUBACUTE CARE

Medical Management

- parenteral fluid and electrolyte replacement
- insulin administration for severe hyperglycemia
- pancreatic enzymes—pancrease to replace pancreatic enzyme function
- antacids—to neutralize gastric secretions
- nasogastric tube placement to suppress pancreatic stimulation
- histamine hydrogen-receptor antagonists—ranitidine (Zantac), cimetidine (Tagemet)—to decrease hydrochloric acid production
- anticholinergics—atropine, Pro-Banthine—to decrease vagal stimulation and decrease gastrointestinal motility
- narcotic analgesics—meperidine (morphine is contraindicated because it may cause spasm of the sphincter of Oddi, which could potentiate pancreatic injury)
- NPO status initially with total parenteral nutrition (hyperalimentation) and lipid administration

Surgical Management

- longitudinal pancreaticojejunostomy (Roux-en-Y)—opening the pancreatic duct and anastomosing it side to side to the proximal jejunum
- subtotal pancreatectomy—attaching a small remnant of the remaining head of the pancreas to the duodenum
- Whipple's procedure (more extensive)—distal third of the stomach, duodenum, common bile duct, gallbladder, and head of the pancreas are removed
- cholecystectomy (excision of the gallbladder) if etiology is gallstone-related

Nursing Management

Medical

- Maintain NG tube and NPO status.
- Monitor intake and output.
- Administer PRN analgesics and assess effectiveness.
- Administer antacids, anticholinergics, and histamine hydrogen-receptor antagonists as ordered.

- Monitor pulse, blood pressure, and hemodynamic parameters for fluid volume changes.
- Monitor heart rhythm for dysrhythmias secondary to electrolyte imbalance.
- Monitor laboratory values—electrolytes, blood sugars, arterial blood gases.
- Encourage prophylactic pulmonary hygiene measures.
- Daily weights.
- Monitor response to oral intake when taking liquids (if oral intake is resumed too soon, re-exacerbation of symptoms may occur).
- Administer pancreatic enzymes (if pancreas severely damaged) as prescribed to replace enzyme deficit and aid in digestion.

Surgical

In addition to routine postoperative care:
- Assess placement and proper function and patency of drains.
- Monitor for manifestations of hypoglycemia and hyperglycemia.
- Administer analgesics as ordered.
- Monitor fluid and electrolyte balance.
- Maintain NG tube and NPO status.
- Administer pancreatic enzyme replacements when no longer NPO.
- See "Cholelithiasis," p. 164.

COMMUNITY AND SELF-CARE

Instruct client regarding:
- medication regime—pancreatic enzyme replacement, insulin replacement (both dependent upon degree of pancreatic damage)
- glucose monitoring, if indicated
- dietary restrictions:
  - — restricting alcohol, tea, coffee, spicy foods, and heavy meals that stimulate pancreatic secretion
  - — eating small, frequent meals
  - — maintaining high-protein, low-fat and moderate to high carbohydrate diet
- symptoms that may indicate recurrence—steatorrhea (fatty-looking stools), severe back or epigas-

tric pain, persistent gastritis, weight loss, symptoms of hyperglycemia, nausea, vomiting, elevated temperature
- wound care if surgery performed
- if alcohol-related, the importance of alcohol abstinence and available community resources
- importance of follow-up visits

(For more information, see pp. 1921–1929 of Black and Matassarin-Jacobs: *Medical-Surgical Nursing: Clinical Management for Continuity of Care,* 5th ed.)

Pancreatitis, Chronic

OVERVIEW

- Chronic pancreatitis is a progressive, inflammatory, destructive disease of the pancreas. It involves progressive fibrosis and degeneration of the pancreas.
- Characteristically, the pancreas is progressively destroyed by repeated exacerbations of usually mild attacks of pancreatitis. This results in scarring and calcification of pancreatic tissue with irreversible damage, affecting both endocrine and exocrine functions.
- Chronic alcoholism is the most frequent cause of chronic pancreatitis. Other causes include hyperparathyroidism, congenital anomalies, and pancreatic trauma.

CLINICAL MANIFESTATIONS

- abdominal pain—dull alternating with severe
- vomiting
- fever
- jaundice
- weight loss (client decreases food intake because food aggravates the pain)
- hyperglycemia (involvement of islet tissue)
- abdominal distention and flatus
- passage of foul, fatty stools (steatorrhea)

ACUTE AND SUBACUTE CARE

Medical Management

- analgesics
- dietary restrictions—low fat, low caffeine, no spicy foods
- insulin therapy, if indicated
- pancreatic enzyme replacement—pancrease
- histamine hydrogen-receptor antagonists—ranitidine (Zantac), cimetidine (Tagamet)

Surgical Management

- pancreatic excision—removal of all or a portion of the pancreas
- pancreaticojejunostomy—pancreatic duct is opened and anastomosed to the jejunum, relieving obstruction
- cholecystectomy (removal of the gallbladder) or choledochotomy (opening of the bile ducts surgically and removing stones)—for underlying biliary disease

Nursing Management

Medical

- Administer analgesics and monitor effectiveness.
- Monitor blood glucose levels.
- Daily weights.
- Monitor intake and output.
- Monitor for signs of delirium tremors, if alcohol-related.
- Administer pancreatic replacement therapy.

Surgical

Postoperative Care

In addition to routine postoperative care:
- Monitor for signs of hyperglycemia.
- Monitor proper function and placement of T-tube, NG tube, etc.
- Administer pancreatic replacement therapy when no longer NPO.

COMMUNITY AND SELF-CARE

Instruct client regarding:

- dietary restrictions
- insulin therapy (if indicated)
- signs of hypoglycemia and hyperglycemia
- pancreatic enzyme replacement therapy
- wound care (if postoperative)
- if alcohol-related, the importance of abstinence and available community resources
- importance of follow-up laboratory and clinic visits

(For more information, see p. 1929 of Black and Matassarin-Jacobs: *Medical-Surgical Nursing: Clinical Management for Continuity of Care,* 5th ed.)

Parkinson's Disease

OVERVIEW

- Parkinson's disease is an idiopathic syndrome characterized by tremor and rigidity.
- Parkinson's disease involves degeneration of dopamine-producing cells in the substantia nigra, which leads to degeneration of neurons in the basal ganglia. Once cell loss in the substantia nigra reaches 80 per cent, symptoms appear. The cause of nigral cell degeneration is unknown.
- Parkinson's disease most often develops in clients after age 60.
- The three cardinal features of Parkinson's disease are tremor, rigidity, and bradykinesia (slowing of the ability to initiate voluntary movement).

CLINICAL MANIFESTATIONS

- generalized feeling of stiffness
- mild, diffuse muscular pain
- hand tremor at rest ("pill-rolling" movement of the thumb against the fingers)
- difficulty initiating voluntary movements (bradykinesia)
- inability to initiate movement (akinesia)

- gait changes:
  — initially—slight stiffness of one leg while walking with corresponding arm held flexed at elbow and abducted at the shoulder; client may drag one foot
  — later—typical shuffling gait with short steps and lack of associated swinging of the arms while walking
- characteristic stance—head, shoulders, and spine flexed forward, giving the appearance of stooped posture
- characteristic facial expression—masklike without expression
- speech pattern —slow, low-volumed, and monotonous in tone with poor articulation
- involuntary drooling
- intellectual ability is usually unimpaired
- decreased lacrimation (tearing)
- constipation
- incontinence
- heat intolerance, excessive perspiration
- difficulty chewing and swallowing

Parkinsonian Crisis

Occasionally, clients experience a parkinsonian crisis as a result of emotional trauma or sudden withdrawal of medications. Symptoms include:

- severe exacerbation of tremor, rigidity, and bradykinesia
- acute anxiety
- diaphoresis
- tachycardia
- hyperpnea

ACUTE AND SUBACUTE CARE

Medical Management

- levodopa therapy—cause the release of dopamine in the central nervous system—Sinemet, Symmetral
- anticholinergics to control symptoms—Cogentin, Artane, Kemadrin

Parkinsonian Crisis

- cardiac and respiratory support

- quiet, subdued environment
- antiparkinson medications

Nursing Management

- Maintain fluid intake of at least 2000 ml/24 hours.
- Establish bowel training program.
- Initiate appropriate safety measures.
- Assess ability to perform activities of daily living.
- Collaborate with Physical and Occupational therapy for adaptive devices for ambulation and self-care activities.
- Allow plenty of time to complete activities.
- Establish a progressive activity/exercise program with adequate rest periods.

COMMUNITY AND SELF-CARE

- Instruct client regarding:
  - — disease process and prognosis
  - — bowel regime
    - regular time for bowel movement
    - fluid intake to 2000 ml/day
    - high fiber diet
    - stool softeners
  - — techniques to enhance voluntary movement
    - to reduce hand tremors—hold small objects in hand, grip arms of chair when seated, etc.
    - to initiate movement—rock back and forth
  - — daily range of motion exercises
  - — importance of good posture to prevent flexion of the neck and shoulders
  - — importance of adequate rest
  - — home safety measures
    - remove loose carpeting and throw rugs
    - place grab bars in bathroom
    - obtain elevated toilet seat
  - — use of adaptive devices for walking and to perform self-care activities
  - — importance of follow-up appointments
- Refer to available community resources.

(For more information, see pp. 878–881 of Black and Matassarin-Jacobs: *Medical-Surgical Nursing: Clinical Management for Continuity of Care,* 5th ed.)

Parotitis (Surgical Mumps)

OVERVIEW

- Parotitis is inflammation of the parotid (salivary) glands. It results from inactivity of the gland due to lack of oral intake or certain medications, such as diuretics. As secretions of the glands diminish, oral bacteria can invade and multiply.

ACUTE AND SUBACUTE CARE

Nursing Management

- Provide frequent oral hygiene.
- Ensure adequate hydration.
- Encourage use of sugarless gum or hard candies to stimulate gland secretion.

(For more information, see p. 1732 of Black and Matassarin-Jacobs: *Medical-Surgical Nursing: Clinical Management for Continuity of Care,* 5th ed.)

Pelvic Inflammatory Disease (PID)

OVERVIEW

- PID refers to ascending pelvic infections; that is, those involving the upper genital tract (beyond the cervix).
- Causative organisms include gonococci, streptococci, staphylococci, and other pus-producing organisms. Infection may spread:
  - — from the endometrium to the fallopian tubes and to the pelvic cavity
  - — via lymphatics across the parametrium to the tubes or ovaries
  - — from the pelvic cavity itself.
- Complications include: pelvic abscess, septic shock, and sterility.
- Chronic PID can occur if treatment is inadequate or the illness did not respond to treatment. Irreversible sterility may result.

CLINICAL MANIFESTATIONS

- malaise, fever, chills, general aching, tachycardia
- anorexia, nausea, vomiting
- sharp, severe aching on both sides of the abdomen or pelvis (pain is worse with defecation)
- heavy, purulent, odoriferous discharge
- chronic PID:
  — chronic pelvic discomfort, menstrual disturbances
  — dysfunctional uterine bleeding
  — constipation
  — malaise
  — periodic return of acute symptoms

ACUTE AND SUBACUTE CARE

Medical Management

- antibiotic therapy for acute or chronic PID

ACUTE AND SUBACUTE CARE

Surgical Management

- laparotomy with removal of infection for acute or chronic PID
- removal of uterus, ovaries, and tubes may be necessary in some cases of acute or chronic PID

Nursing Management

Medical

- Administer antibiotics as prescribed.
- Maintain semi-Fowler's position to promote drainage.
- Administer analgesics and assess effectiveness.
- Provide sitz baths or apply heat to the lower abdomen.
- Document amount, color, odor, and appearance of the drainage.

COMMUNITY AND SELF-CARE

- Provide support (client may feel guilty if disease was sexually transmitted).
- Encourage ventilation of feelings over loss of fertility, if appropriate.

- Instruct client regarding:
  — source of infection, need to have partner treated
  — how to identify recurrences
  — general hygienic measures to prevent recurrences
    - washing perineal area regularly with soap and water, avoid douches
    - wiping front to back
    - changing tampons or pads several times a day during menses
    - washing hands before and after changing tampons and pads and after wiping perineal area
  — maintaining adequate rest, sleep, nutrition
  — when sexual activity can be resumed, safe sex

(For more information, see pp. 2395–2398 of Black and Matassarin-Jacobs: *Medical-Surgical Nursing: Clinical Management for Continuity of Care,* 5th ed.)

Penile Disorders

URETHRAL STRICTURE

- Stricture is caused by urethral scarring or narrowing.
- Urethral stricture may be congenital or caused by untreated or severe urethritis (inflammation of the urethra) or urethral injury (including urologic instrumentation, e.g., cystoscopy).
- Clinical Manifestations
  — narrowed urinary stream
  — over-distended bladder
  — signs of infection
  — dysuria
- Treatment:
  — surgically released by urethral dilation or urethroplasty

PHIMOSIS

- In phimosis, the penile foreskin (prepuce) is constricted at the opening, making retraction difficult or impossible.

- Clinical Manifestations
  - — edema, erythema
  - — tenderness
  - — purulent drainage
- Treatment
  - — control infection, if present, with local treatment and broad-spectrum antimicrobial agents

PARAPHIMOSIS

- Paraphimosis occurs when tight foreskin, once retracted, cannot return to its normal position. Circulation is impeded, and the glans swells rapidly.
- Treatment
  - — manual reduction
  - — surgical incision

PRIAPISM

- Priapism is prolonged, persistent erection without sexual desire.
- Priapism can last hours or days and is usually very painful.
- There is no known cause, although it is sometimes associated with leukemia or sickle cell anemia.
- It is considered an emergency situation because circulation is compromised, and client may not be able to void.
- Treatment
  - — aspiration of blood from the penis followed by injection of phenylephrine intracavernosally in serial injections

(For more information, see pp. 2378–2380 of Black and Matassarin-Jacobs: *Medical-Surgical Nursing: Clinical Management for Continuity of Care,* 5th ed.)

Peptic Ulcer Disease

OVERVIEW

- Peptic ulceration is a break in continuity of esophageal, gastric, or duodenal mucosa.

- Peptic ulcers may form when aggressive factors exceed the defensive resistance of the mucosa. Aggressive factors may be the result of hypersecretion of gastric juices, increased stimulation of the vagus, decreased inhibition of gastric secretions, increased capacity or number of the parietal cells to secrete acid, or increased response of the parietal cells to the stimulator. Defensive resistance depends on: mucosal integrity and regeneration; presence of a protective mucous barrier; adequate blood flow to the mucosa; the ability of the duodenal inhibitory mechanism to regulate secretion; and the presence of adequate gastromucosal prostaglandins.
- Peptic ulcer disease occurs in 10 per cent of the population.
- There are three types of ulcers:
  (1) Duodenal ulcers—occur within 1.5 cm of the pylorus. They are characterized by high gastric acid secretion or sometimes normal gastric acid secretion in conjunction with rapid emptying of the stomach. The cause of more than 90 per cent are due to H. Pylori.
  (2) Gastric ulcers—occur within one inch of the pylorus of the stomach in an area of gastritis. They are most likely caused by a break in the "mucosal barrier" and tend to heal within a few weeks. The cause of more than 70 per cent are due to H. Pylori.
  (3) Stress ulcers—usually occur after an acute medical crisis. They may be caused by:
  — severe trauma or major illness
  — severe burns (sometimes called Curling's ulcers)
  — head injury or intracranial disease (often called Cushing's ulcers)
  — drug ingestion
  — shock
  — sepsis
- Complications of ulcers include hemorrhage, perforation, and obstruction (due to repeated ulcerations and scarring).
- Risk factors include: H. Pylori bacteria, smoking, steroids, aspirin, caffeine, alcohol, Crohn's dis-

ease, Zollinger-Ellison syndrome, hepatic disease, and biliary disease.

CLINICAL MANIFESTATIONS

- aching, burning, cramp-like gnawing pain between the xiphoid cartilage and umbilicus
- pain in upper epigastrium with localization to the left of the midline (gastric ulcers)
- pain in right epigastrium (duodenal ulcers)
- pain associated with food intake and relieved by vomiting (gastric ulcers)
- pain when stomach is empty, relieved by food or antacids (duodenal ulcers)
- gastrointestinal bleeding
- nausea, vomiting

ACUTE AND SUBACUTE CARE

Medical Management

- The treatment for H. Pylori includes: bismuth subsalicylate (Pepto-Bismol), metronidazole (Flagyl), and tetracycline or amoxicillin for 2 weeks.
- hyposecretory agents (cause reduction in acid secretion):
  - H_2 receptor antagonists—block histamine-stimulated gastric secretion (e.g., ranitidine [Zantac], famotidine [Pepcid], cimetidine [Tagamet])
  - prostaglandin analogs—inhibit gastric acid secretion (misoprostal [Cytotec])
  - proton pump inhibitors—suppress secretion of gastric acid (omeprazole [Prilosec])
  - anticholinergics—decrease gastrointestinal motility and inhibit gastric acid secretion by blocking the action of acetylcholine on smooth muscles (e.g., dicyclomine [Bentyl])
  - antacids—generally increase gastric pH to reduce pepsin activity and strengthen the mucosal barrier and esophageal sphincter tone
- mucosal barrier fortifiers (e.g., sucralfate)
  - prevent hydrogen ion back diffusion into the mucosa and stimulate mucous production
- avoidance of coffee, alcohol, and milk
- physical and emotional rest

- stress reduction

Medical Management of Complications Due to Ulcers

hemorrhage

- nasogastric tube to suction with room temperature or cool saline lavage
- arterial administration of vasopressin
- arterial embolization via angiography
- ranitidine and antacids
- replacement of fluid, blood, and electrolytes
- multipolar electrocoagulation (MPEC)—cauterization of the bleeding lesion with a bipolar electric current via endoscopy
- heater probe therapy—application of heat via endoscopy to cauterize the lesion

perforation

- nasogastric tube to suction
- antibiotics
- replacement of fluid, blood, and electrolytes
- surgical intervention, see "Surgical Management" below

Surgical Management

- vagotomy—involves varying degrees of cutting or partially severing the vagus nerves. Eliminates the acid-secreting stimulus to gastric cells.
- vagotomy with pyloroplasty—involves cutting the right and left vagus nerves and widening the existing exit of the stomach at the pylorus. Prevents stasis and enhances emptying.
- gastroenterostomy—creation of a drain in the bottom of the stomach sewn to an opening made in the jejunum. Permits regurgitation of alkaline duodenal contents, thereby neutralizing gastric acid.
- antrectomy—removal of the entire antrum of the stomach, thus excising the cells that secrete gastrin. Reduces the acid-secreting portion of the stomach.
- subtotal gastrectomy—a term referring to any surgery that involves partial removal of the stomach:
  (1) Billroth I—removal of a part of the distal portion of the stomach, including the antrum. The remainder of the stomach is anastomosed to

the duodenum (combined procedure called gastroduoden-ostomy). It decreases the incidence of dumping syndrome that often occurs after a Billroth II procedure.

(2) Billroth II—reanastomosis of the proximal remnant of the stomach to the proximal jejunum (gastrojejunostomy). The duodenum is preserved because pancreatic secretions and bile necessary for digestion continue to be secreted into the duodenum even after gastrectomy, and a route to the intestine must be preserved for them.

- total gastrectomy—removal of the stomach with anastomosis of the esophagus to the jejunum (esophagojejunostomy). The thoracic approach is used. Principal intervention for stomach cancer.

Surgical Management of Complications Due to Ulcers

- hemorrhage—partial gastric resection, excision of the ulcer, vagotomy or pyloroplasty (see above)
- perforation—evacuation of the gastric contents, flushing the peritoneal cavity and patching the perforation with a small piece of omentum
- obstruction—pyloroplasty

Potential Complications Following Gastric Surgery

- marginal ulcers—ulcers at operative site
- hemorrhage
- alkaline reflux gastritis—due to reflux of duodenal contents when the pylorus is bypassed or removed
- acute gastric dilation—postoperative distention of the stomach
- vitamin B_{12} and folic acid deficiency
- reduced absorption of calcium and vitamin D
- "dumping syndrome"—often occurs following a Billroth II procedure. Due to rapid entry of food into the jejunum without proper mixing or duodenal digestive processing. Usually subsides in 6–12 months. See "Nursing Management," p. 548, for signs/symptoms.
- gastrojejunocolic fistula—characterized by fecal vomiting, diarrhea, weight loss, and anorexia
- pyloric obstruction—manifested by vomiting

Nursing Management

Medical

- Administer medications to: eliminate H. Pylori, neutralize gastric acids (antacids), block the release of histamine (H_2-receptor antagonists), and protect the gastric mucosa.
- Monitor gastric pH.
- Encourage rest to reduce peristalsis and gastric secretions.
- Administer antacids with small amounts of water to assure passage beyond the esophagus and into the stomach.
- Use Tylenol instead of aspirin when needed.
- Monitor for signs/symptoms of bleeding/hemorrhage and report to physician: dark, tarry stools (melena) or coffee ground emesis (hematemesis).
- Monitor intake and output.
- Monitor for signs/symptoms of hypovolemia.
- Maintain nasogastric tube to suction.
- Hematest nasogastric drainage and stools.
- If bleeding occurs:
  — monitor vital signs
  — administer fluids, electrolytes, and blood products
  — perform cool saline lavage (do not use iced saline—it causes mucosal damage due to decreased tissue perfusion).
- Monitor for signs/symptoms of perforation and report to physician immediately
  — sudden, sharp, severe pain beginning in the mid-epigastrium, then spreading over entire abdomen
  — abdominal tenderness, hardness, and rigidity
  — client bending over or drawing up knees to decrease tension
- If perforation occurs, prepare for surgery.
- Monitor for signs/symptoms of obstruction and report to physician
  — vomiting
  — feeling of fullness
  — abdominal distention
  — pain at night
- Instruct on small frequent meals and bland diet.

- Instruct on avoidance of milk, alcohol, tobacco, and caffeine.
- Discuss stress reduction, possible alterations in lifestyle, and relaxation techniques.
- Discuss ulcer development, rationale for treatment, and ways to prevent recurrence.

Surgical

Postoperative Care

In addition to routine postoperative care:

- Maintain patent nasogastric or gastrostomy tube to suction to prevent retention of gastric secretions.
- Assess for abdominal distention and report to physician—do not reposition tubes. Irrigate *gently* only if ordered.
- Assess amount and color of nasogastric drainage (should be bright red in immediate postoperative period, but dark red by the end of 24 hours).
- Administer pain medications and assess effectiveness.
- Assess the operative site for excessive drainage—too much fluid in the gastric stump may cause pressure and injury. Report bleeding or hemorrhaging.
- Assess for and report to physician signs/symptoms of gastric dilation (may occur in immediate postoperative period):
  — epigastric pain, tachycardia, hypotension
  — hiccups, complaints of fullness, gagging.
- Assess for alkaline reflux gastritis.
- Assess for gastrojejunocolic fistula (fecal vomiting, diarrhea, weight loss, anorexia).
- Assess for signs/symptoms of pyloric obstruction—vomiting.
- Maintain patency of chest tubes (following total gastrectomy) and monitor output.
- Assist with turning, coughing, deep breathing, and incentive spirometry (pulmonary hygiene is painful due to high abdominal incision).
- Start diet by beginning clear water, 30 ml at a time.
  — Aspirate tube approximately one hour later, to see if fluid retained.

  - Progress to soft foods and eventually to regular diet of 5–6 meals/day.
  - Discuss that progress will be slow—may take up to a year to eat three normal meals daily.
- Discuss nutritionally balanced diet.
- Assess for signs/symptoms of dumping syndrome:
  - vertigo, tachycardia, syncope, sweating, pallor, palpitations, diarrhea, and nausea 5–30 minutes after eating
  - epigastric fullness, abdominal cramping, stomach rumbling, distention, nausea, and a desire to defecate.
- Instruct client on management of dumping syndrome:
  - eat in recumbent or semi-recumbent position
  - lie down after meals
  - increase fat content in diet
  - no fluids 1 hour before, 2 hours after, or with meals
  - take medications as ordered to delay gastric emptying

COMMUNITY AND SELF-CARE

MEDICAL

- Instruct client regarding:
  - need for compliance with therapy (recurrence rate is over 50 per cent if maintenance therapy stopped)
  - need to continue medical regimen even though pain may be gone
  - factors that cause pain and ways to eliminate
  - stress reduction, coping, and relaxation techniques
  - diet and foods/beverages to avoid
  - signs/symptoms of complications and to report these to physician
  - signs/symptoms of recurrence and to report these to physician
  - avoidance of aspirin, aspirin-containing products, and nonsteroidal anti-inflammatory agents as these are ulcerogenic
  - smoking cessation program

SURGICAL

- In addition to the above interventions under "Medical," instruct the client regarding:
  - — signs/symptoms of infection
  - — wound care
  - — adequate nutrition, progression of diet
  - — need for follow-up for pernicious anemia for clients who had gastric resection
  - — management of dumping syndrome
  - — signs/symptoms of complications and to report these to physician

(For more information, see pp. 1764–1781 Black and Matassarin-Jacobs: *Medical-surgical Nursing: Clinical Management for Continuity of Care,* 5th ed.)

Pericarditis, Acute

OVERVIEW

- Pericarditis is a syndrome caused by inflammation of the parietal and visceral pericardium.
- This inflammatory process may develop either as a primary condition or secondary to a number of diseases. It may be acute or chronic.
- Pericarditis may be either exudative or dry (fibrinous). The exudate can accumulate in the pericardial sac causing a tamponade that restricts cardiac filling and emptying. Dry pericarditis can follow a common viral infection, myocardial infarction, tuberculosis, bacteremia, or renal failure. Adhesions form within the pericardial space, along with deposits of serous fibrin and calcification.

CLINICAL MANIFESTATIONS

- chest pain similar to myocardial infarction; at other times mimics pleurisy. Pain is exacerbated with respirations and rotating the trunk but does not radiate. Sitting up frequently relieves the pain.
- pericardial friction rub—a classic manifestation produced by inflamed, roughened pericardial layers that create friction as the surfaces rub together

- fever, chills, malaise, joint pain, anorexia
- dyspnea

ACUTE AND SUBACUTE CARE

Medical Management

- specific treatment for underlying causes
- nonsteroidal anti-inflammatory agents
- analgesia
- pericardiocentesis to drain the pericardial sac is not indicated unless there is evidence of cardiac compression caused by cardiac tamponade

Nursing Management

- Assess for changes in cardiac or respiratory status.
- Assess for cardiac tamponade (paradoxical pulse greater than 10 mmHg, muffled heart sounds, distended neck veins, hypotension, narrowed pulse pressure). See "Cardiac Tamponade," p. 125.
- Treat fever with rest, cooling measures, forced fluids, and antipyretics.
- Administer antimicrobial therapy as prescribed.
- Encourage fluids and well-balanced diet.
- Administer PRN analgesics.
- Provide adequate rest periods.
- Implement progressive activity schedule.

COMMUNITY AND SELF-CARE

Instruct client regarding:

- disease process and treatment regime
- how to monitor pulse and rhythm and to report any sudden changes
- importance of follow-up care

(For more information, see pp. 1335–1337 of Black and Matassarin-Jacobs: *Medical-Surgical Nursing: Clinical Management for Continuity of Care,* 5th ed.)

Pericarditis, Chronic Constrictive

OVERVIEW

- Chronic constrictive pericarditis is an inflammatory condition in which the pericardium changes into a thick, fibrous band of tissue. This tissue encircles, encases, and compresses the heart preventing proper ventricular filling and emptying. Cardiac failure eventually results.
- Chronic constrictive pericarditis usually begins with an initial episode of acute pericarditis characterized by fibrin deposition, often with pericardial effusion.
- Constrictive pericarditis is a progressive disease without spontaneous reversal of symptoms. The majority of clients become progressively more disabled over time.

CLINICAL MANIFESTATIONS

- fatigue on exertion
- dyspnea
- leg edema
- ascites
- low pulse pressure
- distended neck veins
- delayed capillary refill

ACUTE AND SUBACUTE CARE

Medical Management

- digitalis
- diuretics
- sodium restriction

Surgical Management

- excision of the damaged pericardium (pericardiectomy)—should be performed early in the disease

Nursing Management

Medical

- Administer digitalis and diuretics as ordered.

- Monitor intake and output.
- Assess for signs/symptoms of increased cardiac failure.
- Initiate Dietary consult for sodium restricted diet.
- Monitor cardiovascular response to activity and encourage rest periods.

Surgical

- See "Cardiac Surgery," p. 122 for care of the client following cardiac surgery.

COMMUNITY AND SELF-CARE

Instruct the client regarding:
- disease process and treatment regime
- activity restrictions
- dietary restrictions
- signs/symptoms to report
- importance of follow-up care

(For more information, see p. 1337 of Black and Matassarin-Jacobs: *Medical-Surgical Nursing: Clinical Management for Continuity of Care,* 5th ed.)

Peripheral Vascular Disease—Acute Arterial Occlusion

OVERVIEW

- Acute occlusion of a limb's main artery may be caused by trauma, embolism, or thrombosis and may occur in a healthy or diseased artery. About 90 per cent are in the lower limbs.
- Acute occlusion produces a fall in mean and pulse pressures in the distal arteries and a decrease in tissue perfusion and oxygenation.
- Arterial thrombosis is usually due to arterial obstruction by a blood clot that forms in an artery damaged by atherosclerosis.
- In arterial embolism, the wall of the artery is often healthy; the obstruction arises most frequently from a thrombus within the heart. Causitive factors

include atrial fibrillation, myocardial infarction, prosthetic heart valves, and rheumatic heart disease. In the lower extremities, over half of the emboli lodge in either the superficial femoral or the popliteal artery.

CLINICAL MANIFESTATIONS

- pain
- paresthesia
- loss of position sense
- coldness
- paralysis
- pallor progressing to mottled cyanosis
- pulselessness

Muscle necrosis may start as early as 2–3 hours after occlusion. Complete paralysis with stiffness of muscles and joints indicate irreversible damage.

ACUTE AND SUBACUTE CARE

Medical Management

- anticoagulant therapy
- thrombolytic therapy

Surgical Management

- embolectomy — removal of the embolus through an incision
- for thrombus, a reconstructive procedure for revascularization of the limb may be performed. See "Peripheral Vascular Disease: Chronic Arterial," p. 556.

Nursing Management

Medical

- Administer anticoagulant or thrombolytic therapy as prescribed. See "Peripheral Vascular Disease: Chronic Arterial," p. 556.

Surgical

- See Surgical Management, "Peripheral Vascular Disease: Chronic Arterial", p. 556.

(For more information, see p. 1424 of Black and Matassarin-Jacobs: *Medical-Surgical Nursing: Clinical Management for Continuity of Care,* 5th ed.)

Peripheral Vascular Disease—Chronic Arterial

OVERVIEW

- Peripheral arterial occlusive disorders are conditions that involve narrowing of the arterial lumen or damage to the endothelial lining.
- Most of the pathologic changes that occur in peripheral arterial occlusive disease are due to atherosclerosis. Other causes include embolism, thrombosis, trauma, vasospasm, and inflammation.
- Any alteration in blood flow disrupts the balance between oxygen supply and demand. Prolonged reduction of blood flow or the involvement of large areas of decreased perfusion initiates the compensatory mechanisms of vasodilation, collateralization, and utilization of anaerobic pathways for metabolic needs to be met.
- The clinical manifestations of chronic arterial occlusion due to peripheral vascular disease do not appear for 20–40 years. The most common locations for stenosis in a lower extremity are the aortoiliac bifurcation and the femoral bifurcation. These lesions cause narrowing of the arterial lumen and slowly, but critically, reduce blood flow.
- Aortoiliac disorders are characterized by aortoiliac stenosis and occlusion. Femoropopliteal disorder refers to an occlusion in the chief arteries of the proximal leg or thigh.

CLINICAL MANIFESTATIONS

Onset of clinical manifestations is gradual as plaques encroach progressively into the lumen.

- tightening pressure in the calves or buttocks or a sharp, cramplike sensation that occurs during walking and disappears quickly with rest (intermittent claudication)
  - — symptoms are constant and reproducible
  - — as disease progresses, episodes occur more frequently with less exertion
- rest pain, usually at night when client is supine
  - — indicates progressive disease

— described as a dull aching in the toes or forefoot
— hanging the legs over the side of the bed or walking around brings relief
- dependent rubor of affected foot
- weak or absent peripheral pulses
- hypertrophied toenails
- tissue atrophy, ulceration, and gangrene
- paresthesias with exertion

ACUTE AND SUBACUTE CARE

Medical Management

Medical management is recommended for clients with intermittent claudication and, in general, mild to moderate disease. Surgical intervention is reserved for clients who develop rest pain, nonhealing ulcers, or disabling claudication.

- smoking cessation—clients who have quit smoking have been shown to improve their treadmill walking distance
- vascular rehabilitation—daily walking exercise
- dietary management—weight reduction, low cholesterol, low fat, high fiber (beneficial effect on lipid levels)
- pharmacologic management
  — nicotinic acid, fibrin acid derivatives, bile acid resins, meglutol and probucol—decrease lipid levels
  — vasodilators—Trental
- thrombolytic therapy—thrombolytic agents, such as streptokinase and urokinase, are given through a peripheral vein or intra-arterial catheter

Surgical Management

- endovascular interventions
  — percutaneous transluminal angioplasty (PTA, balloon angioplasty)—a catheter with a distal inflatable balloon is used to mechanically dilate stenotic vessels
  — laser-assisted balloon angioplasty (LABA)—uses laser energy and balloon catheter to reverse ischemia by reforming the diseased artery

- peripheral atherectomy—uses a catheter with high speed rotating drill and circular cutters or blades to pulverize the plaque into small particles that are suctioned back through the catheter
- intravascular stents—generally placed after balloon angioplasty, stents are designed to provide a scaffold to maintain the intraluminal structure of the artery
- Following endovascular interventions, clients will take aspirin or dipyridamole as antiplatelet therapy on a long-term basis.

- axillofemoral grafting—graft starts at the axillary artery and travels subcutaneously along the lateral chest wall to the femoral artery
  - reserved for clients who have increased operative risk
  - higher incidence of occlusion than aortofemoral grafts (60–70 per cent at 5 years)
- aortofemoral bypass grafting—use of client's own saphenous vein or synthetic graft to bypass femoral artery and anastomose to the popliteal artery (for above the knee occlusion) or to the posterior tibial, anterior tibial or peroneal arteries (for below the knee occlusion). The patency rates of aortofemerol grafts are 80 to 90 per cent at 5 years.
- arterial reconstruction—using in situ grafting, the client's saphenous vein that is stripped of its valves and anastomosed proximally and distally in area of occlusion

Nursing Management

Medical

- Assess area distal to occlusion for pulses, skin changes, or sensory changes.
- Position the client to maintain tissue perfusion to affected extremity.
  - Place in reverse Trendelenburg position (severe cases).
  - Encourage to sit with feet flat on floor.
- Provide warm environment (chilling can cause vasoconstriction).
  - The use of hot water bottles, heating pads, or hot foot soaks is contraindicated because heat

increases tissue metabolism, and if arteries are unable to dilate, blood flow is inadequate and tissues become necrotic.

- Encourage nicotine and caffeine restriction (cause vasoconstriction).
- Provide restful environment and instruct on relaxation techniques (high emotional levels cause vasoconstriction).
- Keep areas of ulceration clean and free from pressure and irritation.
  - — Debridement and/or whirlpool treatments may be standard interventions.
- Provide meticulous skin and foot care.
- Administer PRN analgesics.
- Implement prescribed exercise program and monitor tolerance.
  - — When assisting with a walking program, make it clear that pain should be the guide to amount of activity. (Intermittent claudication signals that muscles and tissues are not receiving enough oxygen).
- Maintain bedrest as ordered for clients with ulcers, pain at rest, cellulitis, or deep vein thrombosis (even minimal activity can raise oxygen requirements above what damaged arteries can provide).

Postendovascular Intervention

- Assess arterial puncture sites for swelling, bleeding, ecchymosis, or hematoma formation (clients are anticoagulated during procedure).
- Assess peripheral pulses as ordered.
- Maintain bedrest and limb movement restriction as ordered.
- Monitor for signs/symptoms of circulatory compromise, such as sudden change in limb color or temperature, increasing muscle discomfort, pain at rest, and motor or sensory paresthesias.

Thrombolytic Therapy

- Obtain baseline values for partial thromboplastin time, prothrombin time, thrombin time, platelet count, hematocrit, and white blood count (a recent streptococcal infection may diminish the drug's effectiveness).

- Obtain baseline pulses and assessment of affected extremity.
- Assess vital signs, pulses, skin color, movement, and sensation during infusion as ordered.
- Assess for signs of bleeding or hematoma formation at infusion site.
- Assess for clinical manifestations of bleeding from gastrointestinal or genitourinary tracts or into intracerebral or retroperitoneal areas.
- Monitor serial laboratory tests (see above).
- Position affected extremity in straight alignment to facilitate perfusion.
- Avoid intramuscular injections for 24 hours after infusion.

Surgical

Preoperative Care

In addition to routine preoperative care:

- Obtain baseline peripheral pulses and mark area where found to assist in postoperative assessment.
- Administer prescribed preoperative broad spectrum antibiotics (usually for 48 hours)—all infections must be resolved, especially if using a synthetic graft.
- Protect the limb from pressure or trauma and position level or slightly dependent.
- Administer preoperative IV fluids to ensure adequate circulating blood volume to perfuse the graft.

Postoperative Care

In addition to routine postoperative care:

- Monitor anticoagulation therapy (heparin infusion).
- Maintain bedrest with leg flat in bed.
  - Leg is usually wrapped with light dressings or a vascular boot.
  - Leg swelling is commonly related to reperfusion of ischemic muscles and surgical dissection around lymphatic drainage systems.
- Monitor for signs/symptoms of fluid volume deficit related to hemorrhage, hematoma, or third spacing of fluid

- Observe for increase in pulse, decrease in blood pressure, anxiety, restlessness, pallor, thirst, oliguria, and change in level of consciousness.
    - Check dressings for excessive drainage.
    - Assess pulmonary artery pressures and/or cardiac output.
    - Monitor daily weights.
    - Monitor intake and output.
- Monitor patency of graft by checking pedal pulses, skin color, movement, and sensation of extremity as ordered.
- Monitor laboratory findings—arterial blood gases, partial thromboplastin time, hemoglobin, hematocrit, white blood count.
- Monitor for signs of bleeding from anticoagulation therapy (gastrointestinal, retroperitoneal, intracerebral, operative site, etc.).
- Avoid raising knee gatch or placing pillow under the knees.
- Administer broad spectrum antibiotics and monitor for clinical manifestations of infection.
- Assess for signs/symptoms of compartment syndrome—pain, paresthesia, diminished or absent pulses, coolness.
- Administer PRN analgesics.
- Encourage range of motion exercises while on bedrest and progressive ambulation when out of bed activities are permitted.
- Facilitate Physical therapy consult.
- Monitor response to increased activity.

COMMUNITY AND SELF-CARE

Medical

Instruct client regarding:
- disease process and treatment regime
- foot care
    - do not soak feet
    - dry well between toes
    - check bath temperature with thermometer or elbow to prevent burns
    - gently rub corns or calluses, avoid cutting or home surgery
    - use clippers (not scissors) to cut toenails and trim straight across

— never go barefoot
— wear well-fitted shoes
- skin care
  — inspect affected extremity daily
  — report ulcerations, redness, blisters, or cracks
  — use lotion (nonperfumed) to prevent dryness
  — avoid sunburn
  — do not use heating pads, hot water bottles, etc.
  — do not cross legs
- dietary modifications—low fat, low cholesterol, low calorie, no caffeine
- prescribed exercise regime
  — walking is most often prescribed
  — rest if pain occurs and then begin again
  — walk indoors in the winter to prevent injury from falls and avoid vasoconstriction from cold temperatures
  — exercise instruction
- smoking cessation programs
- importance of long-term antiplatelet therapy (aspirin or dipyridamole)
- relaxation techniques
- importance of check-ups (usually every 3 months) to assess progress of disease

SURGICAL

Instruct client regarding:
- wound care
- exercise regime
- foot and skin care (see "Focused Discharge Care," Medical section)
- long-term antiplatelet or anticoagulation therapy
- importance of follow-up visits

(For more information, see pp. 1405–1424 of Black and Matassarin-Jacobs: *Medical-Surgical Nursing: Clinical Management for Continuity of Care,* 5th ed.)

Peritonitis

OVERVIEW

- Peritonitis is inflammation of the peritoneal membrane, which is normally sterile.
- Sources of inflammation may be through the bloodstream, the external environment, or the gastrointestinal tract. Normal flora of the intestine becomes a source of infection if it enters the sterile peritoneal cavity.

CLINICAL MANIFESTATIONS

- pain, usually localized but may be generalized
- abdominal rigidity
- increase in pain with any pressure or motion of the abdomen
- nausea, vomiting, low-grade fever
- shallow respirations
- absence of bowel sounds

ACUTE AND SUBACUTE CARE

Medical Management

- fluid, electrolyte and protein replacement
- long intestinal tube to suction
- intravenous antibiotic therapy

Surgical Management

- incision and drainage of the abscess once it is walled off

Nursing Management

Medical

- Monitor intake and output.
- Assess for adequate hydration
  - — moist mucous membranes
  - — good skin turgor.
- Daily weights.
- Maintain NPO status and administer intravenous fluids.
- Assess for signs/symptoms of sepsis.

- Maintain nasogastric tube to suction.

Surgical

Postoperative Care

In addition to routine postoperative care:

- Monitor for complications of adult respiratory distress syndrome, sepsis or shock.

COMMUNITY AND SELF-CARE

Instruct client regarding:

- signs/symptoms of infection and to report to physician
- wound care
- activity restrictions
- need to finish full course of antibiotics

(For more information, see pp. 1793–1794 of Black and Matassarin-Jacobs: *Medical-Surgical Nursing: Clinical Management for Continuity of Care,* 5th ed.)

Pharyngitis

- Pharyngitis is an inflammation of the pharynx caused by a virus or bacteria and is spread by droplet.
- Chronic pharyngitis occurs in people who use tobacco, alcohol, have a chronic cough, use their voices excessively, and are exposed to dust in the workplace.
- The clinical manifestations include: sore throat, difficulty swallowing, fever, malaise, cough, and elevated white blood cell count.
- The medical management depends on the causative agent but is usually treated with antibiotics.
- The nursing care involves good handwashing techniques, rest, fluids, warm saline gargles, analgesics, and antipyretics as needed.

(For more information, see p. 1079 of Black and Matassarin-Jacobs: *Medical-Surgical Nursing: Clinical Management for Continuity of Care,* 5th ed.)

Pheochromocytoma

OVERVIEW

- Pheochromocytoma is a catecholamine-secreting tumor of the adrenal medulla. Excessive secretion of epinephrine and norepinephrine by the tumor can produce severe symptoms and death.
- Pheochromocytomas are rare and equally common in women and men. The disease most commonly occurs in middle age and rarely after age 60.
- Tumors are typically benign.

CLINICAL MANIFESTATIONS

- hypertension (persistent, fluctuating, intermittent, or paroxysmal in nature)
- pounding headache
- diaphoresis
- apprehension
- palpitations
- nausea and vomiting
- hyperglycemia and glucosuria (excessive catecholamine release results in increased conversion of glycogen to glucose)
- acute attacks are associated with profuse diaphoresis, dilated pupils, and cold extremities
- severe hypertension can precipitate cerebral vascular accident or sudden blindness

ACUTE AND SUBACUTE CARE

Medical Management

- alpha-adrenergic blocking agents for hypertensive crises

Surgical Management

Surgical management is the treatment of choice.

- unilateral or bilateral adrenalectomy (removal of adrenal gland(s))

NURSING MANAGEMENT

Medical

- Administer alpha-adrenergics as prescribed.
- Administer sedatives as ordered.
- Monitor blood pressure closely.
- Assess neurologic status for changes.
- Promote rest.
- Prohibit beverages or food with caffeine.

Surgical

POSTOPERATIVE CARE

In addition to routine postoperative care:

- Assess for signs/symptoms of shock (profound shock can develop as catecholamine levels drop) and hemorrhage (due to high vascularity of the adrenal glands).
- Administer corticosteroids as ordered.
- Prevent shock by:
  - — administration of IV replacement fluids as ordered.
  - — administration of IV pressor agents titrated to blood pressure parameters
  - — monitoring of urine output
- Assess for signs of adrenal insufficiency (profound weakness; severe abdominal, back, or leg pain; hyperpyrexia followed by hypothermia; and coma).

COMMUNITY AND SELF-CARE

Instruct client regarding:

- importance of daily hormonal replacement
- medication injection technique when client not able to tolerate oral medications
- signs of under- and overdosage
- need to call for dosage adjustment if experiencing emotional or physical stress
- need for Medic Alert bracelet and card

(For more information, see pp. 2056–2060 of Black and Matassarin-Jacobs: *Medical-Surgical Nursing: Clinical Management for Continuity of Care,* 5th ed.)

Pituitary Tumors

OVERVIEW

- Pituitary tumors usually occur in the anterior lobe of the pituitary and are benign.
- Hyperpituitarism is defined as oversecretion of one or more of the hormones secreted by the pituitary gland. Syndromes associated with hyperpituitarism are Cushing's syndrome, acromegaly, amenorrhea, galactorrhea, and hyperthyroidism.

CLINICAL MANIFESTATIONS

- visual changes or deficits
- headache
- irregular or absent menstrual cycles and infertility in females
- decreased libido or impotence in males
- galactorrhea—abnormal milk production
- excessive or abnormal growth patterns due to overproduction of growth hormone
- early signs of increasing intracranial pressure

ACUTE AND SUBACUTE CARE

Surgical Management

- transphenoidal hypophysectomy—removal of the tumor via an incision made inside the mouth, at the junction between the upper lip and gum

Nursing Management

Transphenoidal Hypophysectomy

Postoperative Care

Nursing care following transphenoidal hypophysectomy is similar to care following craniotomy (see "Intracranial Tumors," p. 431).

In addition to routine postoperative care:

- Monitor for diabetes insipidus (dilute urine output of 2–15 liters/day—due to a lack of antidiuretic hormone [ADH]).
  - — Accurate intake and output, assessing for polyuria and polydipsia.

— Obtain urine specific gravity every 2 hours, assessing for dilute urine (specific gravity 1.000–1.005).
— Assess for electrolyte imbalance.
— Weigh daily.

- Monitor for signs of cerebral edema and rising intracranial pressure (elevated BP, widened pulse pressure, bradycardia, altered respiratory pattern).
- Monitor for manifestations of target gland deficiencies such as, adrenal insufficiency (sudden penetrating pain in the back, abdomen, or legs, volume depletion, shock) and hypothyroidism (decreased heart rate, decreased BP, somnolence).
- Monitor for signs of meningitis (temperature elevation, severe headache, irritability, nuchal rigidity).
- Assist with frequent oral hygiene with saline rinses and use of foam toothettes (toothbrushes are not used at first as this may disrupt the suture line). Lubricate the lips with petroleum jelly.
- Advance diet and instruct client to avoid rough foods.
- Administer replacement hormones, as ordered.
- Maintain nasal packing to control bleeding (2–5 days). After its removal, observe client for rhinorrhea—can indicate a CSF leak.
- Instruct client to avoid all activities (bending, straining, coughing, sneezing) that may increase intracranial pressure.

COMMUNITY AND SELF-CARE

Instruct client/significant other regarding:

- disease process and treatment regime
- replacement hormone therapy and signs/symptoms of under- or overdose
- correct use of vasopressin (Pitressin), if prescribed for diabetes insipidus
- importance of adequate fluids and how to assess adequate fluid balance (diabetes insipidus)
- signs/symptoms of infection
- need to report persistent postnasal drainage
- oral wound care
- need to avoid sneezing, coughing, and bending from the waist

- need for Medic Alert bracelet or card
- importance of follow-up laboratory tests and visits to physician

(For more information, see pp. 2062–2065 of Black and Matassarin-Jacobs: *Medical-Surgical Nursing: Clinical Management for Continuity of Care,* 5th ed.)

Plastic Surgery

OVERVIEW

- Plastic surgery is the surgical subspecialty concentrating on the restoration of function and form to body structures damaged by trauma, the aging process, disease processes such as skin cancer, and congenital defects.
- Plastic surgery is divided into two major areas:
  (1) aesthetic (cosmetic) surgery—alteration of any physical feature that is already within the "normal" range
  (2) reconstructive surgery—attempt to restore an abnormal body part to normal. The abnormality may be due to injured tissue, disease, or missing tissues.
- Deformities can be actual (that is, objectively measured by others) or perceived (the client is aware of the deformity, but it may not be noticeable to others).
- Plastic surgeons strive for minimal scarring by:
  — making incisions parallel to natural skin lines
  — use of elliptical incisions (the incision lines are longer than the lesion)
  — use of precise suturing techniques.
- Types of surgical modalities
  — microvascular surgery
    - implants—different types of materials are used to augment or replace tissue
    - skin expansion—technique used to increase the amount of local tissue available to reconstruct a defect. An inflatable silicone balloon is implanted under the skin or muscle adjacent to the defect. The expander is inflated

over a period of time to stretch the overlying tissue.
  - lasers—use of a precise beam of light to cause cell destruction with the advantages of reduced bleeding and swelling
- grafts—tissue that is harvested without a blood supply from a donor site. It is transferred to a recipient site, where it develops a new blood supply. A *split-thickness skin graft* is a very thin graft containing epidermis and a very thin layer of dermis. A *full-thickness graft* contains all of the epidermis and dermis. Thinner grafts are more likely to contract during healing, but also are more likely to develop an adequate blood supply. Full thickness grafts are used in areas where contraction would limit function, such as the hand or over joints.
- flaps—tissue that is elevated with its blood supply intact. It may be rotated to reconstruct an adjacent defect or detached from its blood supply at the donor site and reattached to veins and arteries at the recipient site by microvascular anastomosis.

ACUTE AND SUBACUTE CARE

Nursing Management

In addition to routine preoperative care:

- Identify nutritional deficiencies and assist to correct.
- Assist to develop realistic postoperative expectations—report unrealistic expectations to the surgeon.
- Reinforce the fact that the body is naturally asymmetric.
- Instruct client to avoid aspirin and aspirin-containing compounds (interfere with platelet agglutination and promote bleeding and hematoma formation); nicotine (potent vasoconstrictor); and smoking (can result in flap necrosis).

In addition to routine postoperative care:

- Keep graft extremity elevated.
- Assess and document skin color, temperature, sensation; the blanching time of the surgical site; presence of blisters; the presence or absence of

edema or seroma (accumulation of serosanguinous drainage); and any pain, pressure, or bleeding.

— Report cool, pale, or cyanotic skin; prolonged blanching time; and changes in sensation.

— Report any sign of decreased vascularity (blue color, change in temperature, change in size or tightness). Be aware that venous stasis and edema can impair tissue perfusion.

— Report to the physician any blisters (these indicate decreased circulation and impaired tissue viability).

- Assess the client's coping mechanisms.
- Assist client to explore and express feelings.
- Gently assist client to look at and touch surgical site (help client to incorporate it into self-concept and body image).
- Encourage client to take measures (such as taking walks in the halls or accepting visitors) to begin desensitization to reactions of others.
- Encourage client to discuss reaction of others. Support grief reactions.

In addition:

Postoperative Flaps:

- Position client so that the flap is relaxed and elevated.
- Prevent tension on the flap.
- Report pallor or hematoma immediately.
- Discuss leech therapy (use of leeches to relieve venous congestion in replanted or transplanted tissue) if appropriate.

Implants/Skin Expansion:

- Monitor for and instruct client on signs/symptoms of infection or rejection: change in temperature, drainage, increasing edema, redness of skin, and increasing skin temperature.
- Instruct on percutaneous saline injections into the expander, which will be performed to stretch the skin.
- Instruct to keep incision and injection site clean and free of infection.
- Discuss how to camouflage the expander with clothing.
- Discuss sleeping positions that protect the expander from pressure.

Laser Surgery:

- Discuss use of ointment to area for 2–4 weeks.
- Discuss protection from sun exposure to treated area.

COMMUNITY AND SELF-CARE

Discharge teaching depends upon the specific operation and the surgeon's preferences.

(For more information, see pp. 2267–2288 of Black and Matassarin-Jacobs: *Medical-Surgical Nursing: Clinical Management for Continuity of Care,* 5th ed.)

Pleural Effusion

- Pleural effusion is an accumulation of fluid in the pleural space between the visceral and parietal pleura.
- Causes include congestive heart failure; liver or renal failure; infections or tumors in the pleura or pleural spaces; and lymphatic obstruction.
- Clinical manifestations depend upon the amount of fluid present. Dyspnea on exertion, decreased or absent tactile fremitus, and dull or flat percussion notes may be seen or there may be no symptoms at all.
- Thoracentesis is used to remove the fluid. The fluid is analyzed by the laboratory to aid in diagnosis.
- For recurrent pleural effusion with respiratory compromise or persistent pleural pain, obliteration of the pleural space may be performed:
  (1) Pleurectomy—surgically stripping the parietal pleura away from the visceral pleura. This produces an intense inflammatory reaction that promotes adhesion formation between the two layers during healing.
  (2) Pleurodesis—installation of a sclerosing substance (e.g., unbuffered tetracycline, nitrogen mustard, talc) into the pleural space via a thoracotomy tube. This creates an inflammatory

response that scleroses tissue together. The tube will remain clamped for a specified period of time with special positioning changes prescribed.

- Nursing care includes:
  — monitoring respiratory status, especially for dyspnea
  — administering analgesics and assessing effectiveness
  — documenting alleviation or persistence of pleural pain
  — encouraging pulmonary hygiene
  — maintaining closed chest tube drainage system (if appropriate)
  — monitoring for signs/symptoms indicating return of pleural effusion

(For more information, see pp. 1166–1167 of Black and Matassarin-Jacobs: *Medical-Surgical Nursing: Clinical Management for Continuity of Care,* 5th ed.)

Pneumonia

OVERVIEW

- Pneumonia (pneumonitis) is an inflammatory process of lung parenchyma usually associated with a marked increase in interstitial and alveolar fluid.
- In the United States pneumonia is the sixth most common cause of death and one of the most common causes of death in the elderly.
- Pneumonia may occur as a result of bacteria, viruses, mycoplasmas, fungal agents, and protozoa. It also may result from (1) inhalation of toxic or caustic chemicals, smoke, dusts, or gases or (2) aspiration of food, fluids, or vomitus.
- Staphylococcus Aureus is the most common among hospitalized adults.
- Pseudomonas aeruginosa is the most common cause of hospital-acquired gram-negative pneumonia.
- Haemophilus Influenza is the most common in children, smokers, and persons with chronic diseases.

- Streptococcus pneumoniae is the most common cause of community-acquired pneumonia.
- Klebsiella pneumoniae is the most common among the elderly.
- Legionella pneumophilia is the most common in adults and smokers.
- Mycoplasma pneumoniae affects 20–40 per cent of ambulatory clients.
- Risk factors include: smoking, air pollution, upper respiratory infection, prolonged immobility, malnutrition, prolonged debilitating disease, advanced age, AIDS, altered consciousness, and chronic illness.

CLINICAL MANIFESTATIONS

- fever, chills, sweats, pleuritic chest pain
- cough, sputum production, hemoptysis, dyspnea
- headache or fatigue
- crackling breath sounds, whispered pectoriloquy
- increased tactile fremitus over areas of pneumonia

ACUTE AND SUBACUTE CARE

Medical Management

- antibiotic therapy

Nursing Management

- Encourage fluid intake.
- Assess lung sounds and monitor for changes.
- Monitor arterial blood gases and observe for signs/symptoms of hypoxia or hypercapnia.
- Assist with turning, coughing, and deep breathing every 2 hours.
- Instruct on splinting the chest wall for comfort during coughing.
- Administer bronchodilating medications.
- Position to facilitate breathing, i.e., 45 degrees.
- Encourage use of incentive spirometer while awake.
- Administer cough suppressants and analgesics.
- Assess the baseline level of activity and monitor tolerance of activity.
- Schedule activity after treatments or medications.
- Provide adequate rest.

- Instruct on pursed-lip and diaphragmatic breathing.

COMMUNITY AND SELF-CARE

- Instruct client/significant other regarding:
  - — coughing and deep breathing
  - — importance of completing prescribed antibiotics
  - — need for adequate rest and gradual resumption of activity
  - — avoidance of conditions that increase oxygen demand: temperature extremes, weight gain, stress, and smoking
  - — need for adequate nutrition
  - — complications to report to physician: return of fever, chest pain, hemoptysis, chills
- Encourage immunization for the next winter.

(For more information, see pp. 1134–1138 of Black and Matassarin-Jacobs: *Medical-Surgical Nursing: Clinical Management for Continuity of Care,* 5th ed.)

Pneumothorax

- Pneumothorax is the presence of air in the pleural space that prevents complete lung expansion.
- An open pneumothorax is air in the pleural space from a hole in the chest wall or diaphragm. This almost always occurs due to a penetrating chest injury.
- A closed (or spontaneous) pneumothorax is air in the pleural space from a puncture or tear in an internal respiratory structure (bronchus, bronchioles, or alveoli). This may occur spontaneously or be due to a fractured rib, chest surgery, chest trauma, or may be the result of underlying pulmonary disease, such as emphysema, pulmonary neoplasms, or pneumonia.
- Clinical manifestations
  - — moderate pneumothorax—tachypnea; dyspnea; sudden sharp pain on the affected side with chest movement, breathing or coughing; asymmetric chest expansion; diminished or absent

breath sounds on the affected side; restlessness; anxiety and tachycardia
  - severe pneumothorax—all of the preceding along with distended neck veins; PMI (point of maximal impulse of heartbeat) shift; subcutaneous emphysema; decreased tactile and vocal fremitus; tracheal deviation toward the unaffected side; and progressive cyanosis
- Management
  - x-ray confirmation if time permits
  - insertion of an 18-gauge needle into the second or third intercostal space in the midclavicular line (if respiratory distress is too severe to wait for x-ray confirmation)
  - insertion of a chest tube into the pleural space and connection to closed-chest drainage (see "Closed Chest Drainage," p. 178)
  - thoracotomy—surgical opening into the chest cavity. May be done to explore the chest and repair the site of origin of the pneumothorax.

(For more information, see p. 2524 of Black and Matassarin-Jacobs: *Medical-Surgical Nursing: Clinical Management for Continuity of Care,* 5th ed.)

Pneumothorax, Open and Mediastinal Flutter

- An open pneumothorax occurs with "sucking" chest wounds. A traumatic opening in the chest wall is large enough for air to move freely in and out of the chest cavity during ventilation. This abnormal movement of air through the chest wound produces a "slurping" or "sucking" noise.
- Open sucking chest wounds may occur from accidental injuries, surgical trauma, or when a chest drainage catheter is pulled out accidentally.
- Mediastinal flutter may occur with an open pneumothorax. Mediastinal flutter occurs from air rushing in and out of the thoracic cavity on the affected side. On inspiration, the mediastinal structures (heart, trachea, and esophagus) and collapsed

lung are pushed toward the unaffected side. With expiration, these structures move back toward the affected side. This can be fatal if not treated promptly.

- Treatment
  - The wound must be immediately covered with anything available, e.g., a towel. Ask someone to bring a sterile petroleum gauze dressing. Apply this to replace the temporary covering, as soon as possible.
  - When covering the wound, ask the client to take a deep breath and attempt to blow it out while keeping the mouth and nose closed. When the client does this, apply the dressing before the client can inhale. This forces air out of the wound.
- After the dressing is applied, stay with the client. Assess closely for signs/symptoms of tension pneumothorax and mediastinal shift. This may develop if the air leak is in the lung or bronchus, which permits air to escape into the pleural space. In such a situation, closing the chest wound prevents the outflow of escaping air. Thus, an open pneumothorax has been converted into a tension pneumothorax, which is a more dangerous situation. If it appears that a tension pneumothorax is developing after sealing the wound, immediately remove the seal.
- Closed chest drainage will be necessary to remove air from the pleural space to allow lung re-expansion (see "Closed Chest Drainage," p. 178)

Also see "Pneumothorax, Tension and Mediastinal Shift," below

(For more information, see pp. 2524–2525 of Black and Matassarin-Jacobs: *Medical-Surgical Nursing: Clinical Management for Continuity of Care,* 5th ed.)

Pneumothorax, Tension and Mediastinal Shift

- Tension pneumothorax is a serious type of pneumothorax in which air enters the pleural space with each inspiration, becomes trapped there, and is not expelled during expiration. Pressure continues to build in the chest and may collapse the lung on the affected side, which then may cause a mediastinal shift. A mediastinal shift occurs when the contents of the mediastinum (heart, trachea, esophagus, and great vessels) are pushed or "shifted" toward the unaffected side of the chest.

- Mediastinal shift may cause:
  - — compression of the lung opposite the pneumothorax
  - — compression, traction, torsion or kinking of the great vessels
  - — decreased cardiac output and blood pressure
- Common causes of tension pneumothorax are blunt traumatic injuries and flail chest injuries.
- Tension pneumothorax is an emergency requiring prompt assessment and intervention.
- Clinical manifestations include:
  - — marked, severe dyspnea
  - — tachypnea, tachycardia
  - — crepitus (subcutaneous emphysema in the neck and upper chest)
  - — progressive cyanosis
  - — chest pain on the affected side
  - — asymmetric chest wall movement
  - — diminished or absent breath sounds on the affected side
  - — neck vein distention
  - — PMI (point of maximal impulse) shift laterally or medially
  - — muffled heart sounds
  - — laryngeal and tracheal deviation/shift to the unaffected side
- Management

The goal is to convert the tension pneumothorax into an open pneumothorax (a less serious disorder).

- — insertion of an 18-gauge needle on the affected side into the pleural space at the level of the second intercostal space at the midclavicular line to remove air
- — insertion of a chest catheter and connection to a waterseal drainage system after emergency treatment

Also see, "Closed Chest Drainage," p. 178

(For more information, see pp. 2525–2526 of Black and Matassarin-Jacobs: *Medical-Surgical Nursing: Clinical Management for Continuity of Care,* 5th ed.)

Poisoning and Overdose

- Accidental or intentional poisonings (overdoses) requiring emergency care occur frequently.
- Poison Control Centers, the Poison Index, and toxicology texts may be consulted for full information about various toxins.
- Emergency nursing care
  - — Obtain an accurate history.
  - — Assess and stabilize airway, breathing, and circulation.
  - — Start intravenous lines, insert a urinary catheter, initiate an ECG monitor, and obtain appropriate laboratory studies.
  - — Induce emesis *if appropriate.*
    - Client must have an intact gag reflex and be able to cooperate with emetic therapy.
    - Syrup of ipecac is the safest and most effective way to induce emesis (home remedies are often unsafe and ineffective).
    - Syrup of ipecac must be preceded or followed by several hundred milliliters of water or other solutions (juice).
    - Emesis should occur within 15–20 minutes. A second dose may be given, but do not exceed two doses.
    - Emesis is saved for toxicologic analysis; note the presence of any pill particles.
    - Syrup of ipecac in large doses may be cardiotoxic. If the client does not vomit, lavage may be necessary.
    - Reassess the client frequently. If the client becomes more obtunded, gastric lavage may need to be performed because of the risk of aspiration with emesis.
- Gastric lavage may be indicated for clients with a diminished or absent gag reflex; central nervous

system depression; or those unable to cooperate with emetic therapy.
- — Involves placement of a large bore 30- to 36-French Ewald tube (for adults) through the nose or mouth and then washing out the stomach contents by use of normal saline (avoid volumes in excess of 500 ml).
- — Lavage is carried out until return is clear.
- — Bradydysrhythmias, aspiration, and inadvertent pulmonary tube placement are possible complications of this procedure.

- Absorptives, such as activated charcoal, may be used to absorb any remaining particles of the toxic substance.
- Antidotes/antagonists may be used in selected cases for management or diagnosis of the toxic substance. Remember that the half-life of the substance may be longer than the antidote.
- Diuresis, fluid loading, cooling or warming, anticonvulsive therapy, antidysrhythmic therapy, hemodialysis, or exchange transfusions also may be necessary.
- If the overdose was intentional:
  - — Facilitate Psychiatric consult.
  - — Provide empathy and understanding; foster communication.
  - — Implement suicide precautions.
  - — Arrange for someone to stay with the client for the first several days after discharge.
  - — Provide a telephone number for crisis intervention, if the client does not wish to have them contacted while hospitalized.
  - — Provide written instructions for follow-up.
- For accidental overdoses, provide clear instructions for needed follow-up and signs/symptoms to report to physician.

(For more information, see pp. 2537–2539 of Black and Matassarin-Jacobs: *Medical-Surgical Nursing: Clinical Management for Continuity of Care,* 5th ed.)

Polio (Poliomyelitis, Acute Anterior)

- Acute anterior poliomyelitis (polio) is characterized by destruction of motor cells (particularly of the anterior horn cells in the spinal cord and brain stem) and flaccid paralysis of muscles innervated by affected neurons. Poliomyelitis spreads from the gastrointestinal tract to the nervous system. Poliomyelitis is caused by one of three types of poliovirus.
- Paralysis may be spinal or bulbar. Spinal paralysis is flaccid, asymmetric, and scattered in distribution. It tends to be more severe in one extremity (most often a leg). Involvement of the diaphragm and intercostal muscles or damage to the respiratory center involving the reticular activating center in the medulla oblongata may produce respiratory paralysis. Bulbar paralysis involves the muscles supplied by the cranial nerves because bulbar nuclei are affected. These muscles may be paralyzed alone or in combination with spinal musculature. Bulbar paralysis is often unilateral.
- Clinical manifestations include headache, stiff neck, fever, and asymmetric flaccid paralysis without sensory loss.
- Immunization with the trivalent oral poliomyelitis vaccine in infancy is the best means of prevention.
- There is a recently recognized disorder affecting victims of polio called "post-polio syndrome." It is characterized by new onset of progressive muscle weakness, fatigue, decreased endurance, pain in the joints and muscles, and respiratory problems beginning 30 or more years after the original attack. The etiology and pathophysiology are not well understood. Clients with post-polio syndrome need much support.

(For more information, see p. 860 of Black and Matassarin-Jacobs: *Medical-Surgical Nursing: Clinical Management for Continuity of Care,* 5th ed.)

Polycythemia

OVERVIEW

- Polycythemia is defined as an increase in both the numbers of circulating erythrocytes and the concentration of hemoglobin within the blood. Red blood cells may number as high as 8–12 million/mm^3, and the hemoglobin concentration rises to 18–25 g/dl.
- Polycythemia vera is classified as a myeloproliferative disorder (meaning overgrowth of bone marrow). The precise cause remains unknown. The three major hallmarks are: (1) relentless, unrestrained production of erythrocytes; (2) excessive production of myelocytes; (3) overproduction of platelets. This inordinate mass production results in: (1) an increase in blood viscosity; (2) an increase in total blood volume; (3) severe blood congestion of all tissues and organs.
- Polycythemia vera usually develops during middle age, particularly among Jewish men.
- Secondary polycythemia occurs when the body's demand for oxygen increases, and the bone marrow must produce more red cells in order to prevent hypoxia. Polycythemia may be precipitated by conditions that cause prolonged hypoxia, such as:
  - — chronic lung disease
  - — congenital heart disease
  - — prolonged exposure to altitudes of 10,000 feet or more.
- Relative polycythemia occurs when the body loses plasma without losing red blood cells, increasing the concentration of red cells relative to the amount of plasma left. Fluid loss and dehydration as a result of inadequate fluid intake, diarrhea, vomiting, burns, or diuretics may cause relative polycythemia.

CLINICAL MANIFESTATIONS

Polycythemia Vera

- asymptomatic—early stage

- feeling of fullness in the head
- dizziness, headache, tinnitus, visual disturbances
- ruddy complexion
- dusky red mucosa
- hypertension
- shortness of breath, orthopnea (due to congestive heart failure)
- evidence of thrombotic event (cerebral vascular accident, myocardial infarction, peripheral gangrene)
- hemorrhage into capillaries, venules, and arterioles
- enlargement of liver and spleen
- painful, swollen joints (gout)—secondary to increased uric acid

Secondary Polycythemia

- same as polycythemia vera except white blood cell and platelet counts are normal and splenic enlargement is absent

Relative Polycythemia

- same as secondary polycythemia

ACUTE AND SUBACUTE CARE

Medical Management

Polycythemia Vera

- phlebotomy—removal of 500–2000 ml of blood until hematocrit reaches 45 per cent
- myelosuppressive agents—radioactive phosphorus, chlorambucil, busulfan, hydroxyurea
- anticoagulant therapy
- radiation therapy—to decrease the production of red blood cells in the marrow

Secondary Polycythemia

- treatment of underlying disease or condition causing hypoxia

Relative Polycythemia

- re-establishment of fluid and electrolyte balance

Nursing Management

- Assist with phlebotomy and monitor hemodynamic status post procedure.
- Administer prescribed medications.
- Monitor vital signs and breath sounds.
- Assess for signs/symptoms of a thrombotic event.
- Encourage oral intake (to reduce blood viscosity).
- Monitor for signs of bleeding (if on anticoagulant therapy).
- Monitor laboratory findings—CBC, platelet count, prothrombin time.
- Prevent thrombi secondary to circulatory stasis
  — encourage client to ambulate
  — elevate feet when possible
  — instruct to wear support hose
  — turn bedridden client frequently and exercise extremities
- Initiate appropriate safety measures.
- See "Radiation Therapy," p. 605.
- See "Chemotherapy," p. 149.

COMMUNITY AND SELF-CARE

Instruct the client regarding:
- importance of medication regime
- signs/symptoms to report to physician
- safety measures to prevent bleeding if on anticoagulant therapy (soft toothbrush, electric razor, fall prevention, etc.)
- increased fluid intake unless otherwise contraindicated
- importance of regular exercise
- importance of follow-up appointments

(For more information, see pp. 1485–1486 of Black and Matassarin-Jacobs: *Medical-Surgical Nursing: Clinical Management for Continuity of Care,* 5th ed.)

Polyps (Uterine or Cervical)

- Polyps are pedunculated tumors arising from the mucosa and extending into the opening of a body cavity. They occasionally may undergo malignant changes.

- Cervical polyps may bleed following vaginal intercourse and are prone to infection.
- Uterine polyps may cause hypermenorrhea, intermenstrual bleeding, and postmenopausal bleeding.
- Cervical polyps may be removed in the physician's office.
- Uterine polyps may be removed by dilation and curettage as outpatient surgery.

(For more information, see p. 2411 of Black and Matassarin-Jacobs: *Medical-Surgical Nursing: Clinical Management for Continuity of Care,* 5th ed.)

Portal Hypertension

OVERVIEW

- Portal hypertension is a persistent increase in pressure in the portal venous system of the liver as a result of increased resistance or obstruction of the blood flow through the portal venous system.
- The normal flow to and from the liver depends on proper functioning of the portal vein (inflow), hepatic artery (inflow) and the hepatic veins (outflow). Disease processes that damage or alter the flow of blood through the liver or its major vessels are responsible for the development of portal hypertension.
- Cirrhosis is the leading cause of portal hypertension. Hepatic tumors or obstruction of the portal vein by a thrombus are other common causes.
- Complications arising from portal hypertension include:

  (1) hemorrhage — portal pressure causes swollen dilated veins (varices) of the superior rectal veins, abdominal wall veins, and esophago-gastric veins. These varices may rupture and bleed. Portal pressure also causes damage to the spleen. As the spleen enlarges, it tends to de-

stroy blood cells, especially platelets, which increases the risk of hemorrhage and anemia.

(2) hepatic encephalopathy—this may follow a period of bleeding into the gastrointestinal tract. Digestion of this blood takes place in the intestines. Because blood is a protein substance, this process increases ammonia in the gut and bloodstream. Excessive ammonia disturbs brain function.

CLINICAL MANIFESTATIONS

- tortuous epigastric vessels that branch off the umbilicus and lead toward sternum and ribs
- enlarged palpable spleen
- internal hemorrhoids
- ascites
- bruits heard over the upper abdomen

ACUTE AND SUBACUTE CARE

Medical Management

- propranolol (Inderal) to reduce portal pressure
- vasopressin (Pitressin)—directly infused into the superior mesenteric artery to lower portal pressure
- sclerotherapy passing an endoscope into the esophagus and injecting a sclerosing agent that flows to the varices—causes inflammation of the vein wall and then fibrosis
- direct ligation of bleeding varices
- transhepatic embolization of the left gastric vein
- insertion of a Sengstaken-Blakemore or Minnesota tube
  - — the tube is passed into the stomach and then the esophageal and gastric balloons are inflated
  - — the pressure of the balloon against the varices may stop the bleeding

Surgical Management

- creation of a portosystemic shunt—sends portal blood directly into the inferior vena cava bypassing the liver, thus reducing portal hypertension. However, this process increases the incidence of hepatic encephalopathy because the shunted blood is not cleansed of toxic substances.

Nursing Management

Medical

- Monitor daily weights.
- Measure abdominal girth daily.
- Monitor fluid balance.
- Monitor for signs/symptoms of bleeding or hemorrhage.
- Monitor hemoglobin, hematocrit, and blood ammonia levels.
- Monitor for signs/symptoms of hepatic encephalopathy
  — mental confusion
  — impaired memory or attention span
  — decreased concentration or rate of response
  — change in level of consciousness
  — drowsiness with sleep pattern reversal (awake at night, sleepy during the day)
  — change in handwriting or speech
  — asterixis (rapid extension and flexion of the fingers and wrists when the arms are extended and the hands are dorsiflexed—also called "liver flap")
- If hemorrhage occurs, monitor blood pressure, pulse, respirations, and urine output continually and assist with interventions to restore blood volume.
- Maintain Sengstaken-Blakemore/Minnesota tube:
  — Periodically deflate esophageal balloon as ordered to prevent esophageal necrosis.
  — Provide suction to remove secretions and saliva that accumulate above the balloon level to prevent aspiration. (The Minnesota tube has a fourth port for this; if no suction port is present, a nasogastric tube may be passed to the balloon level to allow for suctioning.)
  — Label each port of the balloon.
  — Cleanse and lubricate the nares to prevent erosion of the nares.
  — Keep emergency scissors at the bedside—if airway obstruction occurs, the tube must be cut and pulled out immediately. (Airway ob-

struction can occur if the gastric balloon deflates or breaks and the esophageal balloon migrates up to the oropharynx.)

- Instruct client on factors that may cause rupture of varices and must be avoided.
  - — coughing, straining at stools or any other activities that increase intra-abdominal or intrathoracic pressure
  - — spicy or rough foods that may irritate the esophageal mucosa

Surgical

Portosystemic Shunt Surgery

In addition to routine postoperative care:

- Monitor for postoperative hemorrhage.
- Monitor fluid and electrolyte balance.
- Measure baseline abdominal girth and then daily to assess for increased ascites.
- Monitor cardiovascular function carefully due to the increased venous return to the heart.
- Monitor for hepatic encephalopathy.

COMMUNITY AND SELF-CARE

- Instruct client/significant other regarding:
  - — factors that may rupture varices
  - — signs/symptoms of bleeding
  - — what to do, who to call if hemorrhage occurs
  - — signs/symptoms of hepatic encephalopathy
  - — when to contact physician
  - — shunt care (if performed)
- Refer to alcoholic treatment program or support groups as needed

See also "Hepatic Encephalopathy," p. 337, and "Cirrhosis," p. 174.

(For more information, see pp. 1884–1889 of Black and Matassarin-Jacobs: *Medical-Surgical Nursing: Clinical Management for Continuity of Care,* 5th ed.)

Premenstrual Syndrome (PMS)

- Premenstrual syndrome (PMS) is a disorder that is not well understood but defined as a combination of physical and emotional features that occur in females before and sometimes during menstruation period.
- This disorder occurs mostly in females between the ages of 30 and 40.
- The risk factors include: estrogen-progesterone imbalance; fluid retention; estrogen-progesterone-aldosterone interaction; vasopressin; prolactin; vitamin B_6 deficiency; hypoglycemia; endogenous opiates.
- The clinical manifestations include: altered emotional states, behavioral changes, somatic problems, altered appetite, and motor effects.
- The treatment involves relief of the manifestations, which can include vitamin supplements, progesterone, spironalactone (Aldactone), oral bromocriptine (Parlodel), oral contraceptives, and tranquilizers.
- Nursing care involves support, education, life style changes, reduced salt intake, stress management, and support groups.

(For more information, see pp. 2388–2389 of Black and Matassarin-Jacobs: *Medical-Surgical Nursing: Clinical Management for Continuity of Care,* 5th ed.)

Pressure Ulcers

OVERVIEW

- A pressure ulcer is an alteration in skin integrity that commonly occurs in areas subject to high pressure from body weight or bony prominences, i.e., greater trochanter, heel, sacrum, and ischial tuberosities.
- Continuous pressure on soft tissues between bony prominences and hard surfaces compresses capil-

laries and occludes blood flow. If pressure is relieved, a brief period of rebound capillary dilation occurs and no tissue damage occurs. If pressure is not relieved, microthrombi form in the capillary and completely occlude blood flow. The period of time before breakdown varies between clients; very debilitated clients can have permanent tissue damage in less than 2 hours.

- About 41 per cent of elderly clients in critical care have pressure ulcers and about 60 per cent of quadriplegic clients have pressure ulcers at any given time.
- Risk factors leading to pressure ulcers include:
  — incontinence
  — immobility
  — skin shearing
  — poor nutritional status
  — impaired sensory perception

CLINICAL MANIFESTATIONS

The clinical manifestations of pressure ulcers have been described in four stages

- Stage I—erythema of intact skin. Epidermis remains intact. Is reversible with intervention.
- Stage II—partial thickness loss of skin layers involving epidermis and possibly penetrating into, but not through, the dermis. May present as a blister, abrasion, or shallow crater.
- Stage III—full thickness tissue loss extending through the dermis to involve subcutaneous tissue. Presents as shallow crater unless covered with eschar. Wound base is usually not painful. May include necrotic tissue, undermining of adjacent tissue.
- Stage IV—deep tissue destruction extending through subcutaneous tissue to fascia and may involve muscle layer, joints, and/or bone. Presents as deep crater. May include necrotic tissue, undermining sinus tract formation, exudate and/or infection. Wound base is usually not painful.

ACUTE AND SUBACUTE CARE

Medical Management

- oxygen (hyperbaric oxygen treatments) and vasodilator therapy to restore arterial blood flow

- antibiotics
- dietary modification—high in carbohydrates, fat, protein, iron, and vitamins (it may be necessary to supplement with tube feeding or total parenteral nutrition).
- low-pressure bed

Surgical Management

- debridement—to remove necrotic tissue
  - surgical—surgery is performed to remove the eschar
  - mechanical—use of irrigation or wet-to-dry dressings to accomplish debridement (enzymatic debridement with the use of topical agents)
- surgical repair
  - Stage III—undamaged tissue near wound is rotated to cover the ulcer
  - Stage IV—musculocutaneous flaps are used to cover the ulcer

Nursing Management

Medical

- Analgesics before debridement.
- Use of the Braden Scale (assessment tool) to evaluate risk.
- Assess the client at high risk for developing a pressure ulcer with attention to bony prominences.
- Monitor laboratory findings: hemoglobin, hematocrit, albumin, total protein, and lymphocyte count.
- Cleanse skin using mild cleansing agent if soiling occurs.
- Treat dry skin with moisturizers.
- Avoid massage over bony prominences.
- Minimize skin exposure to moisture due to incontinence, perspiration, or wound drainage.
- Minimize skin injury due to friction and shearing forces through proper positioning, transferring, and turning techniques.
- Facilitate dietary consult.
- Maintain exercise and activity program.
- Reposition every 2 hours using positioning devices to keep bony prominences from direct contact with each other.

- Maintain the head of the bed at lowest degree of elevation tolerated.
- Use lifting devices (trapeze, bed linen) to move client.
- Use low air loss beds, foam mattress, foam chair pad as indicated.
- Wheelchair bound clients should reposition themselves every 15 minutes.

Surgical

Nursing care is dependent upon ulcer stage and surgical intervention selected.

COMMUNITY AND SELF-CARE

- Instruct client regarding:
  — obtaining necessary equipment for home use—proper technique for positioning and transferring (refer to the U.S. Department of Health and Human Services for a patient guide on preventing and treating pressure ulcers)
  — hygiene measures
  — skin inspection
  — maintaining activity and exercise level
  — importance of good nutrition
  — wound care
- Refer to available community resources (home health care).

(For more information, see pp. 2213–2220 of Black and Matassarin-Jacobs: *Medical-Surgical Nursing: Clinical Management for Continuity of Care,* 5th ed.)

Prostate Cancer

OVERVIEW

- Prostate cancer is the most common cancer among men, and the third leading cause of death among men in the United States.

- Most clients with clinically detectable prostate cancer are over age 50. A man's risk of prostate cancer increases with each decade after age 50.
- Typically, the lesions grow slowly and remain confined to the prostatic capsule which delays diagnosis.

CLINICAL MANIFESTATIONS

There may be no symptoms unless benign prostatic hypertrophy is also present because the tumor is usually found in the periphery of the posterior lobe.

- hip or back bone pain—late symptoms caused by metastases
- rectal pressure or obstruction from local tumor growth
- painful ejaculation
- hard nodule in the prostate

ACUTE AND SUBACUTE CARE

Medical Management

- radiation therapy
  — external
  — interstitial—using iodine (^{125}I) seed implants
  — combination of the above two methods
- androgen blockers—block the action or secretion of androgens, which stimulate tumor growth (Eulexin, Zoladex)
- estrogen preparations—suppress the release of pituitary gonadotropin and reduce serum testosterone levels (Diethylstilbestrol [DES])
- chemotherapy—Cytoxan, 5-FU, Adriamycin

Surgical Management

- transurethral prostatectomy (TURP)—for small, well defined tumors or to relieve obstruction
- laser ablation—laser fiber is introduced transurethrally to ablate the lateral lobes of the prostate
- radical prostatectomy—via a perineal or retropubic approach

NURSING MANAGEMENT

Medical

- See "Chemotherapy," p. 149.
- See "Radiation Therapy," p. 605.

Surgical

- See "Benign Prostatic Hyperplasia," p. 76.

(For more information, see pp. 2365–2372 of Black and Matassarin-Jacobs: *Medical-Surgical Nursing: Clinical Management for Continuity of Care,* 5th ed.)

Prostatitis

OVERVIEW

- Prostatitis, inflammation of the prostate gland, may be (1) acute bacterial, (2) chronic bacterial, or (3) nonbacterial.
- Routes of infection include: (1) urethral ascent, (2) descent from the urinary bladder or kidneys, (3) direct extension or lymphatogenous spread from the rectum, and (4) hematogenous spread (via blood).
- Bacterial prostatitis usually is caused by gram-negative rods, especially E. coli and Pseudomonas.

CLINICAL MANIFESTATIONS

- Bacterial
  - — Acute
    - chills and fever
    - low back and perineal pain
    - urinary frequency, urgency, nocturia, and dysuria
    - tender, swollen prostate
    - positive urine cultures identifying the infecting organism
  - — Chronic—less severe inflammation
    - may be asymptomatic but organisms found on routine urinalysis

- urgency, frequency, nocturia, and dysuria
- low back or perineal pain
- myalgia and arthralgia
- prostate on palpation may be normal, feel boggy, or indurated

- Nonbacterial—most common form of prostatitis:
  - same symptoms as bacterial, but no causative organism is identified
  - prostate massage yields abnormal numbers of inflammatory cells

ACUTE AND SUBACUTE CARE

Medical Management

- antimicrobial medications
- anti-inflammatory agents

Nursing Management

Medical

- Administer antibiotics as prescribed.
- Monitor intake and output.
- Encourage oral intake.
- Promote rest.
- Administer PRN analgesics.
- Offer sitz baths.
- Administer stool softeners, as constipation increases the pain of prostatitis.

COMMUNITY AND SELF-CARE

Instruct the client regarding:

- importance of completing antibiotic therapy
- need to maintain oral intake of 2000-3000 ml/day (unless otherwise contraindicated)

(For more information, see pp. 2372–2373 of Black and Matassarin-Jacobs: *Medical-Surgical Nursing: Clinical Management for Continuity of Care,* 5th ed.)

Psoriasis Vulgaris

OVERVIEW

- Psoriasis vulgaris is a chronic, recurrent, erythematous, inflammatory skin disorder. The term "vulgaris" means common.
- Rapidly proliferating epidermal cells form small, scaly patches of skin that develop into erythematous, dry scaling patches of various sizes. Psoriatic patches are covered with silvery white scales.
- The eruptions are usually symmetric and occur on the scalp, elbows, knees, and sacral regions.
- The course of psoriasis is prolonged and unpredictable. Exacerbations and remissions are common, and anxiety and stress often precede flare-ups. Spontaneous clearing is uncommon.
- Nail pitting and arthritis are common.
- The cause is unknown.

ACUTE AND SUBACUTE CARE

Medical Management

- natural sunlight or topical therapy including tar preparations and topical corticosteroids—for mild psoriasis
- injection of small diluted amounts of corticosteroids into or just below the lesion
- topical anthralin to lesions
- tar shampoos with keratolytic agents, followed by topical corticosteroid lotions
- whole body irradiation with ultraviolet light for widespread involvement
- etretinate (Tegison)—a vitamin A derivative used for pustular and erythrodermic psoriasis
- antimetabolites (e.g., Methotrexate) in small doses

Nursing Management

- Instruct client regarding:
  - — use of medications—application and possible side effects
  - — treatment regimen
  - — use of anthralin

- must not be used in women of childbearing age
- avoid contact with normal skin surrounding lesions
- may stain fabric, hair, skin, nails, furniture, and bathroom fixtures

— importance of birth control for clients on antimetabolites

— prevention of infection in open lesions

- Provide psychological support and encourage ventilation of feelings about change in body image (smell of tar preparations or staining of skin may compound feelings).

(For more information, see pp. 2210–2212 of Black and Matassarin-Jacobs: *Medical-Surgical Nursing: Clinical Management for Continuity of Care,* 5th ed.)

Pulmonary Embolism

OVERVIEW

- Pulmonary embolism (PE) is an occlusion of a portion of the pulmonary blood vessels by an embolus. An embolus is a detached intravascular solid, liquid, or gaseous mass that is carried by the bloodstream from its point of origin to a distant site.
- Emboli travel to the lungs and lodge in the pulmonary vasculature. Blood flow is obstructed, resulting in decreased perfusion of that section of the lung. The lung is still ventilated. A ventilation-perfusion mismatch occurs and hypoxemia results.
- Almost all emboli develop from thrombi (clots). Other sources include tumors, air, fat, bone marrow, amniotic fluid, septic thrombi, and vegetations on heart valves that develop with endocarditis.
- The most common source of thrombi originate in the deep calf, femoral, popliteal, or iliac veins.
- 50,000 people die each year from pulmonary embolism in the United States.

CLINICAL MANIFESTATIONS

- chest pain (usually pleuritic)
- dyspnea, tachypnea, apprehension
- cough, hemoptysis, crackles
- split second heart sound, tachycardia
- fever, diaphoresis, syncope

ACUTE AND SUBACUTE CARE

Medical Management

- anticoagulation with heparin to raise the partial thromboplastin time (PTT) to 1.5–2.5 times normal
- initiation of coumadin about 3–5 days before heparin is stopped
- oxygen therapy
- inotropic agents and/or fluids for hypotension
- analgesics
- fibrinolytic therapy (controversial, may dissolve the clot but does not improve the mortality rate)

Surgical Management

- vena cava plication (insertion of an umbrella filter to allow blood flow, but trap emboli)
- embolectomy—surgical removal of emboli from the pulmonary arteries. This is a very high risk surgery.

Nursing Management

- Monitor vital signs frequently until stable.
- Auscultate lung sounds frequently.
- Auscultate heart sounds frequently (assess for murmurs or extra heart sounds).
- Monitor for hypoxemia, respiratory compromise, and hypotension.
- Monitor blood gas values.
- Place in semi-Fowler's position.
- Provide oxygen as ordered.
- Monitor for right-sided heart failure:
  - — peripheral edema
  - — distended neck veins
  - — liver engorgement

- Monitor partial thromboplastin time (PTT) (goal is 1.5–2.5 times the normal value).
- Monitor for excessive anticoagulation: blood in urine or stool, petechiae, bruising, bleeding of gums, change in level of consciousness, flank pain, and coffee ground emesis.
- Use soft toothbrush or foam toothettes for oral care.
- Provide emotional support.

COMMUNITY AND SELF-CARE

Instruct client regarding:
- signs/symptoms of change in respiratory status and to report to physician
- coumadin therapy
  - — measures to prevent bleeding/injury
  - — avoidance of medications/foods that potentiate or interfere with coumadin
  - — notification of all physicians/dentists that client is on anticoagulant therapy
  - — signs/symptoms of overcoagulation or bleeding
  - — importance of follow-up laboratory tests

(For more information, see pp. 1126–1129 of Black and Matassarin-Jacobs: *Medical-Surgical Nursing: Clinical Management for Continuity of Care,* 5th ed.)

Pulmonary Hypertension

OVERVIEW

- Pulmonary hypertension is defined as a prolonged elevation of the pulmonary artery pressure (PAP) above 18 mmHg and systolic PAP above 30 mmHg, which cannot accommodate increased blood flow.
- Risk factors include: chronic hypoxia, acidosis, or both.
- There are two classifications:
  - —Primary (idiopathic)—the cause is unclear but occurs more often in young adults ages 30-40.
  - — Secondary—it is usually associated with underlying heart or lung disease.

- Prognosis is poor in severe disease.

CLINICAL MANIFESTATIONS

- may be asymptomatic
- dyspnea
- fatigue, syncope
- chest pain, palpitations
- muscular weakness
- right ventricular hypertrophy, enlarged pulmonary arteries, prominant hilar vessels per chest x-ray
- elevated PAP, normal pulmonary wedge pressure

ACUTE AND SUBACUTE CARE

Medical Management

- treatment of underlying cause
- vasodilator therapy
- calcium channel blockers
- reduce hypoxemia

Surgical Management

- heart-lung transplant

Nursing Management

- supportive measures
- oxygenation needs
- administration of medications
- nutrition, exercises

COMMUNITY AND SELF-CARE

Instruct client regarding:

- home oxygen
- activity as tolerated
- signs/symptoms of worsening disease

(For more information, see pp. 1129–1130 of Black and Matassarin-Jacobs: *Medical-Surgical Nursing: Clinical Management for Continuity of Care,* 5th ed.)

Pyelonephritis, Acute

OVERVIEW

- Acute pyelonephritis is an inflammation of the renal pelvis caused by a bacterial infection.
- It often occurs after bacterial contamination of the urethra or after instrumentation, such as catheterization or cystoscopy.
- Risk factors include pregnancy, diabetes, hypertension, chronic renal calculi, chronic cystitis, structural abnormalities, stones, indwelling catheters, and mechanical drainage.

CLINICAL MANIFESTATIONS

- high fever, chills, nausea, headaches, and muscular pain
- flank pain on the affected side, often radiating down the ureter or toward the epigastrium
- dysuria, frequency, urgency
- cloudy, bloody, or foul smelling urine
- costovertebral angle tenderness

ACUTE AND SUBACUTE CARE

MEDICAL MANAGEMENT

- parenteral antibiotics (specific to the causative organism) for 3–5 days until the client is afebrile for 24–48 hours, oral administration follows for 2–4 weeks
- elimination of any contributing factors (such as calculi)

SURGICAL MANAGEMENT

- Surgery is done only to correct any underlying defects that caused the pyelonephritis.

NURSING MANAGEMENT

Medical

- Administer antibiotic therapy as prescribed.
- Monitor results of culture and sensitivity tests.
- Monitor intake and output.

- Assess for adequate hydration without overhydrating, as this may dilute the effectiveness of antimicrobials.
- Administer analgesics, anti-emetics, and antipyretics as prescribed.
- Also see, "Urinary Tract Infection," p. 736.

COMMUNITY AND SELF-CARE

Instruct client regarding:

- completing the full course of antibiotic therapy
- need for compliance with follow-up urine cultures, since bacteriuria may be asymptomatic
- ways to prevent further urinary tract infection (see, "Urinary Tract Infection," p. 736)
- signs/symptoms of urinary tract infections and to report these to physician immediately.

(For more information, see pp. 1628–1630 of Black and Matassarin-Jacobs: *Medical-Surgical Nursing: Clinical Management for Continuity of Care,* 5th ed.)

Pyelonephritis, Chronic

OVERVIEW

- Chronic pyelonephritis is an inflammation of the renal pelvis caused by a bacterial infection. It usually occurs with chronic disorders or after chronic obstruction with reflux. Fibrosis and scar tissue develop, altering tubular reabsorption and secretion, which lead to decreased renal function. It is a slowly progressive disease associated with acute attacks.
- Risk factors include: pregnancy, diabetes, hypertension, chronic renal calculi, chronic cystitis, structural abnormalities, stones, indwelling catheters, and mechanical drainage.

CLINICAL MANIFESTATIONS

- no specific symptoms except hypertension

ACUTE AND SUBACUTE CARE

Medical Management

- antibiotics
- antihypertensive medications
- prevention of further renal damage

Surgical Management

- Surgery is done only to correct any underlying defects that caused the pyelonephritis.

Nursing Management

- See "Pyelonephritis, Acute," p. 601.

COMMUNITY AND SELF-CARE

- See "Pyelonephritis, Acute," p. 601.

(For more information, see pp. 1628–1630 of Black and Matassarin-Jacobs: *Medical-Surgical Nursing: Clinical Management for Continuity of Care,* 5th ed.)

Q

Quincy (Peritonsillar Abscess)

- Quincy is an abscess of the peritonsillar area arising from acute streptococcal or staphylococcal tonsillitis.
- Signs/symptoms include drooling (instead of painful swallowing), muffled voice, and thick secretions.
- Treatment involves high-dose antibiotics or an incision and drainage of the area.
- Nursing care involves use of topical anesthetic throat sprays, analgesics, very warm saline throat irrigations, saline mouthwashes, and ice collars.
- Usually a tonsillectomy is performed after resolution of the abscess (usually 1 month).

(For more information, see p. 1080 of Black and Matassarin-Jacobs: *Medical-Surgical Nursing: Clinical Management for Continuity of Care,* 5th ed.)

R

Radiation Therapy

OVERVIEW

- More than 60 per cent of all clients with cancer receive radiation therapy (RT) at some point during their disease course.
- Radiation therapy is the use of high-energy, ionizing rays that destroy the cell's ability to reproduce by damaging the cell's DNA. Rapidly dividing cells, such as some cancer cells, are more vulnerable to radiation than are slower dividing cells. Radiosensitivity (the relative sensitivity of tissues to radiation) depends upon the characteristics of the tissue itself. A highly radiosensitive tumor is one that divides rapidly, is well vascularized, and has a high oxygen content.
- Three treatment modalities for radiation therapy are:
  — primary treatment modality
    - radiation therapy is the only treatment used and provides local cure of the cancer
  — adjuvant treatment modality
    - in conjunction with surgery, either preoperatively or postoperatively to aid in the destruction of cancer cells
    - in conjunction with chemotherapy to treat disease in sites not readily accessible to systemic chemotherapy, such as the brain
  — palliative treatment modality
    - to relieve pain due to obstruction, pathologic fracture, or spinal cord compression
- Types of radiation therapy
  — external radiation therapy
    - administered by high energy x-ray or radioisotope machines
    - the maximum effect of radiation occurs within the tumor, not on the skin surface
  — internal radiation therapy

- placement of radioisotopes directly into or near the tumor itself (sealed source) or into the systemic circulation (unsealed source) by injection or oral route
  - sealed source radiation therapy (brachytherapy) includes:
    - intracavitary
      - radioisotope is placed into an applicator positioned in a body cavity for a calculated time period, usually 24–72 hours
      - used to treat cancers of the uterus and cervix
    - interstitial
      - radioisotope is placed into needles, beads, seeds, ribbons, or catheters and then implanted directly into the tumor
      - used in prostate cancer
  - unsealed source radiation therapy
    - radioisotopes are administered orally, intravenously, or into a body cavity
    - used in thyroid cancer and polycythemia vera

- Factors that determine side effects are:
  - size of the treatment area
  - total dose of radiation
  - area of the body being treated (certain tissues are more sensitive)
- Combined therapy with chemotherapy has the potential for enhanced tumor destruction as well as enhanced side effects. The gastrointestinal, integumentary, and myeloproliferative systems are at greatest risk for damage.
- Interventions to limit side effects
  - fractionating the total dose into small frequent doses
    - increases the probability that tumor cells will be in a vulnerable phase of the cell cycle
    - allows normal cells time to repair themselves
  - alternating the sites of entry (ports) of radiation
  - customized shielding blocks
- In general, skin reactions, fatigue, nausea, and anorexia may occur with RT to any site whereas

other side effects occur only when specific areas are involved in the treatment field. Site-specific manifestations include mucositis, radiation caries, esophagitis, dysphagia, cystitis, alopecia, and bone marrow suppression. Many manifestations do not develop until 10–14 days into treatment, and some do not subside until 2 or more weeks post treatment.

- Radiation safety—consists of three principles to protect caregivers from excessive radiation
  - — distance—greater the distance from the radiation source, the less exposure
  - — time—the less time spent close to source, the less exposure
  - — use of shields —provides a block between radiation source and caregiver

ACUTE AND SUBACUTE CARE

Nursing Management

External Radiation

- Monitor for skin changes over area of radiation.
- Monitor for side effects of radiation therapy (are dependent upon the specific area being irradiated):
  - — nausea, vomiting, diarrhea
  - — cystitis
  - — diminished blood counts
  - — dysphagia
- Monitor blood counts.
- Schedule activities to allow for rest periods.
- Encourage a well balanced diet.

Internal Radiation

Sealed source:

- Place client in a private room.
- Plan care so minimal time is spent in direct contact with the client.
- Use a lead apron or lead shield while in the room.
- Mark the room with appropriate signage.
- Check all linen for presence of foreign bodies.
- Keep long-handled forceps and lead-lined container in client's room.

- Minimize exposure by not exceeding the specified time limitation for the shift.
- Maintain time exposure limitations for visitors and other personnel.
- Maintain bedrest and utilize pressure-relieving devices.
- Check that the applicator is properly placed.
  — if dislodged, use forceps to place in a lead container

Unsealed Source:

- Place client in a private room.
- Maintain and enforce time and distance restrictions and wearing of protective gown, gloves, and shoe covers for yourself, visitors, and other personnel.
- Instruct client to flush toilet several times after use (isotope may be excreted in body fluid).
- Use disposable dishes and utensils.
- Use telephone or intercom to communicate with patient to decrease time of exposure.
- Prior to discharge, the client should be scanned by the radiation safety officer to be certain that the level of radiation has decreased to a safe level.

COMMUNITY AND SELF-CARE

Instruct client regarding:

External Radiation

- skin care
  — keep skin dry
  — do not wash the treatment area until instructed to do so and then only with mild soap and warm water
  — do not remove lines or ink marks placed on skin
  — avoid powders, lotions, creams, alcohol, or deodorants on treated skin
  — do not use tape over treatment area
  — wear loose-fitting clothing to prevent friction
  — shave with an electric razor
  — protect skin from exposure to direct sunlight, chlorinated water, and temperature extremes
- management of side effects
- importance of follow-up appointments

INTERNAL RADIATION

Sealed source:
- perineal care (cervical implant)
- importance of follow-up visits

Unsealed source:
- avoidance of crowds initially
- importance of clinic and laboratory follow-up

(For more information, see pp. 570–573 of Black and Matassarin-Jacobs: *Medical-Surgical Nursing: Clinical Management for Continuity of Care,* 5th ed.)

Raynaud's Disease

OVERVIEW

- Raynaud's disease is characterized by intermittent episodes during which small arteries or arterioles in the extremities constrict, causing temporary pallor and cyanosis of the digits and changes in skin color. These episodes occur in response to cold temperature or strong emotion and are bilateral.
- Raynaud's disease is a primary vasospastic disorder. If the disorder is secondary to another disease or underlying cause, the term *Raynaud's phenomenon* is used. Secondary Raynaud's phenomenon is often associated with connective tissue or collagen vascular disease such as scleroderma, SLE, or rheumatoid arthritis.
- Raynaud's disease appears to be caused by (1) a hypersensitivity of digital arteries to cold, (2) release of serotonin, and (3) congenital predisposition.
- Eighty per cent of clients with Raynaud's disease are women between 20 and 49 years of age.

CLINICAL MANIFESTATIONS

- feelings of cold, numbness, pain, and finally intense redness accompanied by tingling and throbbing of the digits

- color changes of the digits from pallor to cyanosis
- gangrene that is limited to the skin of the tips of the digits

ACUTE AND SUBACUTE CARE

Medical Management

- smoking cessation
- vasodilator therapy

Surgical Management

- sympathectomy—excision of a ganglion in the sympathetic nervous pathway to produce vasodilation

Nursing Management

- Administer vasodilator therapy.
- Provide warm environment.
- Instruct on relaxation techniques.

COMMUNITY AND SELF-CARE

Instruct client regarding:
- disease process and treatment regime
- importance of managing stress
- measures to avoid cold exposure
- smoking cessation programs
- limitation of caffeine and chocolate in diet
- safety measures related to orthostatic hypotension (vasodilator therapy)

(For more information, see pp. 1431–1432 of Black and Matassarin-Jacobs: *Medical-Surgical Nursing: Clinical Management for Continuity of Care,* 5th ed.)

Renal Calculi

OVERVIEW

- Renal calculi are stones formed in the kidney.
- Stones may be of one crystalline type or a combination of types. Types include:

- calcium (due to hypercalciuria)
- oxalate (may be closely related to diet)
- struvite (composed of calcium, magnesium, and ammonium phosphate)
  - cause is bacteria, usually proteus
- uric acid stones (cause is increased urine excretion, fluid depletion, and a low urinary pH)
- xanthine stones (xanthine oxidase deficiency).

- Risk factors include urinary stasis or supersaturation of the urine. Stasis may be caused by immobility; supersaturation may be caused by dehydration or an increase in calcium or other ions. Alteration in purine metabolism (e.g., gout) is a risk factor for uric acid stones. Another factor is previous history of stones.

CLINICAL MANIFESTATIONS

- severe, sharp pain of sudden onset
- renal colic—lumbar pain radiating to bladder (female) or testicles (male)
- ureteral colic—pain radiates to genitalia and thigh
- pain may last minutes to days or be intermittent
- nausea, vomiting, pallor, diaphoresis
- pain also may be dull, aching, or heavy

ACUTE AND SUBACUTE CARE

Medical Management

- cystoscopy with placement of ureteral catheters to drain urine proximal to the stone and dilate the ureter to prompt passage of the stone
- cystoscopy with use of ureteral catheters to mechanically guide stones downward for removal
- chemical irrigation to dissolve the stone
- use of special catheters with loops and expanding baskets through a cystoscope to snare the stone
- extracorporeal lithotripsy—administration of electrically generated shock waves to the area of the stone in order to fracture it
- medications to lower uric acid for uric acid stones (such as allopurinol)
- diet modification if the stone type is identified

Surgical Management

- percutaneous lithotripsy—involves insertion of tubes into the area of stone formation. A contrast dye is injected, and forceps are used to remove the stones. Ultrasonic waves are used to break up stones for easier removal.
- nephroscope—may be used for small stones. The stone is removed by alligator forceps or a stone basket through a nephroscope inserted percutaneously.
- large stones—several methods may be used to break up the stone into smaller pieces (litholapaxy):
  - — a punch lithoclast to fragment the stone into smaller pieces
  - — an ultrasound nephroscope may be inserted into the kidney, and subharmonic sound waves used to shatter the stone
  - — chemolysis—irrigation of the stone with chemical solutions through a nephrostomy tube
- an open surgical procedure is needed if the above measures fail
- When there is extensive kidney damage, sometimes a partial or total nephrectomy is done.

Nursing Management

- Administer antispasmodics and narcotics to control pain and assess effectiveness.
- Strain all urine through a strainer or gauze pad. (Stones may be as small as sand. Rubbing the material of the strainer between two gloved fingers may help detect small stones.)
- Force fluids.
- Monitor intake and output.
- Instruct client to void every two hours.
- If surgery was done: dressing changes over the wound, use of urinary pouch or nephrostomy tubes may be necessary.

COMMUNITY AND SELF-CARE

- Instruct client regarding:
  prevention of recurrence
  - — maintain fluid intake to ensure 2500–3000 ml of urine output daily

— dietary restrictions based on stone analysis:
  - calcium stones—limit calcium and phosphate intake
  - oxalate stones—avoid tea, instant coffee, chocolate, cola drinks, beer, rhubarb, beans, cabbage, apples, grapes, peanuts, peanut butter
  - uric acid stones—low purine diet and avoid wine, cheese, organ meats
— medications to prevent recurrence based on stone analysis
— need to void every 2 hours
— maintain acidic urine
- signs/symptoms of recurrence and to report to physician
- need for follow-up urinalysis and laboratory tests

(For more information, see pp. 1665–1671 of Black and Matassarin-Jacobs: *Medical-Surgical Nursing: Clinical Management for Continuity of Care,* 5th ed.)

Renal Cancer

OVERVIEW

- Renal cell carcinoma (adenocarcinoma) accounts for 90 per cent of all kidney neoplasms.
- Benign kidney tumors are rare; at least 85 per cent of all renal tumors are malignant.
- Common sites of metastasis include: lungs, mediastinum, liver, bone, skin, spleen, and brain.
- The exact cause is unknown. There have been links established to tobacco, lead, cadmium, phosphate, and genetics.

CLINICAL MANIFESTATIONS

Tumor growth may be advanced before the disease is discovered. Signs/symptoms may seem unrelated to the disease (e.g., abdominal mass).

- Hematuria (gross and intermittent), flank pain, and a palpable abdominal or flank mass.

- Less frequent signs/symptoms are fever, weight loss, fatigue, hypertension, anemia, abnormal serum liver profile, hypercalcemia, elevated sedimentation rate.

ACUTE AND SUBACUTE CARE

Medical Management

- radiation therapy may be used in conjunction with chemotherapy and surgery
- irradiation may be used for preoperative preparation of the tumor or postoperatively to destroy residual tumor or to treat lymphatic involvement or metastatic sites
- chemotherapy
  — vinblastine is the most effective single agent
- immunotherapy—use of natural and recombinant interferon

Surgical Management

- nephrectomy (removal of the kidney) is the conventional and principal intervention for renal cancer, although radiation and chemotherapy may be used as adjuncts to surgical removal
- radical nephrectomy (removal of the kidney, adrenal gland, and perinephric fat with the retroperitoneal lymphatics) is the surgical procedure of choice for renal cell carcinoma

Nursing Management

Medical

- For general care during irradiation or chemotherapy, see "Radiation Therapy," p. 605 and "Chemotherapy," p. 149.

Surgical

Postoperative Care

In addition to routine postoperative care:
- Assist with coughing and deep breathing (this is painful for the client due to the close proximity of the incision to the diaphragm).
- Administer analgesics and position comfortably to control pain and facilitate coughing and deep breathing.

- Monitor closely for pneumothorax and paralytic ileus, which may occur postoperatively.
- Monitor intake and output hourly, to ensure the remaining kidney is functioning adequately. Monitor closely for renal failure.
- Provide routine wound care.

COMMUNITY AND SELF-CARE

- depends upon the stage of cancer and the need for further treatment

(For more information, see pp. 1671–1673 of Black and Matassarin-Jacobs: *Medical-Surgical Nursing: Clinical Management for Continuity of Care,* 5th ed.)

Renal Failure, Acute (ARF)

OVERVIEW

- Acute renal failure (ARF) refers to the abrupt loss of kidney function. Over a period of hours to a few days the glomerular filtration rate falls, and serum creatinine and urea nitrogen levels rise.
- Causes are divided into three major categories
  - — Prerenal—interferes with renal perfusion
    - — includes hypotension, circulatory volume depletion, decreased cardiac output, increased vascular resistance, and vascular obstruction
  - — Renal—parenchymal changes from disease or nephrotoxic substances
    - — includes acute tubular necrosis, infectious disease, diabetes, hypokalemia, phosphatemia, and glomerulonephritis
  - — Postrenal obstruction in the urinary tract
    - — includes prostatic hypertrophy, calculi, and tumors
- Risk factors include hypovolemia, hypotension, and nephrotoxic agents.
- ARF has several phases:
  - — Onset phase—from precipitating event to development of renal symptoms

— Oliguric-anuric or nonoliguric phase—this second phase lasts 1–8 weeks and is either oliguric (urine production falls below 400 ml/day) or nonoliguric (urine production may be as much as 2 L/day)
— Diuretic phase—urine output may be 1000 to 2000 ml/day; glomerular filtration returns and leveling of the blood urea nitrogen (BUN) occurs
— Recovery phase—lasts 3–12 months; return to prerenal failure level.

CLINICAL MANIFESTATIONS

- Nonoliguric renal failure
  — urine output up to 2000 ml/day
  — dilute and nearly osmolar urine
  — hypertension
  — tachypnea
  — fluid overload
  — may also see signs of extracellular fluid depletion (dry mucous membranes, poor skin turgor)
- Oliguric renal failure—urine production below 400 ml/day

  The signs and symptoms vary depending upon whether the cause of renal failure is prerenal, renal, or postrenal.

  — Prerenal
    - client has history of precipitating event
    - high specific gravity of urine
    - little or no proteinuria
    - elevated BUN:CR ratio

  — Renal
    - fixed specific gravity
    - high sodium concentration of urine
    - proteinuria
    - weight gain
    - edema
    - hemoptysis
    - anemia
    - hypertension

  — Postrenal
    - fixed specific gravity
    - elevated sodium concentration of urine
    - little or no proteinuria

ACUTE AND SUBACUTE CARE

Medical Management

- dialysis
- fluid replacement
- electrolyte replacement
- diuretic therapy may be used, but is controversial
- high-calorie, low-protein diet, which also may be low in sodium and potassium

Nursing Management

- Strict intake and output.
- Monitor fluid status every 4 hours by assessing mucous membranes, skin turgor, apical pulses, vital signs with postural blood pressures, lung sounds, heart sounds, and mental status.
- Daily or twice per day weights.
- Maintain fluid restriction as ordered and decrease thirst by providing frequent oral hygiene and lip ointment.
- Provide meticulous skin care, frequent turning, and protective mattress as needed.
- Protect from secondary infections and assess for early signs/symptoms of infection.
- Avoid indwelling urinary catheters to decrease the risk of infection.
- Monitor for electrolyte imbalances, especially hyperkalemia.
- Monitor for pericarditis (occurs in 18 per cent of renal failure clients).
- Monitor for anemia; administer packed red blood cells as ordered.
- Monitor for seizures (the seizure threshold is lowered due to the rising BUN).
- Discuss importance of prescribed diet, when appropriate.

COMMUNITY AND SELF-CARE

Instruct client/significant others regarding:

- renal function, signs/symptoms of renal failure, and the need for ongoing treatment
- signs/symptoms of further renal damage or that client has progressed to chronic renal failure
- dietary modifications

- obtaining weights and intake and output
- need for follow-up appointments with nephrologist

(For more information, see pp. 1636–1641 of Black and Matassarin-Jacobs: *Medical-Surgical Nursing: Clinical Management for Continuity of Care,* 5th ed.)

Renal Failure, Chronic (CRF)

OVERVIEW

- Chronic renal failure (CRF) is a progressive reduction of functioning renal tissue such that the remaining kidney mass no longer can maintain the body's internal environment.
- Destruction of nephrons occurs with progressive loss of renal function. It may develop insidiously over many years or can occur as a result of acute renal failure (ARF) from which the client fails to recover.
- The most common causes of chronic renal failure are diabetic and hypertensive nephropathy, glomerulonephritis, and chronic pyelonephritis.

CLINICAL MANIFESTATIONS

- Electrolyte imbalances
  - — hyponatremia is seen initially with hypernatremia in end-stage disease
  - — serum potassium remains normal until late in the disease when hyperkalemia may occur
  - — hypocalcemia, hyperphosphatemia, and elevated magnesium
- Metabolic changes
  - — rising serum BUN/creatinine
  - — proteinuria and serum hypoproteinemia
  - — carbohydrate intolerance
  - — elevated triglycerides
  - — metabolic acidosis
  - — accumulation of uremic toxins leading to pericarditis
  - — impaired insulin production and metabolism

- Hematologic changes
  - — normocytic, normochromic anemia
  - — fatigue, weakness, cold intolerance
- Gastrointestinal changes
  - — anorexia, nausea, vomiting
  - — metallic, bitter, or salty taste in the mouth
  - — esophagitis, gastritis, colitis, gastrointestinal bleeding
  - — stomatitis, gingivitis, parotitis
- Immunologic changes
  - — increased susceptibility to infection
- Changes in medication metabolism
  - — high risk for medication toxicity
- Cardiopulmonary changes
  - — hypertension
  - — volume overload
  - — pulmonary edema
  - — congestive heart failure
- Musculoskeletal changes:
  - — bone demineralization
  - — joint pain
- Integumentary changes
  - — severe pruritus, dry skin, brittle hair and nails
  - — peripheral neuropathy
  - — central nervous system involvement (forgetfulness, inability to concentrate, etc.)
- Reproductive changes
  - — decreased libido
  - — impotence in males
  - — menstrual irregularities in females
  - — hypothyroidism
- Psychosocial changes
  - — personality changes
  - — labile emotions
  - — withdrawal
  - — depression

ACUTE AND SUBACUTE

MEDICAL MANAGEMENT

- conservative interventions include: correction of contributing factors, controlling blood pressure, and adjusting the fluids and diet
- dialysis or renal transplantation eventually is needed by most clients. See "Dialysis," p. 225.

- electrolyte replacement
- diuretics in the early phase
- regulation of fluids and sodium
- sodium bicarbonate to correct acidosis
- erythropoietin—the primary treatment to correct anemia
- antihypertensive therapy
- dietary management depends upon the results of blood chemistries
- calcium preparations
- vitamins and minerals
- topical lotions, antihistamines, and ultraviolet B light for pruritus

Surgical Management

- See "Renal Transplantation," p. 621.

Nursing Management

- Monitor for fluid volume deficit or overload.
  - — obtain daily or twice daily weights.
  - — assess skin turgor, mucous membranes.
  - — monitor vital signs and orthostatic blood pressure.
  - — strict intake and output.
- Monitor for electrolyte imbalances, especially hyperkalemia.
- Monitor blood glucose.
- Monitor for pericarditis and seizures.
- Maintain fluid restriction and instruct on methods to reduce thirst
  - — frequent oral hygiene
  - — lip balms
  - — ice chips or water in a spray bottle with judicious use.
- Arrange for dietary consultation to discuss dietary modifications.
- Implement measures to alleviate nausea, vomiting, and stomatitis to improve appetite.
- Instruct on use of bran and stool softeners to relieve constipation.
- Discuss importance of balancing rest and activity.
- Provide and instruct client on meticulous skin care and measures to reduce dry skin and pruritus.

- Encourage client and significant other to discuss feelings regarding coping with long-term illness, changes in body image, and uncertain future.
- Maintain safety precautions if changes in mentation are present.
- Protect from infection.
- See also "Dialysis," p. 225 and "Renal Transplantation," below.

COMMUNITY AND SELF-CARE

- Instruct the client/significant other regarding:
  - how to monitor fluid status and signs/symptoms to report to physician
  - how to do daily weights and how to interpret relationship of weight loss/gain to need for sodium and water
  - how to take blood pressure
  - prevention of infection
  - need for meticulous skin and oral care
  - safety precautions if change in mentation present
  - medications and changes in medication metabolism
  - dietary regimen
  - importance of follow-up laboratory and physician appointments
  - also see information in "Nursing Management" above
- Provide referrals for patient and significant other for support and assistance in coping.

(For more information, see pp. 1641–1660 of Black and Matassarin-Jacobs: *Medical-Surgical Nursing: Clinical Management for Continuity of Care,* 5th ed.)

Renal Transplantation

OVERVIEW

- Renal transplantation is the surgical implantation of a human kidney as an intervention for irreversible kidney failure. Kidneys may be obtained from

living related donors (which have a higher graft survival rate) or cadaver renal donors.
- Complications of transplantation may include graft rejection, infection, urinary tract complications, noninfectious hepatitis, cirrhosis, peptic ulcer disease, hypertension, osteoporosis, myopathy, fluid and electrolyte imbalances, pneumonia, increased incidence of gynecologic cancers, and skin carcinomas.
- The overall mortality rate 2 years post-transplant is approximately 10 per cent.

ACUTE AND SUBACUTE CARE

Nursing Management

Preoperative Care

In addition to routine preoperative care:
- Provide preoperative teaching and prepare donor and recipient for psychological reactions that may occur postsurgically. (The donor may feel anger over need to protect the remaining kidney or abandonment when the focus shifts to the recipient.)
- Instruct that infections will be eradicated preoperatively; dialysis will be performed, and immunosuppressive therapy started.

Postoperative Care

In addition to routine postoperative care:
- Monitor fluid status and maintain circulatory function.
  - — Obtain weights as ordered.
  - — Strict intake and output, hourly or half-hourly.
  - — Monitor laboratory results, particularly electrolytes, BUN, creatinine, hemoglobin/hematocrit, WBC, and platelets.
  - — Monitor vital signs, watch closely for hypertension.
- Monitor for signs/symptoms of graft rejection (fever, graft tenderness, anemia, and malaise).
- Monitor for urinary tract complications, cardiac dysrhythmias, and congestive heart failure.
- Protect from infection
  - — cough, turn, and deep breathe every 2 hours

— strict aseptic technique for wound or line care
— meticulous oral care and antifungal mouthwashes as prescribed.

- Administer immunosuppressants as prescribed.
- Assess for signs/symptoms of complications due to immunosuppressive therapy
  — increased risk of infection—urinary tract infections, pneumonia, and sepsis are most commonly seen. Oral and esophageal infections also may occur.
  — increased risk of malignancies (especially skin carcinomas)
  — degenerative bone disease
  — steroid induced diabetes mellitus
- Perform postoperative dialysis until kidney is functioning properly.
- Provide emotional support to assist client to incorporate new kidney as part of whole being.
- Provide education and counseling to client/significant other to assist with lifestyle and role changes. Make referrals as needed.

COMMUNITY AND SELF-CARE

- Instruct client/significant other regarding:
  — medications—purpose, dosage, administration, side effects, and toxic effects
  — signs/symptoms of infection and rejection—report to physician if they occur
  — information about the transplant to give to dentists and other physicians
  — prevention of infection
  — signs/symptoms of other complications to report to physician
  — importance of compliance with follow-up appointments/laboratory tests
- Provide referrals as needed for psychosocial support.
- See also "Renal Failure, Chronic," p. 618.

(For more information, see pp. 1660–1665 of Black and Matassarin-Jacobs: *Medical-Surgical Nursing: Clinical Management for Continuity of Care,* 5th ed.)

Retinal Detachment

OVERVIEW

- Retinal detachment is the separation of the retina from the pigment epithelium.
- Retinal detachment (secondary to a tear in the retina) is characterized by a retinal hole, liquid in the vitreous with access to the hole, and a subsequent fluid accumulation between the retina and the pigment epithelium. The liquid seeps through the hole and separates the retina from its blood supply, causing it to lose its ability to function. The retina may become increasingly detached over a period of hours to years.
- The risk of detachment increases after the fourth decade and most often occurs between the ages of 50 and 70.
- Predisposing factors to retinal detachment include:
  — cataract extraction
  — aging
  — trauma
  — degeneration of the retina
  — family history of retinal detachment

CLINICAL MANIFESTATIONS

- sudden onset that may be accompanied by a burst of black spots or floaters (indicates bleeding has occurred)
- description of a shadow falling across the field of vision
- experiences flashes of light
- no pain

ACUTE AND SUBACUTE CARE

Medical Management

None

Surgical Management

A retinal detachment is an ophthalmic emergency. The goal of surgical repair is to place the retina back in contact with the choroid and to seal accompanying holes and breaks.

- cryopexy (use of a freezing probe) or photocoagulation—used to seal hole if it has not progressed to detachment.
- scleral buckling—procedure used to place the retina back in contact with choroid. The sclera is depressed from the outside by a sponge or band sutured in place permanently.
  - in addition to the buckling, an intraocular injection of air and/or a sulfahexafluoride (SF6) gas bubble may be used to apply pressure on the retina from the inside of the eye. The air/gas bubble is slowly absorbed.

Nursing Management

Preoperative Care

In addition to routine preoperative care:
- Maintain activity restrictions dependent upon size and location of detachment.
- Administer preoperative eye drops to dilate the pupil.
- Administer preoperative sedatives.

Postoperative Care

In addition to routine postoperative care:
- Maintain eye patch in place.
- Position as ordered if air/gas bubble injected (so that bubble can apply maximal pressure on the retina by the force of gravity). The position, usually head down and to one side, is maintained for several days.
- Administer PRN analgesics.
- Monitor for signs/symptoms of increased intraocular pressure (pain, nausea).
- Apply either warm or cold compresses for comfort.
- Administer postoperative medications:
  - IV Diamox to reduce increased intraocular pressure
  - antibiotic-steroid combination eye drops to prevent infection and reduce inflammation
  - cycloplegic agents to dilate the pupil and relax ciliary muscles
- Assist with ambulation and activities of daily living.

COMMUNITY AND SELF-CARE

Instruct client regarding:

- eye care
- measures to avoid increasing intraocular pressure
  - — no lifting of heavy objects
  - — no bending at the waist
  - — no straining with stool
  - — avoidance of coughing and vomiting
- technique for instilling eye drops
- signs/symptoms of increased intraocular pressure (pain, nausea, decreased vision)
- signs/symptoms of infection (redness, swelling, drainage, blurred vision, or pain)
- need to wear eye protection (shield or glasses)
- need to avoid air travel initially (if air/gas bubble injected) because air or gas will expand at high altitudes
- need for follow-up appointments

(For more information, see pp. 961–964 of Black and Matassarin-Jacobs: *Medical-Surgical Nursing: Clinical Management for Continuity of Care,* 5th ed.)

Rheumatic Fever

OVERVIEW

- Rheumatic fever is a diffuse inflammatory disease. It is a delayed response to an infection by group A beta-hemolytic streptococcus. Although these infections remain common, the incidence of rheumatic fever has declined dramatically in the United States.
- Rheumatic fever produces a diffuse, proliferative, and exudative inflammatory process. There is involvement of the heart, joints, subcutaneous tissue, central nervous system, and skin. Although the pathogenesis is not clear, it is probably through an abnormal humoral and cell-mediated response to streptococcal cell membrane antigens. The inflammatory process often produces permanent and severe heart damage. There may be Aschoff

bodies, minute nodules with localized fibrin deposits surrounded by areas of necrosis in the myocardium. Endocardial inflammation causes swelling of the valve leaflet and vegetations form on the valve tissues. The damaged valve may become narrowed and stenosed, or the valve leaflets may become so short that they cannot close completely. Both valvular stenosis and regurgitation eventually cause heart failure.

- Rheumatic fever develops in only a relatively small percentage of clients (3 per cent), even after a virulent bout of streptococcal infection.
- Poor hygiene and crowding are risk factors for acute rheumatic fever. If appropriate antibiotic therapy for group A beta-hemolytic streptococcal infections is given within the first 9 days of an infection, rheumatic fever will usually be prevented.
- Complications of rheumatic fever include valvular disorders, cardiomegaly, and congestive heart failure.

CLINICAL MANIFESTATIONS

- arthritis—painful and migratory. It most often affects the larger joints.
- carditis with significant murmur, chest pain, cardiomegaly, friction rub, and signs/symptoms of congestive heart failure
- fever
- erythema marginatum—rash seen primarily on the trunk. Lesions are crescent-shaped and have clear centers.
- subcutaneous nodules—small, painless, firm nodules that adhere loosely to the tendon sheaths (especially in the knees, knuckles and elbows)
- abdominal pain—may be related to liver engorgement
- weakness, malaise
- weight loss, anorexia

ACUTE AND SUBACUTE CARE

Medical Management

- oral antibiotics—penicillin or erythromycin
- salicylates

- corticosteroids
- cardiac glycosides and diuretics (if congestive heart failure present)
- bedrest

Nursing Management

- Administer antibiotics as ordered.
- Administer PRN analgesics and assess effectiveness.
- Maintain bedrest initially, followed by progressive activity program.
- Assess cardiac status for signs of congestive heart failure or carditis.
- Monitor temperature.
- Encourage well-balanced diet.
- Daily weights.

COMMUNITY AND SELF-CARE

Instruct the client regarding:

- disease process and treatment regime
- importance of completing course of antibiotics (client typically takes prophylactic agents for rheumatic fever for 5 years after initial attack)
- adequate rest with progressive resumption of activity
- importance of good care of teeth and gums to prevent caries and gingivitis
- prophylactic antibiotics prior to any dental work or minor surgery
- need to avoid people who have upper respiratory infection or recent streptococcal infection
- need to notify the physician if any of the symptoms of streptococcal pharyngitis develop—fever, chills, sore throat, enlarged, painful lymph nodes

(For more information, see pp. 1327–1331 of Black and Matassarin-Jacobs: *Medical-Surgical Nursing: Clinical Management for Continuity of Care,* 5th ed.)

Rheumatoid Arthritis

OVERVIEW

- Rheumatoid arthritis (RA) is an autoimmune connective tissue disease (collagen disease) that most commonly causes inflammation of the joints with subsequent joint deformity.
- A combination of factors seems to be responsible for the onset of RA. It seems that RA occurs in genetically predisposed persons, and it appears to be triggered by some unknown infectious agent or endogenous antigen.
- Altered B-cell regulation leads to a nonspecific polyclonal immunoglobulin G (IgG) response that causes lymphocyte production of antibodies that recognize the host as foreign and attacks them. The altered antibodies are called rheumatoid factors and they form immune complexes with IgG that are deposited in synovial membranes where they stimulate inflammation.
- Joint deformity occurs from repeated episodes of inflammation. The damage to the joint occurs in four distinct phases: (1) the initiation phase, (2) the immune response phase—cartilage is destroyed, (3) inflammatory phase—swelling damages tiny blood vessels in the synovial membrane and thickened fibrous scar tissue (called "pannus") is formed, and (4) destruction phase—fibrous tissue becomes calcified leading to joint fusion with permanent deformity.
- The incidence of RA is 1 per cent of the worldwide population. Women are affected with rheumatoid arthritis two to three times more often than are men until the age of 65. Women are most likely to develop clinical manifestations during the menopausal years.
- Since RA is a systemic disease, clinical manifestations may occur in other organs. They include skin changes, pulmonary disease, cardiac disease, ocular disease, and neurologic disease. However, the joints are generally affected first.
- RA is a disease of remissions and exacerbations. The most common course is repeated periods of

inflammation of varying degrees throughout the course, leading to progressive debilitation.

CLINICAL MANIFESTATIONS

- increasing fatigue, accompanied by diffuse musculoskeletal pain
- stiffness after inactivity such as sleep (morning stiffness) or prolonged sitting
- red, warm, swollen, stiff, and tender joints
- low-grade temperature
- guarded movement, limited range of motion and strength
- malaise and weight loss
- paresthesias of the hands and feet
- symptoms are worse in the morning
- firm, nontender subcutaneous nodules at wrist, knee, finger, and elbow joints
- chronic deformities of the hands and feet
- muscle spasms
- skin changes secondary to vasculitis
- depression and early afternoon fatigue

ACUTE AND SUBACUTE CARE

Medical Management

- analgesics and anti-inflammatory agents
  - — salicylates
  - — nonsteroidal anti-inflammatory medications—ibuprofen (Motrin), naproxen (Naprosyn), indomethacin (Indocin), sulindac (Clinoril)
  - — corticosteroids
  - — gold salts
- immunosuppressive (cytotoxic) agents—Cytoxan, Leukeran
- prescribed rest
- physical therapy
- occupational therapy
- heat/cold compresses to inflamed joints

Surgical Management

- tendon transfer—prevents progressive deformity caused by muscle spasms
- synovectomy—removal of synovial tissue in elbow, wrist, finger, or knee joints

- arthrodesis—bony fusion of a joint
- osteotomy—excising or cutting through the bone in a joint or limb to relieve pressure
- joint replacement—implants composed of stainless steel and polyurethene are used to replace affected joints in the hip, knee, shoulder, fingers, toes, or elbow

Nursing Management

Medical

- Administer analgesics and anti-inflammatory agents as ordered.
- Maintain bedrest during acute episodes.
- Position client to prevent contractures.
- Perform activities and exercises as outlined by physical therapy.
- Consult Physical and Occupational therapy for adaptive devices.
- Encourage warm shower in A.M. to decrease stiffness.
- Monitor response to activity.
- Provide adequate rest periods.
- Apply cold/heat to inflamed joints.

Surgical (Shoulder Arthroplasty)

Postoperative Care

In addition to routine postoperative care:

- Assess nerve function and circulation of the operative arm every 4 hours.
- Elevate head of bed 30 degrees to reduce swelling.
- Administer analgesics.
- Apply ice to shoulder as ordered.
- Position shoulder for comfort.
- Assist to perform rehabilitative exercises as ordered.

Surgical (Elbow Arthroplasty)

Postoperative Care

In addition to routine postoperative care:

- Elevate the arm above the shoulder.
- Assess neurovascular function of the operative arm every 4 hours.

- Administer analgesics as ordered.
- Assist to perform rehabilitative exercises as ordered.

Surgical (Hand Arthroplasty)

Postoperative Care

In addition to routine postoperative care:

- Elevate hand off of the bed.
- Perform neurovascular assessment every hour for several hours.
- Encourage patient to exercise the fingers 10 times every hour.

Surgical (Total Hip/Total Knee)

Preoperative Care

In addition to routine preoperative care:

- Teach the client how to use crutches and/or walker and encourage practice.
- Assist to practice transfer technique from bed to chair.
- Instruct and assist to practice postoperative exercises.

Postoperative Care

In addition to routine postoperative care:
Total Hip Replacement

- Maintain affected leg in abducted position and straight alignment while recumbent.
- Encourage and supervise prescribed exercises.
- Prevent hip flexion greater than 90 degrees when positioning or transferring.
- Assess nerve function and circulation in affected leg every 1–2 hours.
- Institute measures to prevent thrombophlebitis:
  — support stockings
  — low-dose Heparin
  — in-bed exercises.
- Monitor white blood count, temperature, and incision site for signs of infection.
- Administer prophylactic antibiotics as prescribed (steroid therapy, cytotoxic therapy, and implantation of a foreign object put the client at risk for infection).

- Administer PRN analgesics.
- Monitor for signs of adrenocortical insufficiency (clients on steroid therapy prior to surgery may exhibit signs of insufficiency secondary to the stress of the surgery)
  - — tachycardia
  - — hypotension
  - — diaphoresis
  - — decreasing level of consciousness
- Monitor for signs/symptoms of a pulmonary embolism or fat embolism
  - — respiratory distress
  - — tachycardia
  - — hypertension
  - — tachypnea
  - — fever
- Initiate weight bearing and ambulation as ordered.

Total Knee Replacement

- Maintain knee in maximum extension.
- Monitor use of continuous passive motion machine (CPM). The CPM should be used at all times except when not lying supine. The initial CPM setting is at 30 degrees of flexion and full extension. The degree of flexion is slowly increased each day, until 90 degrees of flexion is reached.
- Encourage and supervise prescribed exercises.
- Institute weight bearing and ambulation as ordered.
- Monitor for possible complications: thrombophlebitis, pulmonary embolism, fat embolism, infection, and adrenal insufficiency.

COMMUNITY AND SELF-CARE

Instruct the client regarding:

- techniques to reduce stress to joints, tendons, and ligaments
  - — monitor response to activity—carry out activities only to the point of fatigue or discomfort
  - — alternate between light and heavy tasks
  - — use larger, stronger joints to perform tasks (i.e., lift with palm and forearm instead of fingers)
  - — plan rest periods
  - — change position frequently
  - — assess the joints—avoid doing activities (other than gentle ROM) when joints are inflamed

— maintain good posture
- importance of controlling emotional and physical stress
- importance of medication regime
  — advise to take salicylates and nonsteroidal anti-inflammatory drugs with food or antacids
- prescribed exercises
- application of heat/cold compresses to inflamed joints

Surgical Management—total hip

- importance of not flexing hip greater than 90 degrees and avoiding extremes of internal rotation for 6 months to 1 year
- importance of not crossing one leg over the other
- importance of prescribed exercises
- avoidance of sitting continuously for longer than 1 hour
- avoidance of actions that place a strain on the hip joint—excessive bending, heavy lifting, jogging, and jumping
- avoidance of sitting in low, reclining, or rocking chairs
- use of adaptive devices (crutches/walker) until full weight bearing is allowed
- driving restrictions

(For more information, see pp. 655–674 of Black and Matassarin-Jacobs: *Medical-Surgical Nursing: Clinical Management for Continuity of Care*, 5th ed.)

Rhinitis

- Rhinitis is an inflammation of the nasal mucosa.
- The four classifications include: (1) acute, (2) allergic, (3) vasomotor, and (4) medicmentosa.
- The clinical manifestations include nasal drainage—usually clear unless the infection has spread to the sinuses and then the drainage will be yellow or green.
- Medical management includes:
  — decongestants
  — analgesics

- antibiotics
- allergy evaluation for allergic rhinitis
- antihistamines, steroids, mast-cell stabilizing nasal spray (for allergic rhinitis)

- Nursing management involves administering the medications and educating the client regarding side effects and the proper use of nasal sprays to avoid overuse. Over-the-counter nasal sprays should only be used for 3 days.
- Rhinitis should only last 5–7 days and follow-up with the physician is advised.

(For more information, see pp. 1080–1081 of Black and Matassarin-Jacobs: *Medical-Surgical Nursing: Clinical Management for Continuity of Care,* 5th ed.)

Rhinoplasty

- Rhinoplasty is the surgical correction of external nose deformities. The incisions are made inside the nose.
- Types of procedures performed may include reshaping the bony dorsum of the nose, the tip of the nose, and/or cartilage along the nares.
- Rhinoplasty usually is performed as day surgery under local anesthesia and sedation or general anesthesia.
- Discharge teaching—instruct the client on the following:
  - sleep with the head of bed elevated for 1 week
  - do not remove the external splint or nasal packing
  - do not blow the nose
  - sneeze only with the mouth open
  - remain on a soft diet for 2 days
  - avoid decongestant nasal sprays
  - it will take approximately 3 months before the client will be able to tell the final results of the surgery

(For more information, see pp. 2274–2275 of Black and Matassarin-Jacobs: *Medical-Surgical Nursing: Clinical Management for Continuity of Care,* 5th ed.)

S

Sarcoidosis

OVERVIEW

- Sarcoidosis is an inflammatory condition of widespread granulomatous lesions that affect many body systems.
- Lung involvement occurs in over 90 per cent of the cases, which can progress to fibrosis and restrictive lung disease.
- The onset occurs between the ages of 20 and 40 and is 14 times more common in blacks than whites.
- Involvement may be seen with the lymphatic system, skin, liver, eyes, spleen, bones, salivary glands, joints, and heart.

CLINICAL MANIFESTATIONS

- one-third of the clients are asymptomatic
- dry cough, hemoptysis, shortness of breath
- chest pain
- pneumothorax
- fatigue, weakness, malaise
- weight loss, fever

ACUTE AND SUBACUTE CARE

Medical Management

- determined by the degree of involvement
- on-going assessment of disease progression
- systemic corticosteroids
- bronchoscopy

Surgical Management

- open lung biopsy

Nursing Management

- Assess for side effects from the medications.

- Assess for signs of progress such as: increased tolerance to exercise; improved pulmonary function; improved oxygenation.
- If symptoms worsen document and notify the physician.

COMMUNITY AND SELF-CARE

Instruct client regarding:

- possible side effects of steroids such as weight gain, mood changes
- exercise and pulmonary rehabilitation
- when to notify the physician

(For more information, see pp. 1149–1150 of Black and Matassarin-Jacobs: *Medical-Surgical Nursing: Clinical Management for Continuity of Care,* 5th ed.)

Scleroderma

OVERVIEW

- Scleroderma, also called progressive systemic sclerosis (PSS), is a connective tissue disorder characterized by fibrosis and degenerative changes of the skin, synovium, digital arteries, and small arteries of the internal organs.
- Scleroderma is classified into two categories: localized—the less severe form affects primarily the skin, and generalized—involves skin and many internal organs such as the kidneys, lungs, heart, digestive system, and joints. There are two forms of PSS: (1) CREST syndrome and, (2) progressively fatal PSS.
- The cause of scleroderma is unknown. Excess deposition of collagen is the characteristic feature. Vascular changes include fibrosis of the endothelium of small arterioles. This damage and cell death activates platelets and causes more inflammation.

CLINICAL MANIFESTATIONS

Crest Syndrome

- calcinosis—small white calcium deposits beneath the skin
- Raynaud's phenomenon—vasospasms of small peripheral arteries
- esophogeal dysfunction—impaired motility
- scleroderma of the digits
- telangiectasia—spider-like hemangiomas

Progressively Fatal PSS

- subcutaneous edema
- fever
- malaise
- thick, hide-like skin with loss of normal skin folds
- ulcerations around the fingertips
- polyarthritis and polyarthralgias
- dysphagia (secondary to esophageal dysfunction)
- hypermotility and malabsorption (secondary to fibrosis and atrophy of the gastrointestinal tract)
- low oxygen diffusing capacity (secondary to pulmonary fibrosis and decreased lung compliance)
- hypertension (secondary to renal involvement)
- mild anemia

ACUTE AND SUBACUTE CARE

Medical Management

Medical treatment is supportive and symptomatic.

- steroid therapy
- immunosuppressants

Nursing Management

- Provide measures to prevent skin breakdown.
- Administer analgesics.
- Initiate progressive activity program and monitor client response.
- Implement dietary modifications for dysphagia.
- Monitor laboratory results—renal profile, nutritional panel, blood counts, arterial blood gases.
- Provide restful environment.

COMMUNITY AND SELF-CARE

Instruct client regarding:

- importance of medication regime
- skin breakdown prevention measures
- avoidance of activities that trigger pain associated with Raynaud's phenomenon and joint pain:
  - — respond to pain that lasts for more than 1–2 hours by stopping that particular activity
  - — alternate light and heavy tasks
  - — plan for rest
  - — if joints are red or swollen, use them as little as possible
  - — avoid extreme cold, wear gloves when hands are exposed to cold
  - — eliminate smoking
- dietary modification
- importance of follow-up visits

(For more information, see pp. 677–678 of Black and Matassarin-Jacobs: *Medical-Surgical Nursing: Clinical Management for Continuity of Care,* 5th ed.)

Sclerosing Cholangitis

OVERVIEW

- Sclerosing cholangitis is an inflammatory disease of the bile ducts that causes fibrosis and thickening of their walls and multiple, short, concentric strictures.
- The cause has been linked to altered immunity, toxins, and infectious agents.
- The disease is progressive and gradually causes cirrhosis, portal hypertension, and death from hepatic failure. It may also predispose the client to the development of cholangiocarcinoma.
- Approximately two-thirds of cases occur in clients under the age of 45, and the male-to-female ratio is 3:2.

CLINICAL MANIFESTATIONS

- fatigue
- anorexia and weight loss
- jaundice

- pruritus
- vague upper abdominal pain

ACUTE AND SUBACUTE CARE

Medical Management

- corticosteroids
- antibiotics
- immunosuppressants
- bile acid-binding agents—colchicine, penicillamine
- cholestyramine (Questran)—binds with bile salts in the intestines, removing excess bile salts and reducing itching

Surgical Management

- limited due to progressive nature of the disease and recurrent cholangitis
- liver transplantation—most definitive treatment

Nursing Management

Medical

- Administer antibiotics and corticosteroids as ordered.
- Monitor liver enzymes.
- Assess for signs of hepatic failure.

Surgical

- See care of client following liver transplantation, "Liver Transplant," p. 453.

COMMUNITY AND SELF-CARE

Instruct client regarding:
- importance of medication regime
- signs/symptoms of liver failure
- importance of follow-up appointments
- see "Liver Transplant," p. 453.
- see "Portal Hypertension," p. 585, and "Cirrhosis," p. 174.

(For more information, see p. 1920 of Black and Matassarin-Jacobs: *Medical-Surgical Nursing: Clinical Management for Continuity of Care,* 5th ed.)

Scoliosis

OVERVIEW

- Scoliosis is defined as an abnormal lateral curvature of the spine when viewing from the posteroanterior view. Adult scoliosis is a spinal curvature existing after skeletal maturity.
- A curve may be present in any area of the spine—cervical, thoracic, thoracolumbar, and lumbar. There is usually a second compensatory curve in the opposite direction.
- Adult scoliosis occurs in individuals aged 40 years or older.
- If an individual has a positive family history of scoliosis, the risk for occurrence is greater.
- Curves of less than 40 degrees, without symptoms, generally remain stable and do not require intervention.
- The prevalence of scoliosis in the general population ranges from 2–4 per cent.

CLINICAL MANIFESTATIONS

- shortness of breath and fatigue (thoracic spine curve)
- back pain
- decreased height
- cosmetic deformity

ACUTE AND SUBACUTE CARE

Medical Management

- pain management

Surgical Management

- application of spinal instrumentation:
  - Cortel-Dubousset system
  - Harrington rod system
  - Luque rod system
  - Dwyer cable instrumentation
- bone grafted fusions

Nursing Management

Medical

- Administer analgesics as ordered.

Surgical

Postoperative Care

In addition to routine postoperative care:
- Nursing care will depend on the type of surgical procedure.
- Consult Physical Therapy for activity/exercise instructions.

COMMUNITY AND SELF-CARE

Instruct client regarding:
- pain management
- management of postoperative immobilization device
- progressive ambulation

(For more information, see pp. 2120–2121 of Black and Matassarin-Jacobs: *Medical-Surgical Nursing: Clinical Management for Continuity of Care,* 5th ed.)

Sexual Assault, Alleged

OVERVIEW

- "Alleged sexual assault" is the term health care providers are required to use when caring for clients who may be victims of rape. The client should be advised of this, to avoid the perception that the health care provider is insensitive.
- The goal of emergency care for these clients is to provide sensitive, thorough physical care, coupled with empathetic psychosocial support, and to carefully gather vital information and evidence that is usually legally evaluated.
- Sexual assault victims often experience both acute and long-term physical and psychological trauma. The psychological trauma, known as rape-trauma

syndrome, may last only a few days to weeks or may last many years.

ACUTE AND SUBACUTE CARE

Nursing Management

- Assess and maintain airway, breathing, and circulation. Assess for trauma to the larynx or mandible.
- Ensure privacy and explain to the client not to wash, gargle, or douche until all necessary specimens are obtained.
- Obtain a detailed history and physical examination after explaining the need for detail.
- Perform thorough assessment, recording extent, location, and treatment of all injuries. Pictures may be included.
- Provide emotional support throughout gynecologic examination.
- Obtain specimens for laboratory studies, including cultures for gonorrhea; hanging drop analysis and smears for the presence of sperm and their motility; acid phosphatase of vaginal secretions; analysis of foreign pubic hairs by the police laboratory, HIV screen, and serologic fluorescent treponemal antibody studies.
- Ask the client's permission to contact a sexual assault counselor. Be aware that relative calmness or seeming unconcern does not mean that the client is handling it well.
- Note the condition of the client's clothing and document tears, stains, or dishevelment. Make arrangements for clean clothes to be brought to the client and place torn clothes in a bag for the police.
- Administer antibiotics and agents to prevent pregnancy as ordered.
- Suggest that someone stay with the client several days for support.
- Document carefully the history, assessment, interventions, and discharge teaching.

COMMUNITY AND SELF-CARE

Instruct client regarding:

- follow-up care in 4–6 weeks for test results, pregnancy test, and psychosocial support
- the name and number of rape counseling resources if the client is unable or unwilling to use counseling resources at the time of emergency treatment (the client may later desire this information)
- possible emotional responses to this type of trauma
- menses should start within 7 days after completion of treatment; if this does not occur, dilation and curettage is arranged
- reinforcement of information on referral services and information provided by sexual assault counselor

(For more information, see p. 2432 of Black and Matassarin-Jacobs: *Medical-Surgical Nursing: Clinical Management for Continuity of Care,* 5th ed.)

Shock

OVERVIEW

- Shock is defined as failure of the circulatory system to maintain adequate perfusion of vital organs. Inadequate tissue perfusion can be caused by various disorders that result in decreased oxygenation at the cellular level.
- Inadequate oxygenation leads to an abnormal physiologic state in which there is altered cellular metabolism and accumulated waste products in cells. If the condition is untreated, cell and organ death occurs.
- For adequate blood circulation to occur, three factors must function effectively together:
  - — circulating blood volume
  - — vascular tone or the resistance of the blood vessels
  - — cardiac pump or pumping action of the heart.

  When these three components are functioning properly, mean arterial pressure (MAP) is maintained at normal levels and tissues are adequately perfused. If one of the three components fail, compensatory mechanisms are initiated. For example, vasoconstriction and increased cardiac output may be used to compensate for decreased volume. Thus, as long as two of these factors can maintain a satisfactory compensatory action, adequate blood circulation can be sustained. However, if compensatory mechanisms fail or if more than one of the three factors necessary for adequate circulation malfunction, circulatory failure results, and shock develops.

- Shock is commonly discussed in three major categories:
  (1) hypovolemic shock—due to inadequate circulating blood volume
    — common causes:
      - hemorrhage
      - burns—shift of plasma from the vascular space to the interstitial space or loss of plasma through the surface of the burn
      - dehydration

  (2) cardiogenic shock—due to inadequate pumping action of the heart, as a result of impaired muscle action or mechanical obstruction of blood flow to and from the heart
    — common causes:
      - myocardial infarction
      - valvular insufficiency
      - dysrhythmias
      - obstructive conditions—pulmonary embolism, pericardial tamponade, tension pneumothorax

  (3) distributive shock (vasogenic shock)—results from inadequate vascular tone. The blood volume remains normal, but the size of the vascular space increases dramatically because of massive vasodilation.

  Three types:
    — anaphylactic shock—severe hypersensitivity reaction resulting in massive systemic vasodilation
    — neurogenic shock—interference with nervous system control of blood vessels, such as spinal cord injury, spinal anesthesia, or severe vasovagal reactions due to pain or emotional trauma

— septic shock—resulting from massive sepsis and the release of toxins or vasoactive substances

- Risk factors include:
  - — major trauma
  - — previous myocardial damage
  - — immunosuppressive therapy
  - — exposure to allergen
- Stages of shock:
  (1) compensated stage—cardiac output is slightly decreased
    (a) blood moves from tissues into the vascular system increasing circulating volume
    (b) sympathetic nervous system stimulation causes vasoconstriction and tachycardia
    (c) the body's compensatory mechanisms are able to maintain BP within normal to low-normal range and are able to maintain tissue perfusion to the vital organs
  (2) decompensated stage
    (a) persistent vasoconstriction causes capillary dilation, decreased venous return, and decreased circulation of reoxygenated blood
    (b) lactic acidosis occurs as a result of anaerobic metabolism
    (c) acidosis causes increased capillary permeability, and blood "pools" in the capillaries further decreasing venous return
    (d) mean arterial pressure and cardiac output decrease
    (e) decrease in circulating volume and capillary flow does not allow adequate perfusion and oxygenation of vital organs and tissues
  (3) progressive stage—occurs if the cycle of inadequate tissue perfusion is not interrupted. Cellular ischemia and necrosis lead to organ failure and death of the client.

CLINICAL MANIFESTATIONS

- rapid, shallow breathing
- rapid, weak, thready pulse
- hypotension
- narrowing pulse pressure (the difference between systolic and diastolic pressure readings)—during shock, the pulse pressure is more significant than

the blood pressure because it tends to parallel cardiac stroke volume

- restlessness, anxiety, and irritability during early stages
- decreased level of consciousness
- weakness
- dizziness or faintness when sitting up from horizontal position
- decreased urinary output
- diaphoresis
- ashen pallor progressing to cyanosis
- flat neck veins
- slow capillary refill and collapse of superficial veins in extremities
- dilated pupils
- thirst, dry mucous membranes
- cold, clammy skin, "goosebumps"
- nausea, vomiting
- decreased bowel sounds
- hypothermia

Specific clinical manifestations for each type of shock:

Hypovolemic

- cool, clammy skin
- marked diaphoresis
- cyanosis
- increased urine osmolality and specific gravity initially (due to sodium and water reabsorption)

Cardiogenic

- jugular venous distention, increased CVP
- tachycardia, pulmonary edema, crackles in the lungs, increased pulmonary capillary wedge pressure (PCWP)
- cold, clammy skin

Distributive

- anaphylactic
  — initially, feeling of uneasiness or doom
  — complaint of headache
  — severe anxiety, dizziness, disorientation, and loss of consciousness
  — feeling of a "lump in the throat"

- — coughing, dyspnea, stridor
  - — wheezing and prolonged expiratory phase
  - — pruritus and urticaria
  - — edema of the eyelids, lips, or tongue (angioedema)
- neurogenic
  - — bradycardia and hypotension (loss of ability to vasoconstrict)
  - — below level of injury, skin temperature takes on same temperature as room (poikilothermia)
  - — dry skin (inability to sweat)
- septic
  - — warm, dry, flushed skin (early stage secondary to massive vasodilation)
  - — cold, clammy, mottled skin (later stage)
  - — hypothermia
  - — crackles and wheezes (secondary to pulmonary congestion)
  - — drowsiness, stupor, progressing to coma

ACUTE AND SUBACUTE CARE

Medical Management

- blood loss management
  - — external bleeding—application of direct pressure, pressure dressing, or surgical intervention
  - — intra-abdominal or retroperitoneal bleeding—MAST suit (see below), gastric lavage, surgical intervention
- respiratory support
  - — supplemental oxygen
  - — chest physiotherapy
  - — mechanical ventilation
  - — endotracheal intubation
- circulatory support
  - — MAST (medical antishock trouser suit)—encases the lower part of the body in a one-piece, three-chambered (two leg and one abdominal chamber) suit from the lower costal margin to the ankles. The suit is inflated, causing increased vascular resistance and decreased diameter of the blood vessels in the abdomen and legs. This results in impedance of blood flow and decreases leakage into the tissues. Cardiac output

increases and arterial blood pressure improves (most often used in trauma settings).
  - IABP (intra-aortic balloon pump)—(used primarily in cardiogenic shock)—a balloon-tipped catheter is placed in the descending thoracic aorta. It inflates during diastole and deflates just before systole. This counterpulsation displaces blood back into the aorta and improves coronary artery circulation.
  - external counterpulsation device—legs are encased in air or water-filled tubular bags connected to a pumping unit. Pressure is applied to the legs during diastole and released in systole.
  - Swan-Ganz catheter placement for hemodynamic monitoring
- positioning—to promote venous return without compressing the abdominal organs against the diaphragm
  - modified Trendelenburg's position with lower extremities elevated about 30–45 degrees, knees straight, trunk horizontal or slightly raised, and neck comfortably positioned with head level to chest or slightly higher
  - not used in cardiogenic shock when there is already circulatory overload
- fluid therapy—fluid replacement should be administered through large-bore peripheral lines, central lines, or both. Fluid replacement therapy must replace blood lost from the circulation and fluid lost from the interstitial space.
  - crystalloid or balanced salt solutions—normal saline, Ringer's lactate, half-normal saline
  - colloid solutions—contain proteins too large to exit normally at the capillary, thus remain in the vascular compartment, increasing osmotic pressure helping to retain fluid there
    - plasma
    - dextran
    - hetastarch
    - albumin
  - blood transfusion—when hemorrhage is the primary cause of shock, the rapid administration of large volumes of packed cells or whole blood may be necessary
- pharmacologic management

- vasoconstrictors—elevate systemic blood pressure and increase blood flow to the brain and heart in severely hypotensive states
  - high dose dopamine (Inotropin)
  - norepinephrine (Levophed)
  - phenylephrine (Neo-Synephrine)
- vasodilators—induce vasodilation of blood vessels or inhibit vasoconstriction so that blood can be redistributed
  - amrinone (Inocor)
  - dobutamine (Dobutrex)
  - epinephrine (Adrenalin)
  - isoproterenol (Isuprel)
  - nitroprusside (Nipride)
  - low-dose dopamine (Inotropin)
- vasoconstrictor/vasodilator combination—to offset profound effects of some vasoconstrictors or to provide the benefit of both types of drugs
- antibiotics—for hypovolemic shock (secondary to trauma with open wounds) or septic shock
- steroids—in neurogenic shock, reduce edema in the spinal cord
- Heparin therapy—to prevent or treat some complications of shock (pulmonary embolism, deep vein thrombosis, disseminated intravascular coagulation) and in cardiogenic shock to prevent thrombi formation near the area of infarction
- calcium replacement—needed for normal functioning of nervous and cardiovascular systems
- stress ulcer prophylaxis—histamine hydrogen-receptor antagonists
  - cimetidine
  - famotidine
  - ranitidine
- antihistamine therapy—anaphylactic shock
  - diphenhydramine hydrochloride (Benadryl)
- cardiotonic medications
  - digitalis—used if evidence of cardiac failure to strengthen inotropic action of the heart
  - antidysrhythmics—to improve cardiac efficiency

- atropine—to treat bradycardia, which predisposes to cardiogenic shock

- renal support
  - diuretics for low urine output
  - fluid replacement
  - correction of metabolic acidosis
- thermoregulation—even though client feels cold and clammy, do not apply heat to the skin—will dilate vessels and draw blood away from vital organs and will increase metabolism and oxygen demand. The environment is kept warm to prevent chilling, which also increases energy demands.
- nasogastric suction—early response in shock is decreased splanchnic circulation, causing inadequate tissue perfusion and delayed gastric emptying; thus, increasing vomiting and aspiration potential
- Summary of the Management of Hypovolemic Shock:
  - stop external bleeding
  - decrease intra-abdominal or retroperitoneal bleeding by applying MAST suit
  - administer crystalloids
  - transfuse with fresh whole blood, packed cells, plasma
  - administer plasma expanders (albumin, hetastarch, dextran)
- Summary of the Management of Cardiogenic Shock:
  - fluid challenge to rule out hypovolemia (unless congestive heart failure or pulmonary edema is present)
  - insert central venous pressure or pulmonary artery catheter
  - administer fluids to maintain left ventricular filling pressure
  - administer dopamine or dobutamine
  - administer vasodilators
  - administer diuretics
  - administer cardiotonics
  - IABP or external counterpulsation device if unresponsive to therapies
  - pericardiocentesis, if tamponade present
  - thrombolytic or anticoagulant therapy
  - treat dysrhythmias
- Summary of Management of Distributive Shock

- anaphylactic shock
  - airway management
  - epinephrine administration
  - vasopressor therapy (norepinephrine, high-dose dopamine)
  - Benadryl administration (antihistamine)
  - theophylline administration
  - IV steroids
  - gastric lavage to remove ingested antigen
  - ice pack to injection or sting site
- septic shock
  - identify origin of sepsis
  - IV fluid resuscitation
  - antibiotic therapy
  - dopamine or dobutamine therapy
  - temperature control
- neurogenic (spinal) shock
  - treat bradycardia with atropine
  - vasopressor administration
  - fluid replacement therapy
- vasovagal shock
  - place patient in head-down or recumbent position
  - administer atropine if bradycardic
  - eliminate pain

Surgical Management

Surgery may be performed to control sources of bleeding.

Nursing Management

- Assess cardiac, respiratory, and neurologic status.
- Administer and monitor fluid therapy replacement to prevent fluid overload.
- Provide respiratory support:
  - supplemental oxygen
  - mechanical ventilation
- Monitor vital signs and hemodynamic values.
- Monitor urinary output.
- Continuous cardiac monitoring.
- Place patient in modified Trendelenburg's position (unless in cardiogenic shock).
- Administer and monitor ordered vasoactive drug therapy:

- Vasoconstrictors
  - Monitor arterial blood pressure; watch for undesirable blood pressure elevation.
  - Titrate IV medications to obtain desirable blood pressure.
  - Monitor IV administration sites closely to detect infiltration early.
- Vasodilators
  - Monitor blood pressure and central venous pressure for severe hypotension.
  - Keep patients lying relatively flat to prevent orthostatic hypotension.
- Administer epinephrine (to stop the release of histamine) and Benadryl (to relieve symptoms) in anaphylactic shock.
- Administer analgesia to control pain. Narcotics, which cause vasodilation resulting in hypotension are never given without first knowing if the blood volume is adequate.
- Administer electrolyte replacement therapy.
- Monitor laboratory values—arterial blood gases, electrolytes, hemoglobin, oxygen saturations.
- Maintain nasogastric tube to suction.
- Monitor nasogastric aspirant for blood and pH value to assess for development of a stress ulcer.
- Administer histamine hydrogen-receptor antagonists and antacids.
- Administer antibiotics as ordered (septic shock or open trauma wounds).
- Administer cardiotonic medications as ordered (to improve contractility).
- Monitor for complications of immobility (pulmonary embolism, deep vein thrombosis, pressure sores, etc.).

COMMUNITY AND SELF-CARE

- Shock must be fully resolved before a client is discharged. Instruction will center on managing the care of any complication that developed or surgical intervention involved.

(For more information, see pp. 497–531 of Black and Matassarin-Jacobs: *Medical-Surgical Nursing: Clinical Management for Continuity of Care*, 5th ed.)

Sinusitis

OVERVIEW

- Sinusitis is an infection of one of the paranasal sinuses. It occurs when ostia in the nose are obstructed or ciliary action is impaired, causing mucous accumulation and infection.

CLINICAL MANIFESTATIONS

- pain in the sinus area, worsened with bending
- pain or numbness in the upper teeth
- purulent or discolored nasal discharge

ACUTE AND SUBACUTE CARE

Medical Management

- antibiotics to treat infection
- decongestants to reduce edema
- steroid nasal sprays to reduce mucosal inflammation
- humidification to prevent nasal crusting and to moisten secretions
- antral or sinus lavage if the above measures are not effective

Surgical Management

- Functional endoscopic sinus surgery (FESS) is often the first surgical technique performed to reestablish sinus ventilation and mucociliary clearance. Small sinus endoscopes are passed through the nasal cavity and into the sinuses. Diseased tissue is removed, and sinus ostia enlarged.
- Caldwell-Luc is another surgical procedure for maxillary sinusitis. The diseased mucous membrane is removed through an incision into the gingival buccal sulcus above the lateral incisor teeth. An opening also may be created between the maxillary sinus and lateral nasal wall (nasal antral window) to increase aeration of the sinus and permit drainage into the nasal cavity.
- External sphenoethmoidectomy is a surgical procedure to remove diseased mucosa from the sphe-

noid or ethmoid sinuses. A small incision is made over the ethmoid sinus and diseased mucosa is removed.

Nursing Management

Surgical

Functional Endoscopic Sinus Surgery (FESS)

Postoperative Care

In addition to routine postoperative care:

- Monitor placement of nasal packing (usually removed within several hours of procedure).
- Apply ice compresses to the nose and cheek to minimize edema and control bleeding.
- Monitor amount of nasal bleeding; change drip pad as needed.
- Monitor for increased bleeding, respiratory distress and edema for the first 24 hours after surgery.
- Monitor for visual changes; blindness can occur, though rarely from intraorbital hematoma formation or direct injury to the optic nerve.
- Maintain semi-Fowler's to high-Fowler's position for 24–48 hours after surgery to minimize edema.

Caldwell-Luc

Postoperative Care

In addition to routine postoperative care:

- Monitor placement of nasal and maxillary sinus packing. Nasal packing generally is removed the morning after surgery; antral packing remains in place for 36-72 hours. Assess oral cavity for blood or dislodged packing that may obstruct the pharynx.
- Assess for increased bleeding, respiratory distress, and edema for the first 24 hours after surgery.
- Assess for any numbness of the upper teeth due to interruption of the sensory nerves from the incision (this may last several weeks).
- Apply ice compresses to the nose and cheek to minimize edema and control bleeding.
- Maintain semi-Fowler's to high-Fowler's position for 24-48 hours after surgery to minimize edema.
- Administer mild analgesics as prescribed.

- External sphenoethmoidectomy—same as for Caldwell-Luc procedure except an eye pressure pad is worn to decrease periorbital edema.

COMMUNITY AND SELF-CARE

Functional Endoscopic Sinus Surgery (FESS)

Instruct client regarding:
- increasing fluids to moisten secretions
- avoidance of blowing the nose for 7-10 days
- using nasal saline sprays as recommended (usually started 3-5 days postoperatively)
- avoidance of strenuous activity, lifting, or straining for 2 weeks
- importance of follow-up to physician's office for removal of crusts and debris

Caldwell-Luc

- Same as for FESS procedure above.

(For more information, see pp. 1077–1078 of Black and Matassarin-Jacobs: *Medical-Surgical Nursing: Clinical Management for Continuity of Care,* 5th ed.)

Skin Cancer

OVERVIEW

- Skin cancer is a malignant condition caused by uncontrolled growth and spread of abnormal cells in a specific layer of skin.
- There are several kinds of skin cancer:
  - — Basal cell cancer—malignant epithelial tumor of the skin that arises from basal cells in the dermis; almost never metastasizes.
  - — Squamous cell cancer—tumor of the epidermal keratinocytes; usually found on rim of the ear, the face, the lips and mouth, and the dorsa of the hands. It may metastasize to the lymph nodes and be subsequently fatal. It rarely occurs in dark-skinned clients.

— Malignant melanoma—deadliest form of skin cancer. The incidence and mortality have risen by 7–15 per cent per year in countries populated with fair-skinned whites. The tumor can metastasize, usually to the brain, lungs, bones, liver and skin. It is universally fatal.

- Skin cancer is the most common cancer in the United States. More than 90 per cent of skin cancers are either basal cell or squamous cell cancer. Both have an excellent cure rate of 95 per cent or greater with treatment.
- The cause of skin cancer is prolonged or intermittent exposure to ultraviolet radiation from the sun, especially when it results in sunburn and blistering.
- Clients with red, blonde, or light-brown hair with light complexions or freckles, many of Celtic or Scandinavian origin, are most susceptible.
- Danger signals suggesting malignant changes in pigmented nevi are:
  - — changes in color (especially red, white, and blue)
  - — change in diameter
  - — change in outline
  - — change in surface characteristics
  - — change in consistency
  - — change in symptoms
  - — change in shape
  - — change in surrounding skin.

CLINICAL MANIFESTATIONS

Basal Cell Carcinoma

- painless and slow-growing lesions appearing on sun-exposed skin, face, ears, head, neck, or hands
- lesions with "pearly" texture

Squamous Cell Carcinoma

May present in any of the forms below. These tumors are poorly marginated with the edge blending into the skin.

- ulcer
- flat red area
- cutaneous horn

- indurated plaque
- hyperkeratotic papule or nodule

Malignant Melanoma

- lesion with shades of brown and black plus red, white, or blue coloration
- bleeding of a mole or change in color, size, or thickness
- notching or indentation of the border of a lesion

ACUTE AND SUBACUTE CARE

Surgical Management

Treatment of skin cancer requires removal of the lesion. The tumor removed needs to have a specified margin free of tumor to guarantee full removal of the tumor.

- Moh's surgery for basal cell and squamous cell carcinoma—a special surgical technique used for the removal of skin malignancies. The technique is based upon a series of excisions. Careful microscopic tissue assessment "maps" the presence or absence of malignant cells within each specimen.
- excision of basal cell or squamous cell carcinoma and closure of the area with a skin flap
- wide local excision with a 1–3 cm margin of normal skin is the initial treatment for malignant melanoma
- possible radiation therapy, surgical removal of metastatic lesions, chemotherapy and local hyperthermia for metastatic melanoma

Nursing Management

- Instruct client/significant other regarding:
  - — wound care after surgical removal
  - — need for regular self inspection
  - — signs/symptoms of recurrent skin cancer
  - — avoidance of excessive exposure to the sun
  - — use of sunscreen and other sun protection
  - — importance of follow-up
- Malignant melanoma:
  - — signs/symptoms to report to physician
- See "Chemotherapy," p. 149.
- See "Radiation Therapy," p. 605.

- Provide emotional support to client and significant other.
- Make referrals to cancer support groups, home health care agencies, and community resources as appropriate.

(For more information, see pp. 2225–2230 of Black and Matassarin-Jacobs: *Medical-Surgical Nursing: Clinical Management for Continuity of Care,* 5th ed.)

Sleep Apnea

- Sleep apnea is characterized by recurrent periods of breathing cessation for 10 seconds or longer occurring at least five times per hour during sleep. Sleep apnea can be differentiated as obstructive sleep apnea or central sleep apnea syndrome.

Obstructive Sleep Apnea

- In obstructive sleep apnea (OSA), the client makes respiratory efforts, but they are ineffective against a collapsed or obstructed upper airway. As hypoxia ensues, the client eventually awakens to breathe. This causes frequent awakenings, which impair the normal sleep cycle and cause excessive daytime sleepiness.
- Affects over 1 per cent of the adult population and up to 5 per cent of middle-aged men.
- A small number of clients may progress to Pickwickian syndrome, characterized by obesity, severe sleep apnea, daytime hypercapnia, and cor pulmonale.
- OSA is common among obese males with short, thick necks who are heavy snorers.
- Mild OSA may be treated through weight reduction and avoidance of sleeping on the back. For other clients, referral to a sleep disorders center or use of continuous positive airway pressure (CPAP) during sleep may be needed.
- A uvulopalatopharyngoplasty (resection of the uvula, posterior soft palate, tonsils and any exces-

sive pharyngeal tissue) may be performed for OSA. A tracheostomy may be required for some clients.
- Oral or dental appliances are being used more often as a treatment.
- The nurse should instruct clients to avoid hypnotics, benzodiazepines, or alcohol.

Central Sleep Apnea Syndrome

- This syndrome is characterized by apneic periods during which there is no apparent respiratory effort. It may be seen with central nervous system lesions, but most commonly is mixed with obstructive sleep apnea. Cheyne-Stokes respirations are common.
- The usual treatment is CPAP, but use of diaphragmatic pacemakers or mechanical ventilation may be required in severe cases.
- The nurse should instruct the client to avoid hypnotic or sedative drugs and alcohol.

(For more information, see pp. 401–402 of Black and Matassarin-Jacobs: *Medical-Surgical Nursing: Clinical Management for Continuity of Care,* 5th ed.)

Sleep Disturbances, Hospital Acquired

OVERVIEW

- There are a variety of disturbances in sleep that may occur during hospitalization:
  - sleep-onset difficulty—difficulty getting to sleep, usually due to anxiety and strange environment
  - sleep maintenance disturbance—waking frequently with difficulty getting back to sleep. Causes include: sustained use of or withdrawal from medications; internal factors, such as pain, discomfort or the urge to void; and external stimuli, such as noise, light, temperature, and equipment.
  - early morning awakening—frequently seen among the elderly. This also may be an indication of depression.

— sleep deprivation—may occur due to frequent caregiver interruptions, noise level, and 24-hour lighting. This is of particular concern in critical care units. This may be a major contributing factor to postoperative psychosis.

ACUTE AND SUBACUTE CARE

Nursing Management

- Obtain an initial history of the client's usual sleep habits and recent sleep quality.
- If sleep quality is reported to be poor, explore the nature of the disturbance in detail, including:
  — usual activities prior to retiring
  — caffeine intake
  — use of alcohol, sleeping pills, and other medications
  — consistency of rising time
  — frequency and duration of naps
  — number and perceived cause of awakenings.
- Follow usual bedtime routine as much as possible during hospitalization.
- Provide techniques to mimic nighttime and promote relaxation at usual bedtime:
  — offer milk before sleep if condition allows (contains tryptophan, which promotes sleep)
  — external warmth and extra blankets
  — dim lights and provide quiet environment
  — analgesia
  — back massage or music
  — hypnotics (such as benzodiazepine triazolam [Halcion])—these should be a last resort measure. If given, be aware that safety measures should be in place as most hypnotics cause some anterograde amnesia and cognitively intact clients may experience some disorientation.
- If the client's sleep must be interrupted, schedule assessments and interventions to allow 90–120 minutes of uninterrupted sleep. Assess if the client is in REM sleep (manifested by rapid eye movements, erratic respirations, changes in heart rate, and very low muscle tone) prior to interruption. Avoid awakening during REM sleep and allow progression to next stage of sleep if at all possible.

(For more information, see pp. 406–409 of Black and Matassarin-Jacobs: *Medical-Surgical Nursing: Clinical Management for Continuity of Care,* 5th ed.)

Spinal Cord Injury

OVERVIEW

- Injury to the spinal cord can range in severity from mild flexion-extension "whiplash" injuries to complete transection of the cord with quadriplegia. Trauma to the cord can occur at any level but most commonly occurs in the cervical and lower thoracic-upper lumbar vertebrae. These segments of the spine are the most mobile and, thereby, most easily injured.
- Each year approximately 10,000 individuals sustain a spinal cord injury. Most of these individuals are males under the age of 40.
- Trauma is the most common cause of spinal injury. Traumatic spinal injury may be due to automobile or motorcycle accidents, gunshot or knife wounds, falls, or sporting mishaps. Disorders that may result in spinal cord injury include:
  - — cervical spondylosis—producing spinal canal narrowing, causing injury to the cord and roots
  - — myelitis
  - — osteoporosis—causing compression fractures of the vertebrae
  - — syringomyelia—cavitation of the cord
  - — tumors—both infiltrative and compressive
  - — vascular disease—infarction or hemorrhage
- Pathophysiology:
  - — SCIs (spinal cord injuries) most often occur as a result of injury to the vertebrae. The cord is injured as a result of acceleration, deceleration, or impact. The forces injure the spinal cord by compressing, pulling, or tearing the tissues. Microscopic bleeding occurs immediately after injury, primarily in the gray matter of the cord. Within the first hour, edema develops and often spreads along the length of the cord. Cord edema peaks within 2–3 days and subsides

within the first 7 days after injury. The edema leads to temporary loss of sensation and function. Therefore, immediately after injury, it is not easy to determine the degree of permanent impairment.

— Mechanism of injury
  (1) flexion-rotation, dislocation, or fracture dislocation
    — most common spinal injuries are flexion injuries; the spine is forced into acute hyperextension
    — occurs in cervical spine (C_5 and C_6)
    — rupture of the posterior ligaments results in forward dislocation of the vertebrae. Blood vessels may be damaged leading to ischemia of the cord.
  (2) hyperextension
    — the anterior ligament is ruptured with fracture of the posterior elements of the vertebral body
    — complete transection of the cord can occur
  (3) compression
    — caused by falls or jumps in which the individual lands directly on the feet, head, or sacrum
    — force of impact fractures the vertebrae, compressing the cord. Disc and bone fragments may be propelled backward into the spinal cord.
    — lumbar and lower thoracic vertebrae are most commonly injured

CLINICAL MANIFESTATIONS

Initial clinical manifestations of acute spinal cord injury depend upon the level and extent of injury. Below the level of injury or lesion there is loss of (1) voluntary movement, (2) sensation of pain, temperature, pressure, and proprioception, (3) bowel and bladder function, and (4) spinal and automatic reflexes.

- Level of injury
  — injury to the cervical spine and cord produces quadriplegia

— injuries above C_4 may be fatal due to loss of innervation to the diaphragm and intercostal muscles
— injuries to the thoracic or lumbar spine produce paraplegia

- Changes in reflexes
  — reflexes are absent in early SCI because of spinal cord edema. Blood pressure and temperature in denervated areas fall markedly and respond poorly to reflex stimuli.
  — after edema subsides, some body functions may return by reflex but may be initiated by atypical stimuli. For example, scratching the skin may cause vasodilation, sweating, urination etc.
- Muscle spasms
  — muscle spasms vary from mild muscular twitching to vigorous mass reflex states that may throw the patient out of bed
  — muscle spasms may be aggravated by cold weather, prolonged sitting, or emotionally upsetting events. Reflex spasms may be triggered by visceral stimuli, such as a distended bladder or cutaneous stimulation (i.e. tickling, stroking, or pinching).
- Autonomic Dysreflexia
  — a life-threatening syndrome, is a cluster of clinical manifestations that results when multiple spinal cord autonomic responses discharge simultaneously
  — syndrome is observed in as many as 85 per cent of clients with injury above T-7. It often resolves after 3 years but may reoccur.
  — The manifestations result from an exaggerated sympathetic response to a noxious stimulus below the cord lesion. Common stimuli are bladder and bowel distention, pressure ulcers, bladder stones, ingrown toenails, etc.
  — exaggerated sympathetic responses cause the blood vessels below the lesion to constrict causing hypertension, a pounding headache, flushing, nasal stuffiness, diaphoresis, piloerection, dilated pupils with blurred vision, bradycardia, restlessness, and nausea
- Syndromes causing partial paralysis

(1) central cord syndrome
- produces more weakness in upper extremities than lower
- weakness is caused by edema and hemorrhage

(2) anterior cord syndrome
- complete motor function loss and decreased pain sensation
- touch, position, and vibration sensation remain intact

(3) Brown-Sequard syndrome
- lateral hemisection of the cord (lesion cuts or affects only half of the cord)
- ipsilateral motor paralysis, loss of vibratory and position sense
- contralateral loss of pain and temperature sensation

- Complete transection
  - results in immediate loss of all sensation and voluntary movement in areas below the transection
  - initially, all reflex activity is lost, but recovery does occur, although reflexes may be hyperactive
  - spinal shock (post traumatic areflexia)
    - complete loss of skeletal muscle function, bowel and bladder tone, sexual function, and autonomic reflexes
    - loss of venous return and hypotension
    - hypothalamus cannot control temperature, and client assumes the ambient temperature (temperature of surrounding air)
    - may last 7 days to 3 months
    - return of reflexes, development of hyperreflexia rather than flaccidity, and return of reflex emptying of the bladder indicate shock is resolving

ACUTE AND SUBACUTE CARE

Medical Management

- spinal cord immobilization
- respiratory support
- hemodynamic monitoring—heart rate, blood pressure, respirations, temperature, fluid balance

- shock therapy—vasopressors, fluid replacement
- skeletal traction (cervical injuries)
- steroid therapy—to decrease inflammation

Surgical Management

- decompressive laminectomy—lamina of vertebrae are removed to minimize pressure on the spinal cord—controversial
- fusion—insertion of metal plates and screws for stabilization—controversial
- immobilization in a brace or halo jacket—a ring is fixed to the skull with pins and then attached to a jacket by rods for cervical fracture stabilization

Nursing Management

- Monitor respiratory status.
- Monitor hemodynamic status.
- Maintain traction as ordered.
- Monitor sensory/motor status.
- Encourage to cough, deep breathe, and to use incentive spirometer.
- Monitor arterial blood gas results and oxygen saturations.
- Suction PRN.
- Initiate aspiration precautions.
- Provide frequent oral care.
- Provide measures to maintain skin integrity:
  - — reposition as ordered
  - — assessment of skin and pressure points
  - — pressure reducing beds or mattresses
  - — Stryker frame—allows turning from back to abdomen and vice versa while keeping immobilized
  - — Roto Rest bed—keeps body aligned while oscillating from side to side
- Provide nutritional support—dietary supplements, tube feedings, etc.
- Monitor the client for indications of autonomic dysreflexia:
  - — severe hypertension
  - — throbbing headache
  - — profuse diaphoresis
  - — flushing of the skin above the lesion
  - — nasal stuffiness

— blurred vision
— nausea
— bradycardia

- Intervene if autonomic dysreflexia occurs:
  — Monitor blood pressure closely.
  — Elevate head of bed to sitting position.
  — Notify physician.
  — Check for possible sources of irritation (kinked or clogged catheter, distended bowel or bladder, and pain).
  — Remove stimulus.
  — Administer antihypertensives as ordered.
- Initiate safety measures to prevent injury secondary to muscle spasms.
- Avoid unnecessary stimulation of areas that elicit reflex spinal automatisms—flexion and contraction of muscles of the limbs and abdomen, evacuation of bladder and bowel, sweating and flushing below the lesion.
- Accurate intake and output.
- Encourage up to 3000 ml/day unless otherwise contraindicated.
- Assess bladder control.
- Implement measures to preserve bladder capacity and muscle tone.
- Establish and maintain a routine pattern of bowel elimination.
- Assure urinary catheter patency (obstruction may cause autonomic dysreflexia).
- Observe for signs of urinary infection.
- Assess for indications of constipation or paralytic ileus.
- Maintain nasogastric tube and NPO status, if paralytic ileus present.
- Institute measures to prevent constipation and impaction:
  — forced fluids
  — diet high in bulk and roughage
  — stool softeners
  — routine daily pattern of elimination.
- Administer PRN analgesics and antispasmodics; evaluate effectiveness.
- Monitor for complications of decreased venous return (secondary to loss of muscle contractions

in lower extremities)—pulmonary embolus, deep vein thrombosis.

- Institute measures to decrease venous pooling and clot formation:
  - — passive/active range of motion exercises
  - — antiembolic stockings
  - — sequential compression devices
  - — subcutaneous Heparin as ordered.
- Institute measures to prevent complications from immobility:
  - — frequent position changes
  - — proper positioning of joints
  - — use of splints and removable casts
  - — intermittent turning to a prone position
  - — positioning of upper extremities away from the body
  - — draping bed linens
  - — keeping knees flexed at 15° when supine
  - — use of active and passive conditioning exercises.
- Collaborate with Physical Therapy for exercise program, transfer techniques, use of brace or corset, and weight-bearing activities.
- Moisten the cornea with natural tears for the client with altered blinking reflexes.
- Monitor for orthostatic hypotension when changing position (secondary to venous pooling).
- Encourage independence in activities of daily living within physical limitations.
- Collaborate with Occupational/Physical Therapy for adaptive devices.
- Assist the client/family in working through the grief process and to develop adaptive coping strategies.

COMMUNITY AND SELF-CARE

Most spinal cord injured clients are transferred from an acute care hospital to a rehabilitation facility. After functional capabilities are maximized, the client is discharged home.

Instruct the client regarding:

- measures to prevent skin breakdown in desensitized and paralyzed areas:
  - — repositioning techniques
  - — daily inspection of pressure areas

  - pressure relieving devices for bed/chair
  - meticulous skin care.
- exercise regime
- safety measures related to sensory loss:
  - avoid wearing ill-fitting shoes
  - avoid use of heating pads or hot water bottles
  - tepid bath water
  - shifting of body weight while sitting
  - regular foot and nail care.
- bladder training program:
  - intermittent catheterization (by client or caregiver)
  - methods to empty bladder without catheterization:
    - Credé Maneuver—client makes a fist and presses directly over bladder and down towards pubic area with a kneading motion
    - Valsalva Maneuver—client inhales deeply, holds breath, and bears down as if for a bowel movement
    - rectal stretch—client inserts finger into rectum; when sphincter relaxes, the client gently pulls on the sphincter to relax the perineal floor
    - reflex stimulation—tapping the suprapubic area, stroking the glans penis, thigh, or vulva, etc.
  - maintain an established elimination schedule
  - fluids to 3000 ml/day
- bowel training program:
  - maintain an established elimination schedule
  - fluids to 3000 ml/day
  - dietary modification—high bulk, increased roughage
- use of adaptive devices and ambulation aids
- factors that may precipitate muscle spasms:
  - cold temperature
  - prolonged sitting
  - emotional upset
  - cutaneous stimulation (tickling, stroking, or pinching)
- pulmonary hygiene
  - cough, deep breathe
  - incentive spirometry

- factors that may precipitate autonomic dysreflexia and necessary interventions
- measures to prevent deep vein thrombosis:
  — antiembolic stockings
  — passive range of motion exercises
  — assess for signs of deep vein thrombosis
- Refer to community resources.

(For more information, see pp. 890–915 of Black and Matassarin-Jacobs: *Medical-Surgical Nursing: Clinical Management for Continuity of Care,* 5th ed.)

Spinal Tumors

OVERVIEW

- Spinal tumors are most common in young or middle-aged adults and most often involve the thoracic region.
- Spinal tumors may occur outside the spinal cord (extramedullary) or within the substance of the spinal cord (intramedullary). Neurofibromas and meningiomas are the most common spinal tumors. Both are benign and operable and may not produce permanent damage if removed early enough. Spinal cord compression is the most common pathologic feature of all tumors within the spinal canal, because there is little room for expansion.

CLINICAL MANIFESTATIONS

Extramedullary Tumors

Early

- pain
- sensory loss
- muscle weakness and wasting

Progressive

- spastic weakness below level of lesion
- decreased sensation
- hyper-reactive reflexes

Severe

- paraplegia and quadriplegia

Intramedullary Tumors

- high cervical involvement—spastic quadriplegia and sensory changes
- lower areas of spinal cord produce motor and sensory changes appropriate to function at that level

ACUTE AND SUBACUTE CARE

Surgical Management

Treatment of Choice

- tumor removal
- partial resection of the tumor followed by radiation therapy (complete surgical removal of an intramedullary tumor is rare)

Nursing Management

See "Herniated Intervertebral Disc," p. 346.

(For more information, see pp. 915–916 of Black and Matassarin-Jacobs: *Medical-Surgical Nursing: Clinical Management for Continuity of Care,* 5th ed.)

Squamous Cell Carcinoma of the Oral Cavity

OVERVIEW

- Squamous cell carcinoma is the leading type of oral cancer. It is a malignant growth arising from tiny flat squamous cells that line mucous membranes. It most often is seen on the lower lip and tongue.
- The primary cause is chronic irritation of the mucous lining of the mouth and oral cavity.
- Squamous cell cancer of the tongue has a poor prognosis due to the extensive vascular and lymphatic supply of the tongue.

- Cancer of the lip has a high cure rate.
- Risk factors include alcohol and tobacco overuse, poor oral hygiene, or chronic chemical or thermal trauma.
- Basal cell carcinoma can also occur on the lips and is the second most common oral cancer. The cause is usually due to excessive sunlight exposure.

CLINICAL MANIFESTATIONS

- sore or lesion in the oral cavity
- irritation of the tongue
- sore throat, tongue, or ear pain
- trouble wearing dentures

ACUTE AND SUBACUTE CARE

Medical Management

Treatment depends upon the site and staging of the tumor.

- external beam radiation
- interstitial radiation (implanting radioactive seeds for small lesions that have not infiltrated surrounding tissue)
- chemotherapy

Surgical Management

- local excision or laser therapy of small tumors
- local excision and reconstruction with a split thickness skin graft for small tumors in the anterior floor of the mouth
- extensive surgical excision and possible removal of associated lymph nodes for invasive tumors:
  - — glossectomy—removal of the tongue
  - — hemiglossectomy—removal of part of the tongue
  - — mandibulectomy—removal of the mandible
  - — radical neck dissection—removal of all tissue under the skin, from the jaw down to the clavicle, and from the anterior border of the trapezius muscle to the midline

Nursing Management

Medical

- Discuss prevention of further oral lesions:

— Avoid chemical, physical, and thermal oral trauma.
— Perform oral hygiene at least three times a day.
— See a dentist for ill-fitting dentures.
— See a physician for any mouth lesions that do not heal in 2–3 weeks.

- Discuss "Radiation Therapy," see p. 605.
- Discuss "Chemotherapy," see p. 149.
- Promote and encourage adequate nutrition:
  — Provide analgesics 30–45 minutes before meals.
  — Encourage small frequent meals.
  — Provide/encourage oral care before and after meals.
  — Provide artificial saliva and administer pilocarpine, as ordered for xerostomia (dryness of the mouth) due to radiation therapy. Sugarless gum or candy and frequent oral rinses also will provide moisture.

Surgical

Preoperative Care

In addition to routine preoperative care:

- Discuss purpose and care of tracheostomy (temporary/permanent) and feeding tube as appropriate.
- Make referrals to assist with coping with changes in appearance.

Postoperative Care

Nursing care required depends upon the extent of the surgery.

In addition to routine postoperative care:

Local Excisions

- Monitor the amount of drainage.
- Monitor intactness of dressing and packing.
- Instruct the client on gentle oral care.
- Instruct on oral rinses every 4 hours of half-strength hydrogen peroxide and water or saline (after removal of dressings and packing).

Extensive Surgery

- Maintain a patent airway.
  — Maintain semi- to high-Fowler's position.
- Monitor for hemorrhage.
- Protect suture lines from trauma.

- No oral hygiene or suctioning until approved by the physician.
- Monitor condition of donor and graft sites if a skin graft was performed.
- Provide tracheostomy care, see "Tracheostomy," p. 705.
- Monitor pulse oximetry.
- Maintain adequate hydration by IV. Begin tube feedings as ordered when bowel sounds return.
- Provide means of communication if tracheostomy present.
- Resume oral feedings as prescribed when adequate healing has occurred.
  — Assess swallowing ability.
  — Instruct that there is decreased sensation in the oral cavity.
  — Instruct to avoid putting food directly on surgical site.
  — Instruct to perform oral hygiene after meals.

If a radical neck dissection was performed, also see "Laryngeal Cancer," p. 439.

COMMUNITY AND SELF-CARE

- Instruct client regarding:
  — diet
  — signs/symptoms of complications and to report these to physician
  — oral care
  — wound care
  — tracheostomy care (as appropriate)
  — tube feedings (as appropriate)
- Provide referrals to home health care agency for assistance with respiratory support (home oxygen), nutritional support, and wound care.
- Provide referrals to support groups for coping with cancer or change in body image.

(For more information, see pp. 1727–1732 of Black and Matassarin-Jacobs: *Medical-Surgical Nursing: Clinical Management for Continuity of Care,* 5th ed.)

Subclavian Steal Syndrome

OVERVIEW

- Subclavian steal syndrome produces arm ischemia secondary to altered blood flow from subclavian artery blockage. The arm is perfused from the carotid artery as blood is taken from the brain to supply the arm.

CLINICAL MANIFESTATIONS

- difference in blood pressure between arms
- dizziness
- syncope
- arm paresthesias

ACUTE AND SUBACUTE CARE

Surgical Intervention

- carotid-subclavian bypass
- transluminal dilation of the subclavian artery
- endarterectomy of the subclavian artery

(For more information, see p. 1430 of Black and Matassarin-Jacobs: *Medical-Surgical Nursing: Clinical Management for Continuity of Care,* 5th ed.)

Substance Abuse

- According to the *Diagnostic and Statistical Manual of Mental Disorders* (*DSM-IV*), substance use is classified as: taking a drug of abuse; the adverse effects of the medication; exposure to toxic substances. *DSM-IV* identifies eleven types of substances: alcohol; amphetamines; inhalants; caffeine; cannabis; cocaine; hallucinogens; inhalants; nicotine; opioids; phencyclidine (PCP); sedatives, hypnotics, or anxiolytics. They also include substance-related disorders, toxins, or prescribed and over the counter medications.

- The severity of symptoms depend on the dose of the drug and the length of use.
- Theories of substance abuse:

BIOLOGIC THEORIES

- Substance abuse may be physiologic conditions due to:
  - — genetic predisposition—e.g., as in alcohol abuse
  - — defects in metabolism, neurobiologic abnormalities, or abnormal levels of chemicals in the body

PSYCHOSOCIAL THEORIES

- Certain personality features may interplay with genetic susceptibility and individual biologic response to chemical substances. These include low self-esteem, emotional immaturity, low frustration tolerance, and unwillingness or inability to endure and cope with tension.
- Seek gratification of needs through behaviors such as drinking.
- Parental lack of emotional warmth, parental rejection, and parental overprotection may be factors leading to the addiction process. Substance abuse can be one way to feel better about themselves and meet emotional needs.

SOCIOCULTURAL THEORIES

- Social conditions and contexts may help create and sustain substance abuse:
  - — social and cultural norms within various groups in society
  - — factors in a person's background
  - — values, beliefs, spiritual orientation
  - — family standards, social environment
  - — ethnicity, sex
- Substances that may be abused include: alcohol, narcotics, depressants, stimulants, hallucinogens, and cannabis derivatives.
- Nurses may screen for substance use/abuse by assessing from the client or significant others:
  - — past and present habits of substance use, including the amount, frequency,and type of substance used

— situations in which the substance is used
— self-perception of substance-using behavior and effects on daily life
— use of screening tools to identify clients who abuse drugs

- If substance abuse is known or suspected, nurses must know the time of the last dose, information about past withdrawal episodes, signs/symptoms of withdrawal, and treatment for withdrawal.
- If substance abuse is not detected and treated, a person may progress to a severe state of withdrawal that may be hard to manage.
- A thorough mental exam is performed.
- Components of a drug and alcohol history include:
  — how often the drug was used (past and present)
  — age at first use and last use
  — method of use, quantity used
  — reactions to drugs
  — how drug was obtained
  — client's perception and related health problems
- Nurses need to be aware of slang terms used for substances.
- Nurses may need to discuss substance abuse programs and refer clients to these as appropriate.
- Several potentially abusive substances, their effects and management are listed below.

ALCOHOL

- Alcohol is a central nervous system depressant.
- Psychophysiologic disturbances from chronic alcohol abuse include:
  — nutritional deficits, malabsorption syndrome
  — peripheral neuropathies
  — Wernicke-Korsakoff syndrome:
    - symptoms of the Wernicke component: ocular disturbances, horizontal nystagmus on lateral gaze; palsy of the sixth cranial nerve (which results in diplopia); wide, reeling gait, difficulty standing
    - Korsakoff's psychosis—disturbance in memory function (especially recent events); confusion; and confabulation (filling in memory gaps with imaginary experiences)

- cerebral atrophy (difficulty with abstraction, problem solving, new learning, memory, and perceptual-motor speed)
- alcoholic liver disease (begins with fatty liver, progresses to alcoholic hepatitis, and finally cirrhosis)
- ascites, portal hypertension, hepatic encephalopathy
- esophageal varices (due to portal hypertension from cirrhosis)
- gastric ulcers
- alcoholic pancreatitis
- cardiomyopathy, congestive heart failure, arrhythmias, hypertension
- higher incidence of chronic obstructive pulmonary disease (COPD)
- pneumonia, tuberculosis
- fluid and electrolyte imbalances
- interferes with absorption of vitamin B_{12}, thiamine, and folic acid
- anemia, thrombocytopenia, leukopenia, spider nevi, capillary fragility
- myopathy (damage to skeletal muscle)
- lowered serum testosterone levels
- altered immune system
- cancer of the oropharynx, larynx, and esophagus; possible cancer of the pancreas and prostate

- The effects of alcohol may include:
  - altered judgment, self-control, speech, and motor coordination
- Alcohol intoxication may lead to:
  - confusion, stupor
  - coma, death

It is important to note that in a tolerant drinker, blood levels may be high without obvious impairment.

Withdrawal

- First 24 Hours:
  - anorexia
  - anxiety, insomnia, tremor, restlessness
- The next 2–3 days:
  - elevated heart rate, blood pressure, and temperature

- disorientation, nightmares, abdominal pain, nausea, diaphoresis
- grand mal convulsive seizures may occur during the first 48 hours of withdrawal
- delirium tremors (DTs), which denotes serious withdrawal, may occur 3 days to 4 weeks after cessation of drinking
  - characterized by cardiac arrhythmias, confusion, disorientation, frightening hallucinations, delusions, severe psychomotor agitation, and increased autonomic activity; that is, fever, tachycardia, hypertension, profuse diaphoresis, and tachypnea

Nursing Management of Withdrawal

- Monitor pulse and blood pressure frequently for the first 24 hours or until stable.
- Assess for signs/symptoms of withdrawal, including tremors, diaphoresis, pulse, and blood pressure. Notify physician of any signs/symptoms of withdrawal.
- Administer benzodiazepines, such as chlordiazepoxide (Librium), diazepam (Valium), lorazepam (Ativan), or oxazepam (Serax) as ordered.
- Maintain a quiet environment.
- Provide reassurance and support.
- Provide a calm, safe, and comfortable environment.
- Be aware that some clients are placed on disulfiram (Antabuse),which can help discourage drinking. If the client drinks alcohol while on this medication the following symptoms can occur: blurred vision, chest pain, confusion, dizziness, palpitations, flushing, diaphoresis, nausea, vomiting, headache, and dyspnea. If the client drinks large amounts of alcohol, seizures, myocardial infarction, and death can occur.

STIMULANTS

- The three types of stimulants are: cocaine, caffeine, amphetamines.
- Nicotine is also considered a CNS stimulant.
- Amphetamines usually are taken orally. People take them to stay awake, increase their ability to perform tasks, or to produce euphoria.

- Cocaine stimulates the CNS and the cardiovascular system. Cocaine may be swallowed but usually is inhaled. It also may be smoked in a concentrated freebase form called "crack."
- Behavioral changes seen with stimulant use:
  - — hyperalertness, labile emotions, sleep disturbances, anxiety, talkativeness, impaired judgment, euphoria, hyperactivity, and overenthusiasm
  - — sustained stimulant use may lead to a toxic psychosis manifested by delusions, hallucinations, and suspiciousness
  - — formication (sensation of bugs crawling on skin) with cocaine and amphetamine abuse.
- Physiologic reactions include:
  - — gastrointestinal disturbances from caffeine use
  - — diaphoresis, tremors, tachycardia, hypertension, hypotension, mydriasis
  - — cardiac arrhythmias
  - — malnutrition, weight loss from appetite suppression
  - — thinned, ulcerated, or even a perforated nasal septum in persons who have been snorting cocaine
  - — possible myocardial infarction with cocaine use
- Overdose of cocaine causes tremor, seizures, and delerium. Death can also occur from cardiac and/or respiratory failure.
- Psychological dependence is high.

Withdrawal

- Abrupt cessation of amphetamines can cause: agitation, severe depression, hyperphagia, and hypersomnolence.
- Abrupt withdrawal of cocaine results in an exhausted state known as "crashing." The signs and symptoms include: profound depression, memories of euphoria, and cravings for the drug. The client can also be hospitalized with severe depression and the risk of suicide.

Nursing Management of Withdrawal

- For clients with symptoms of stimulant abuse:
  - — Intervene to prevent adverse effects of withdrawal.

- Provide environmental safety measures.
- Assess for emotional and physical changes.
- Set realistic limits on their behavior and use a calm approach.

Nursing Management of Overdose

- Assess for signs/symptoms of overdose: chest pain, panic, hostility, diaphoresis, vomiting, hyperpyrexia, and convulsions.
- Handle cardiovascular collapse or respiratory distress with pharmacologic interventions as appropriate.
- Monitor pulse, heart rhythm, blood pressure, and temperature closely.
- Assist in development of effective coping skills.
- Provide support and education for the client and family.

CANNABIS DERIVATIVES

- Marijuana is a cannabis derivative and is the most widely used illegal drug in the United States.
- Behavioral changes and initial physiologic reactions include:
  - euphoria, elation, relaxation, feeling of well-being
  - ataxia, tremor
  - rapidly changing emotions, memory impairment
  - tachycardia, elevated blood pressure
  - dry mouth

Nursing Management

- The nurse is most likely to encounter an intoxicated cannabis user in the context of an adverse reaction to the drug experience.
- The initial effects will disappear in 4–6 hours, but the effects of drug intoxication may last as long as 5 days.
- Care is supportive, and reassurance is given to the client that this is temporary.
- After the initial period, nurses provide education regarding cannabis and its adverse effects:
  - causes lung disease
  - chronic sinusitis and pharyngitis
  - lowered testosterone level

HALLUCINOGENS

- Produce hallucinations, delusions, and alterations in thought, perception, and feeling.
- An example is lipergic acid diethylamide (LSD).
- The user experiences euphoria, dilated pupils, anxiety, increased respirations, blood pressure, and pulse.
- With intoxication the client experiences panic attacks, paranoia, confusion, and hallucinations. These clients are also at risk for suicide, homicide, and acts of violence.
- Severe overdose can cause seizures, high temperatures, and cardiac distress.
- Nursing care focuses on providing a safe, nonstimulating environment.

INHALANTS

- Inhalants are chemicals that give off fumes or vapors that pass the blood–brain barrier. These include: glue, gasoline, nail polish remover, lighter fluid, paint thinner, aerosols, and anesthetics.
- These clients experience giddiness and euphoria with decreased inhibition, bradycardia, slowed respiratory rate, and decreased mental activity.
- With intoxication they experience: delerium; cardiac arrhythmias; irritation of the nose and mouth; cough; depression of the brain waves.
- Continuous use can cause major organ failure and sudden death.

OPIOIDS

- Opioids cause feelings of well being.
- Overdoses are life threatening.
- Nursing management requires emergency care and constant monitoring.
- Methadone program for severe withdrawal.

PHENCYCLIDINE (PCP)

- PCP is a synthetic drug with stimulant, depressant, and hallucinogenic properties.
- The symptoms include: tachycardia, hypertension, increased respiratory rate, diaphoresis, drooling,

pupillary constriction, lack of coordination, slurred speech, nystagmus, euphoria, and disorientation.
- The client may also be confused, violent, hostile, and paranoid.
- Nursing care involves management of changes in vital signs, level of consciousness, gastric lavage, acidification of the urine, and withrawal symptoms.

SEDATIVES, HYPNOTICS, AND ANXIOLYTICS

- CNS depressants.
- Nursing care involves monitoring vital signs and gastric lavage with possible emergency intervention.
- It is also necessary to promote rest, safety, and treatment of emotional and physical symptoms.

(For more information, see pp. 2479–2499 of Black and Matassarin-Jacobs: *Medical-Surgical Nursing: Clinical Management for Continuity of Care,* 5th ed.)

Syndrome of Inappropriate Antidiuretic Hormone (SIADH)

OVERVIEW

- SIADH is a disorder associated with excessive amounts of antidiuretic hormone (ADH) secreted by the posterior pituitary gland, resulting in a water imbalance.
- SIADH is the opposite of diabetes insipidus. Key features of ADH excess are: (1) water retention, (2) hyponatremia, and (3) hypo-osmolality. A continual release of ADH causes water retention from renal tubules and collecting ducts; extracellular fluid volume increases with dilutional hyponatremia; hyponatremia suppresses renin and aldosterone secretions causing a decrease in proximal tubule reabsorption of sodium.
- Risk factors include:
  — treatment of diabetes insipidus with vasopressin
  — a variety of malignancies

CLINICAL MANIFESTATIONS

- weight gain without edema
- central nervous system dysfunction (secondary to hyponatremia)
  - — alterations in level of consciousness
  - — decreased deep tendon reflexes
  - — fatigue
  - — headache
  - — seizures
  - — coma
- tachycardia, tachypnea
- anorexia, nausea

ACUTE AND SUBACUTE CARE

Medical Management

- fluid restriction
- replacement of sodium chloride
- administration of diuretics and demeclocycline (a tetracycline that increases free-water clearance)

Nursing Management

- Maintain fluid restriction.
- Monitor intake and output.
- Assess cardiovascular status for signs of overload.
- Daily weights.
- Assess neurologic status.
- Maintain dietary modifications (low sodium).

COMMUNITY AND SELF-CARE

Instruct the client regarding:

- need for fluid and sodium restrictions
- daily weights—report gain of 2 pounds or more per day

(For more information, see pp. 2067–2068 of Black and Matassarin-Jacobs: *Medical-Surgical Nursing: Clinical Management for Continuity of Care,* 5th ed.)

Syphilis

OVERVIEW

- This systemic, infectious disease is caused by the spirochete, *Treponema pallidum.*
- The organism enters the body through intact mucous membranes or abraded skin almost exclusively by direct sexual contact (acquired syphilis). Sexual transmission occurs when the mucocutaneous lesions of primary and secondary syphilis are present. After entry, the organisms multiply locally and disseminate through the lymphatics and the bloodstream.
- Syphilis has become dramatically less prevalent with the advent of antibiotics but has not been eradicated. It is the third most commonly reported communicable disease in the United States.
- Adolescents, young adults, and homosexual males are at the greatest risk.
- The infection can be passed transplacentally from mother to fetus (congenital syphilis).
- Syphilis can progress to irreversible blindness, mental illness, paralysis, heart disease, and death.

CLINICAL MANIFESTATIONS

Syphilis is characterized by well-defined stages that occur over a period of of years: primary, secondary, latent, and late or tertiary.

- Primary Stage
  - — appearance of chancre—an oval ulcer with a raised border that does not bleed readily and is painless unless infected. The chancre is at the site of inoculation, usually the genitalia, anus, or mouth. If untreated, a chancre disappears after 4–6 weeks.
  - — regional lymphadenopathy—local lymph glands at the chancre swell painlessly
- Secondary Stage (if untreated, begins 6–8 weeks after infection)
  - — generalized skin rash—a maculopapular and nonpruritic rash appears on the palms and soles of the feet

— generalized lymphadenopathy
— mucous patches—gray, superficial patches on mucous membranes in the mouth
— Condylomata lata—broad-based, flat papules develop in warm, moist body areas, most commonly the labia, anus, or at the corners of the mouth. Condylomata are highly contagious.
— generalized flu-like symptoms
— patchy hair loss from eyebrows and scalp
— secondary stage symptoms usually disappear after 2-6 weeks, and the latency period begins

- Latent Stage (begins 2 or more years after primary lesion)
  — typically no symptoms
  — patient is seroactive but shows no other evidence of the disease
  — disease is not transmitted by sexual contact during this phase. However, transmission through the bloodstream or placenta can occur.
  — about two-thirds of infected clients remain in this phase without further problems
- Late (Tertiary) Stage
  — if untreated, in 1–35 years about one-third of infected patients will enter this stage
  — chronic bone and joint inflammation
  — cardiovascular problems (e.g., valve involvement, aneurysms)
  — granulomatous lesions on any part of the body
  — central nervous system problems (including mental illness, slurred speech, ataxic gait, paralysis, judgment loss, and senility)
  — not infectious during this stage

ACUTE AND SUBACUTE CARE

Medical Management

All sexual contacts should be evaluated and treated.

- penicillin
  — primary, secondary, and early latent—benzathine penicillin G (IM), single dose
  — late latent stage: benzathine penicillin G IM, weekly for 3 weeks
  — neurosyphilis: aqueous penicillin (IV) every 4 hours for 10–14 days

- follow-up cultures

All stages respond to antibiotic therapy, but the structural changes present in late syphilis are irreversible.

Nursing Management

- Administer antibiotics as ordered.
- Monitor cardiac and neurologic changes in late stages.

COMMUNITY AND SELF-CARE

Instruct the client regarding:

- the importance of completing the antibiotic regime and follow-up
- the importance of abstaining from sexual contact for at least 1 month after treatment for primary or secondary syphilis
- the importance of treating all sexual contacts
- information about transmission, reinfection, early detection, treatment, and follow-up
- if pregnant, the possibility of infecting the baby

(For more information, see pp. 2470–2472 of Black and Matassarin-Jacobs: *Medical-Surgical Nursing: Clinical Management for Continuity of Care,* 5th ed.)

Systemic Lupus Erythematosus

OVERVIEW

- Systemic lupus erythematosus (SLE) is a chronic, inflammatory autoimmune disease characterized by a wide array of clinical manifestations in vascular and connective tissue. SLE has an insidious onset and is characterized by remissions and exacerbations.
- There are two types of lupus erythematosus: systemic lupus erythematosus, and discoid lupus. Discoid lupus is a mild form of the disorder that involves only the skin. The face, neck , and upper chest are usually affected.
- The primary autoantibodies produced in SLE are directed at the cell nuclei and are called anti-

nuclear antibodies, or ANAs. Normally, the T suppressor cells prevent autoantibody formation. In SLE, a defect in these cells prevents this protective process. When the cells die, the nuclei are released and bind to the ANA. The immune complex formed triggers an inflammatory response. The complexes deposit in the kidney, heart, brain, the lining of blood vessels, and joints. The leading cause of death in clients with SLE is renal failure.

- SLE is relatively rare, occurring in 1 in 2000 persons. SLE is 10 times more common in women than men and occurs between the ages of 15 and 40 years.
- The exact cause of SLE is unknown. Causes of exacerbations include exposure to sunlight or other forms of ultraviolet light, physical and emotional stress, and pregnancy.
- There is a form of drug-induced SLE associated with adverse reactions to some drugs including procainamide (Pronestyl) and hydralazine (Apresoline). Phenytoin (Dilantin), Quinidine, and Captopril may also produce an SLE-like syndrome.

CLINICAL MANIFESTATIONS

Chronic SLE

Manifestations depend on the organs involved.

- severe hemolytic anemia
- fever, malaise, weight loss
- thrombocytopenic purpura
- pericarditis
- tachycardia
- abdominal pain, nausea, and vomiting
- peripheral vascular syndrome (e.g., Raynaud's phenomena)
- hypertension
- ulcerative mucous membrane lesions
- hepatic dysfunction
- generalized lymphadenopathy
- glomerulonephritis
- psychosis and coma
- cutaneous discoid LE lesions
- erythema of exposed skin

Acute SLE

- pleural effusion
- fever
- musculoskelatal aches and pains
- butterfly rash on the face
- generalized lymphadenopathy
- basilar pneumonia
- pericarditis
- tachycardia
- hepatosplenomegaly
- delirium, convulsions
- coma

ACUTE AND SUBACUTE CARE

Medical Management

- nonsteroidal anti-inflammatory agents—aspirin, ibuprofen
- antimalarial drugs (for cutaneous manifestations)
- corticosteroids
- cytotoxic agents—cyclophosphamide, azathioprine
- plasmapheresis—removes circulating autoantibodies and immune complexes
- additional therapies based on organ systems involved

Nursing Management

- Administer anti-inflammatory agents as ordered and monitor side effects.
- Monitor laboratory findings—renal profile, nutritional panel, blood counts.
- Assess cardiopulmonary status and response to activity.
- Provide physiologic support to prevent skin breakdown.
- Encourage nutritionally balanced diet.
- Minimize the risk of opportunistic infections.
- Maintain quiet, restful environment.
- Provide emotional support to the client facing a chronic, potentially fatal disease.

COMMUNITY AND SELF-CARE

Instruct the client regarding:

- disease process and treatment regime
- importance of medication regime
  - — advise to take anti-inflammatory agents with food or antacids
- importance of pneumococcal pneumonia vaccine and yearly influenza vaccine
- measures to decrease exposure to sunlight or ultraviolet light
- signs and symptoms to report
- importance of avoiding emotional or physical stress that may trigger an exacerbation
- need for yearly eye exams to monitor side effects of antimalarial therapy
- risk factor modification for hypertension and coronary artery disease
- importance of follow-up appointments

(For more information, see pp. 674–677 of Black and Matassarin-Jacobs: *Medical-Surgical Nursing: Clinical Management for Continuity of Care,* 5th ed.)

T

Testicular Disorders

TESTICULAR TORSION

- Testicular torsion occurs when a testicle is mobile, and the spermatic cord twists, cutting off the blood supply.
- Torsion is the most common testicular disorder in children.
- Clinical manifestations—arise suddenly
  - — scrotal swelling
  - — severe scrotal pain
- Treatment
  - — emergency surgery to untwist spermatic cord and immobilize the testicle by suturing it to the scrotum.

ORCHITIS

- Orchitis is an acute testicular inflammation.
- Orchitis may be associated with trauma or an infection elsewhere in the body, such as mumps, pneumonia, tuberculosis, and syphilis.
- Clinical manifestations
  - — edematous and tender testicles
  - — reddened scrotal skin
  - — fever
- Treatment
  - — bedrest
  - — scrotal support
  - — local heat
  - — analgesics

HYDROCELE

- Hydrocele is a painless collection of clear, yellow fluid along the spermatic cord.
- Treatment
  - — aspiration or surgical drainage

HEMATOCELE

- Hematocele is a collection of blood in the tunica vaginalis.
- Treatment:
  — aspiration or surgical drainage

SPERMATOCELE

- Spermatocele is a collection of milky fluid and spermatozoa originating in the epididymis.
- Treatment
  — aspiration or surgical drainage

VARICOCELE

- Varicocele is dilation and varicosity of the network of veins supplying the testicles.
- Clinical manifestations
  — pulling sensation
  — dull ache or scrotal pain
- Treatment
  — scrotal support
  — surgery if varicocele is thought to contribute to infertility

UNDESCENDED TESTES (CRYPTORCHIDISM)

- Cryptorchidism is the most common congenital testicular condition.
- One or both testicles are arrested in the abdomen, inguinal canal, low pelvis, or high scrotum.
- Cryptorchidism is associated with infertility.
- The incidence of testicular cancer is high in men with undescended testes if not corrected by surgery.
- Treatment
  — orchiopexy—testicle(s) are brought down and sutured to the scrotum

EUNUCHOIDISM

- Eunuchoidism is a congenital condition in which puberty does not occur; genitals and prostate remain infantile; the voice is high-pitched; axillary and pubic hair is scant; and skeletal proportions are abnormal.

- Treatment
  — hormone replacement

(For more information, see pp. 2377–2378 of Black and Matassarin-Jacobs: *Medical-Surgical Nursing: Clinical Management for Continuity of Care,* 5th ed.)

Testicular Tumors

OVERVIEW

- Testicular cancer is the most common and serious solid tumor cancer in males between the ages of 15 and 35.
- The major risk factor is cryptorchidism (undescended testicles). It is now recommended that any child born with an undescended testicle have an orchiopexy as soon as possible after birth. The longer the testicles are left undescended, the greater the risk of testicular cancer.

CLINICAL MANIFESTATIONS

- painless enlargement, noted as heaviness in the testicles
- findings suggesting metastasis include back pain, vague abdominal pain, nausea and vomiting, anorexia, and weight loss

ACUTE AND SUBACUTE CARE

Medical Management

- radiation therapy
- chemotherapy—Cisplatin

Surgical Management

Primary treatment for testicular cancer:

- radical orchiectomy—removal of the testis, epididymis, and vas deferens. The amputated testicle can be replaced with a testicular prosthesis.
- radical orchiectomy with retroperitoneal lymph node dissection—major complication is impotence because many of the autonomic nerves necessary for ejaculation are located in this area

- radical orchiectomy followed by a course of chemotherapy for known lymph node involvement or as prophylaxis

Nursing Management

Medical

- Administer ordered chemotherapy. See "Chemotherapy," p. 149.
- Monitor for and intervene if side effects develop.
- Provide emotional support.

Surgical

- Provide routine postoperative care.

COMMUNITY AND SELF-CARE

Instruct the client regarding:

- management of side effects if receiving chemotherapy
- wound care for postoperative client

(For more information, see pp. 2373–2377 of Black and Matassarin-Jacobs: *Medical-Surgical Nursing: Clinical Management for Continuity of Care,* 5th ed.)

Tetanus

- Tetanus is caused by the anaerobic spore-forming rod *Clostridium tetani.* The spores produce a toxin when introduced into a wound. The toxin suppresses spinal and brain stem inhibitory neurons and may act on skeletal muscle at the point of entry.
- Clinical manifestations include:
  - — painful muscular spasms and contractions in the affected extremity
  - — spasms of the jaw muscles
  - — spasms of muscles of the neck, trunk, limbs, and the respiratory and pharyngeal muscles
  - — seizures
  - — impaired respiration

- Interventions
  — surgery to debride wound
  — single dose of tetanus immune globulin
  — 10-day course of penicillin G or alternate agents
  — respiratory support (possible mechanical ventilation)
  — chlorpromazine, meprobamate, or diazepam to control muscle spasms
  — nasogastric feeding, if the client has dysphagia
  — prophylactic anticoagulation to prevent thrombus formation
- The mortality rate is 25–50 per cent.
- The best prevention is immunization with regular booster doses of toxoid.

(For more information, see p. 857 of Black and Matassarin-Jacobs: *Medical-Surgical Nursing: Clinical Management for Continuity of Care,* 5th ed.)

Thalassemias

OVERVIEW

- The thalassemias are a group of inherited, chronic, hemolytic anemias.
- The severity of the anemia depends upon whether the afflicted client is homozygous or heterozygous for the trait. Thalassemia major and intermedia, both characterized by profound anemia, appear in homozygotes. Thalassemia minor, characterized by a mild anemia, develops in heterozygotes.
- The outlook for clients with thalassemia major is poor. Many fail to live through puberty. Thalassemia minor, on the other hand, does not affect life expectancy.
- Areas of prevalence include the Mediterranean, West Africa, Southeast Asia, India, Turkey, Sudan, and Israel.

CLINICAL MANIFESTATIONS

Thalassemia Major

- jaundice (accumulation of bilirubin)

- cholelithiasis (excess bilirubin from red blood cell breakdown causes gallstones)
- enlarged spleen
- chronic fatigue
- pallor
- mongoloid faces and thickening of the cranium (bone hyperactivity)

Thalassemia Minor

- asymptomatic except for mild anemia
- diagnosis made on blood smear

ACUTE AND SUBACUTE CARE

Medical Management

Thalassemia Major

- transfusion therapy on a monthly or bimonthly basis

Surgical Management

- splenectomy if the transfused cells are being rapidly destroyed by the spleen

Thalassemia Minor

Treatment usually not required; however, clients who carry the trait should have genetic counseling.

Nursing Management

- Administer transfusion therapy as ordered. See "Blood Component Transfusion," p. 88.
- Monitor laboratory findings—CBC.
- Monitor response to activity and provide rest periods.

COMMUNITY AND SELF-CARE

Instruct client regarding:

- importance of treatment regime
- need for follow-up appointments

(For more information, see pp. 1482–1483 of Black and Matassarin-Jacobs: *Medical-Surgical Nursing: Clinical Management for Continuity of Care,* 5th ed.)

Thoracic Outlet Syndromes

OVERVIEW

- Thoracic outlet syndromes are a group of disorders caused by compression or mechanical irritation of the brachial plexus, subclavian artery, or subclavian vein as these structures pass through the thoracic outlet.

CLINICAL MANIFESTATIONS

Neurologic Type

- aching or throbbing pain of the neck or upper limb
- paresthesias

Arterial Type

- absent or weak pulse
- pallor and cyanosis
- coolness
- paresthesias and pain

Venous Type

- sudden swelling
- pain
- cyanosis of the upper extremity

ACUTE AND SUBACUTE CARE

Medical Management

Neurologic Type

- physical therapy

Venous Type

- arm elevation
- anticoagulation or thrombolytic therapy
- thrombectomy

Surgical Management

- removal of anatomic abnormality and emboli (arterial type)

(For more information, see p. 1430 of Black and Matassarin-Jacobs: *Medical-Surgical Nursing: Clinical Management for Continuity of Care,* 5th ed.)

Thromboangiitis Obliterans (Buerger's Disease)

OVERVIEW

- Thromboangiitis obliterans is a vasculitis of small and medium-size veins and arteries in the extremities of young adults.
- The cause remains unknown. Almost all clients are moderate to heavy smokers.
- The disease process starts distally and progresses cephalad, involving both upper and lower extremities.
- The disease occurs in the second to fourth decade and is seen predominantly in men.

CLINICAL MANIFESTATIONS

- intermittent claudication—occurs in the arch of the foot or calf of the leg
- rest pain with persistent ischemia of one or more digits
- cold sensitivity
- paresthesias
- weak or absent peripheral pulses
- abnormally red or cyanotic extremity (advanced cases), particularly when dependent
- color or temperature changes involving only one extremity, certain digits, or portions of digits (advanced cases)
- ulceration and gangrene
- edema of the leg
- changes in skin and nails

ACUTE AND SUBACUTE CARE

Medical Management

- smoking cessation
- pain control

- vasodilators—calcium channel blockers, prazosin

SURGICAL MANAGEMENT

- sympathetic ganglionectomy—produces vasodilation
- amputation if conservative measures fail

NURSING MANAGEMENT

Medical

- Administer analgesics.
- Administer vasodilators.
- Provide measures to increase body warmth.

Surgical

- See "Amputation," p. 32.

COMMUNITY AND SELF-CARE

Instruct client regarding:

MEDICAL

- disease process and treatment regime
- importance of avoiding exposure to cold
- signs/symptoms of advancing disease
- smoking cessation program
- pain control

SURGICAL

- See "Amputation," p. 32.

(For more information, see pp. 1430–1431 of Black and Matassarin-Jacobs: *Medical-Surgical Nursing: Clinical Management for Continuity of Care,* 5th ed.)

Thyroid Cancer

OVERVIEW

- The incidence of malignant tumors of the thyroid is rising. They account for three to four new cases per 100,000 population per year. Thyroid cancer has peak incidence in the sixth decade of life. The rate of females to males is 4:1.

- Clients receiving large doses of radiation to the head and neck and clients with a thyroid nodule (less than 20 years of age and greater than 60) are at the greatest risk of developing thyroid cancer.
- Other risk factors include: female, genetic, and family and/or history of thyroid cancer.

CLINICAL MANIFESTATIONS

- hard, irregular, painless nodule in an enlarged thyroid gland
- palpable lymph nodes
- respiratory difficulty and dysphagia

ACUTE AND SUBACUTE CARE

Medical Management

- chemotherapy
- radioiodine treatment with ^{131}I.

Surgical Management

- thyroidectomy—removal of all or part of the thyroid
- neck resection may be done for metastases

Nursing Management

Medical

- Administer chemotherapy as ordered; monitor for side effects. See "Chemotherapy," p. 149.
- Maintain radiation precautions for patients receiving ^{131}I. See "Radiation Therapy," p. 605.
- Encourage nutritionally balanced diet.
- Monitor activity tolerance, promote rest periods.

Surgical

- For care of client undergoing thyroidectomy, see "Hyperthyroidism," p. 389.

COMMUNITY AND SELF-CARE

Instruct client regarding:

- postoperative home care
  - — importance of taking thyroid replacement hormone (total thyroidectomy)
  - — wound care
  - — symptoms of thyroid deficiency and excess
- chemotherapy
  - — management of side effects
- radioiodine treatment
  - — necessary radiation precautions

(For more information, see pp. 2027–2029 of Black and Matassarin-Jacobs: *Medical-Surgical Nursing: Clinical Management for Continuity of Care,* 5th ed.)

Thyroiditis

OVERVIEW

- Thyroiditis is an inflammation of the thyroid gland.
- There are three basic forms: (1) acute suppurative; (2) subacute granulomatous and subacute lymphocytic; (3) chronic thyroiditis (Hashimoto's).
- Acute thyroiditis is more common in females ages 20–40.
- There is a genetic predisposition to subacute disease.
- Hashimoto's thyroiditis is the most common with the incidence being greater in women than in men.

CLINICAL MANIFESTATIONS

Acute Thyroiditis

- abrupt onset of unilateral anterior neck pain that might radiate to the ear or mandible
- fever, diaphoresis

Subacute Thyroiditis

- pain in granulomatous thyroiditis but lymphocytic is usually painless
- myalgia, low-grade fever
- lassitude, sore throat
- thyrotoxicosis

- hyperthyroidism and goiter in lymphocytic

Chronic Thyroiditis

- painless asymmetrical enlargement of the gland
- dysphagia, respiratory distress
- euthyroid

ACUTE AND SUBACUTE CARE

Medical Management

- parenteral antibiotics
- supportive with granulomatous thyroiditis
- salicylates, nonsteroidal anti-inflammatory agents, and oral glucocorticoids
- beta-adrenergic blockers with subacute thyroiditis

Surgical Management

- incision and drainage of the gland—if no response to medical therapy
- fine-needle biopsy to rule out malignancy

Nursing Management

- administration of medications for treatment
- supportive therapy

COMMUNITY AND SELF-CARE

Instruct client regarding:
- medications
- thyroid function monitoring

(For more information, see pp. 2025–2027 of Black and Matassarin-Jacobs: *Medical-Surgical Nursing: Clinical Management for Continuity of Care,* 5th ed.)

Tonsillectomy

OVERVIEW

- Tonsillectomy is removal of the tonsils, which are almond-shaped lymphoid tissue located in the ton-

sillar fossa of the oropharynx. A snarelike or blunt dissection instrument is used to remove the tonsillar tissue, and cautery is applied to bleeding vessels.
- Tonsillectomy is indicated in clients who have repeated episodes of tonsillitis and usually is done under a general anesthetic.
- An adenoidectomy may be performed in conjunction with the tonsillectomy.

ACUTE AND SUBACUTE CARE

Nursing Management

Postoperative Care

In addition to routine postoperative care:
- Inspect the oropharynx and mouth frequently for fresh blood during the first several postoperative hours (hemorrhage most often is seen during the first 12–24 hours).
- Monitor vital signs and instruct the client to report any increased swallowing.
- Encourage cool oral fluids; progress to soft diet; avoid any spicy foods.
- Administer analgesics for throat pain and otalgia.

COMMUNITY AND SELF-CARE

Instruct the client regarding:
- soft diet and cool fluids
- avoidance of rough or sharp foods (e.g., potato chips)
- reporting to physician any bleeding, increased swallowing or signs/symptoms of infection

(For more information, see pp. 1079–1080 of Black and Matassarin-Jacobs: *Medical-Surgical Nursing: Clinical Management for Continuity of Care,* 5th ed.)

Total Parenteral Nutrition

OVERVIEW

- Total parenteral nutrition (TPN) is the intravenous administration of amino acid-dextrose solutions (usually in conjunction with fat emulsions) in order to provide sufficient nutrients in clients who are unable to ingest, digest, or absorb sufficient nutrients to maintain themselves in a state of positive nitrogen balance.

- Indications for TPN include:
  - debilitating diseases, such as malabsorption of the bowel
  - inability to eat adequate nutrients
  - gastric cancer or cancer cachexia
  - chemotherapy or radiation therapy
  - anorexia nervosa
  - excessive metabolic needs (extensive burns or draining wounds)
  - need to rest the gastrointestinal tract
- TPN is usually administered through an indwelling subclavian catheter, right atrial tunnelled catheter, or subcutaneous port.

ACUTE AND SUBACUTE CARE

Nursing Management

- Initiate TPN via an infusion pump at a slow rate. Gradually increase rate as ordered.
- Monitor catheter insertion site for redness, tenderness, drainage, or edema.
- Never abruptly discontinue TPN as hypoglycemia can occur.
  - If the next TPN bag is unavailable, administer a 10 per cent dextrose solution until the TPN is available.
  - When TPN is to be discontinued, the rate is gradually decreased over a period of time.
- Monitor blood sugars every 6 hours.
- Monitor for signs/symptoms of hypoglycemia and hyperglycemia.
- Monitor for signs/symptoms of infection and increased temperature.
- Monitor intake and output.
- Obtain daily weights.
- Monitor laboratory values—BUN/creatinine, electrolytes, minerals, nutritional panel.
- Monitor for venous thrombosis: neck vein distention (unilateral); unilateral edema of the arm, neck or face; shoulder pain.

- Maintain strict aseptic technique when performing bag and tubing changes.
- Change the TPN solution every 24 hours.
- Perform dressing and tubing changes as outlined by healthcare facility policy.

(For more information, see pp. 1754–1756 of Black and Matassarin-Jacobs: *Medical-Surgical Nursing: Clinical Management for Continuity of Care,* 5th ed.)

Tracheostomy

OVERVIEW

- A tracheostomy is the surgical creation of a stoma from the trachea to the overlying skin for airway management.
- Indications for a tracheostomy are:
  — need for long-term artificial airway
  — upper airway obstruction
  — upper airway bleeding
  — inability to clear lower airway secretions
  — altered level of consciousness with inability to protect the lower airway
  — need for continuous mechanical ventilation
  — prolonged endotracheal tube insertion
  — sleep apnea
- Types of tracheostomy tubes
  — universal or standard tracheostomy tube (e.g., Shiley)—consists of three parts: an outer cannula, an inner cannula, and an obturator. The outer cannula fits in the client's tracheostomy stoma to keep it open. The inner cannula is locked inside the outer cannula and maintains airway patency. The obturator is used for insertion and is immediately replaced by the inner cannula after insertion.
  — single-cannula tracheostomy tube—has only one cannula. Not appropriate for clients producing secretions.
  — fenestrated tracheostomy tube—similar to a universal tracheostomy tube, except it has an opening on the curvature of the posterior wall

of the outer cannula. When the inner cannula is in place, the tube functions as a universal tracheostomy tube. If the inner cannula is removed, air flows through the upper airway and allows speech and more effective coughing. When the inner cannula is replaced with a short decannulation stopper (tracheostomy plug), all airflow passes through the upper airway. When plugged, the person can speak, cough, and breathe deeply. If the tube is cuffed, the cuff must be deflated before plugging the tracheostomy, so that air can pass to the lungs. If this is not done, asphyxiation results.

— talking tracheostomy—this is a one-way valve in a plastic T-piece attached to the 15-mm end of the inner cannula of a universal tracheostomy tube. It permits talking without the need to plug the tracheostomy tube. The cuff of the tracheostomy tube must always be deflated before using a talking tracheostomy adapter. Otherwise, suffocation (from inability to exhale) can result.

— Communitrach—this tube allows speech but involves coordination on the client's part to occlude the distal end of an airflow tube. Speech will not sound normal.

— metal tracheostomy (e.g., Jackson)—most often used following a permanent tracheostomy or laryngectomy. The inner and outer cannulas lock together and are made of sterling silver or stainless steel.

— permanent tracheostomy—this is usually an uncuffed tracheostomy with a low-profile inner cannula that lies flush with the neck. This minimizes the tracheostomy's appearance and allows clothing to be arranged to conceal the tracheostomy.

— tracheostomy button—a short, straight tracheostomy tube that fits into a tracheostomy's stoma, but is not deep enough to enter the tracheal lumen. May be used during weaning as an intermediate device between the standard tracheostomy tube and complete extubation.

- Tracheostomy cuffs—a tracheostomy tube may be cuffed or uncuffed. Inflated cuffs protect the lower airway by creating a seal between the upper and lower airways. When inflated, they seal the area between the outer cannula and tracheal wall. They do not hold the tube in place. A pilot balloon reflects the absence or presence of air in the cuff, but cannot be an absolute indicator of cuff inflation. Most tracheostomy cuffs are designed to exert a low pressure against the tracheal wall, yet accept a high volume of air (high volume-low pressure cuffs). Low cuff pressure is necessary to prevent tracheal mucosal damage. Cuff pressures should not exceed 20 cm H_2O. Cuff pressures above 42 cm H_2O will stop circulation to the tracheal mucosa and precipitate necrosis.

- Complications due to prolonged contact between tube cuffs at high pressure and the tracheal wall include: obstruction, cuff inflation problems, tracheoesophageal fistula, and malposition of the tube. Other potential problems that may occur with tracheostomy tubes are:
  - tube displacement—the tracheostomy tube should lie 1–2 cm above the carina. If the tube is not properly placed, it may be in the soft tissues of the neck, or in the right main bronchus (allowing only ventilation of the right lung).
  - accidental extubation (tube removal)—dislodgement of the tube from the stoma, which may occur if the tube is not properly secured
  - airway obstruction—due to: misalignment of the tube (the tube tip is against the tracheal wall); cuff over-inflation; or occlusion of the tube with excessive or dried secretions
  - infection—bronchopulmonary infection or stoma site infection may occur
- Weaning from a tracheostomy tube—usually begins by plugging the tracheostomy tube's opening with a tracheostomy plug (decannulation stopper). At first, the plug is inserted for only short times and then the time is gradually lengthened. When plugging a cuffed tracheostomy, the cuff must be deflated, otherwise ventilation cannot occur and respiratory arrest will result.
- Tracheostomy removal (extubation)—performed only after successful tracheostomy plugging and

when the client's respiratory status and function are stable.

- Tracheostomy tubes ideally should be changed every 6–8 weeks, or more frequently if the client is at risk for tracheobronchial infections. Protocols vary between health care facilities.
- If respiratory arrest occurs, emergency mouth-to-tracheostomy or mouth-to-stoma resuscitation may be necessary. Ventilation is first attempted by attaching a manual self-inflating bag to the standard 15-mm adapter on the inner cannula. On cuffed tracheostomies, the cuff should be inflated. For uncuffed tracheostomies, more forceful, rapid ventilation may compensate for some volume loss that occurs. If inadequate ventilation continues to be a problem, or tube malfunction is suspected, remove the tube and perform mouth-to-stoma ventilation (the nose and mouth are kept closed to prevent air from escaping from the upper airway).

ACUTE AND SUBACUTE CARE

Nursing Management

Maintain a Patent Airway

- Following a tracheostomy, frequently assess:
  - — vital signs
  - — mucous membrane color
  - — for signs/symptoms of shock, hemorrhage, or respiratory insufficiency.
- Suction PRN. Provide oxygen and hyperinflate the client's lungs by delivering five or six breaths with a manual resuscitation bag before and after suctioning. Instill artificial saline to thin secretions if necessary.
- Provide adequate hydration and humidification.
- Change the client's position frequently.
- When deflating a tracheostomy cuff, give a deep manual inflation with a resuscitation bag, simultaneously deflating the cuff (this allows secretions trapped at the cuff to be blown up into the mouth, preventing them from falling into the lower airway).
- Monitor oxygen saturations or arterial blood gas analysis.

Prevent Infection

- Maintain aseptic technique for all care directly involving the tracheostomy.
- Inspect skin around the stoma and the stoma itself for irritation, inflammation, skin breakdown, and purulent drainage.
- Assess color, quantity, and odor of sputum production.
- Change tracheostomy dressings when damp, and do not use plastic-backed dressings.
- Cleanse the skin around the stoma using hydrogen peroxide and cotton-tipped applicators. Rinse the area with normal saline using cotton-tipped applicators. Use 4x4 gauze sponges to dry.

Provide Adequate Nutrition

- Assess for a tracheoesophageal fistula before permitting oral feedings (to assess, give client a "test swallow" of water with blue dye added). If severe coughing occurs, or if blue fluid is suctioned from the tracheostomy, do not give other foods or fluids and call physician.
- Sit client upright to feed.
- Offer foods and fluids with texture (such as pudding), which are easier to swallow.
- Tip the client's chin to the chest to aid in swallowing.
- If the client is receiving nutrition via a G-tube, inflate the tracheostomy cuff one hour before feeding. Suction above the cuff before deflating again.

Provide a Method of Communication

- Ensure that the client has an emergency call system to summon help. Ensure that the staff know the client cannot speak.
- Provide a method agreeable to the client to communicate needs (i.e., picture board, paper and pen, etc.).

Prevent Injury

- Ensure that the tracheostomy tube always is secured and ties knotted (two fingers should be able to slide under the ties to ensure it is not too tight). Do not place the knot over the carotid artery or spine.
- Drain water and condensate in tubing away from the tracheostomy.

- Support ventilator and aerosol tubing to prevent pulling on the tracheostomy tube.
- Do not allow smoking or the use of aerosol cans in the client's room.
- Do not shake bedding or create dust clouds in the room.
- Cover the tracheostomy with a thin cloth during shaving.
- Use only manufactured pre-sewn dressings around the trach (cut dressings may have loose edges that could be aspirated into the tracheostomy).
- Monitor tracheostomy cuff pressure and use the minimal leak technique to inflate the cuff.
- Keep the obturator taped above the head of the bed and keep tracheal dilators (spreaders) in the room.
- Use caution when changing tracheostomy ties to prevent extubation.
  - Hold the tube with two fingers.
  - Use two people, or only change one tie at a time.
  - If accidental extubation occurs and the stoma is less than four days old:
    - call for help immediately
    - maintain ventilation and oxygenation by bag and mask
    - if ventilation is impossible, reinsert the tube:
      - deflate the cuff
      - remove the tube's inner cannula
      - insert the obturator in the outer cannula
      - elevate the client's shoulders with a pillow and gently hyperextend the neck
      - use tracheal dilators (spreaders) as needed to hold the stoma open
      - insert the outer cannula into the client's neck and immediately remove the obturator
      - auscultate for breath sounds; if present, insert the inner cannula and reconnect to oxygen and ventilation equipment
      - if the tracheostomy cannot be reinserted within 1 minute, call a code for respiratory arrest. An emergency cricothyroidectomy may be necessary.

If accidental extubation occurs greater than 4 days following a tracheostomy, the same procedure is used, although it is generally easier. If bleeding occurs or the airway is obstructed, emergency measures are indicated.

Maintain Oral Mucosa Integrity

- Provide oral hygiene every 2 hours.

Prevent Constipation

- Be aware that the client is predisposed to constipation due to inability to perform the Valsalva's maneuver (the glottis and the vocal cords are bypassed with a tracheostomy).
- Use ordered stool softeners, laxatives as needed.

Reduce Fear and Anxiety

- Provide emotional support and reassurance.
- Frequently check the client.
- Explain all procedures and equipment.

COMMUNITY AND SELF-CARE

- Instruct client/significant other regarding:
  - — tracheostomy care and safety measures
  - — suctioning, use of a manual resuscitation bag, hyperoxygenating
  - — aerosol therapy
  - — airway maintenance
  - — signs/symptoms of infection
  - — clothing to disguise tracheostomy
- Refer to support groups.
- Refer to home health care agency for follow up.
- Involve a pulmonary nurse specialist if appropriate.
- Also see, "Laryngeal Cancer," p. 439.

(For more information, see pp. 1061–1076 of Black and Matassarin-Jacobs: *Medical-Surgical Nursing: Clinical Management for Continuity of Care,* 5th ed.)

Traction

OVERVIEW

- Therapeutic traction is accomplished by exerting a pull in two directions, the pull of traction and the pull of countertraction. Traction (pull) usually is produced by weights. Countertraction is produced by other weights or the weight of the person's own body. Forces also are exerted by the position of the client (e.g., flexion of the knee and hip). It is imperative that the position of the pulleys and the angle of splints not be adjusted without physician order.

- The goal of traction is to return bone fragments to their normal position or to treat muscle sprain, strain, and spasm.
- If traction is applied to a long bone, the direction of traction is in line with the bone's long axis. When applied to the head or pelvis, the pull is in line with the person's spinal column.
- Methods of applying traction:
  - Continuous—a constant pull is maintained. Used to treat certain fractures and dislocations.
  - Intermittent—periodic pull relieved by releasing the weight. Used to reduce flexion contractures.
  - Running traction (straight traction)—exerts a direct pull on the affected part without a hammock or splint to provide balanced support. It may be applied to the skin or skeleton.
  - Suspension traction (balanced traction)—exerts a pull on the affected part and also supports the extremity in a hammock or splint held in place by balanced weights attached to an overhead bar. It may be either skeletal or skin traction.
  - Skin—traction is applied to the underlying skeletal system and other structures using foam slings or by encircling a body part with a halter, corset, or sling.
  - Skeletal—traction is accomplished by surgically inserting metal wires (Kirschner wires) or pins (Steinmann pins) through bones or by anchoring metal tongs (such as Crutchfield, Gardner-Wells, etc.) in the skull. Kirschner wires or Steinmann pins are round stainless steel rods typically inserted with a drill, perpendicular to and completely through bones.
  - Cervical—traction applied via a head halter to hold the head in extension to treat muscle sprain, strain, and spasm. It can also be used to

stabilize fractures or dislocations of the cervical or upper thoracic spine.

— Pelvic—application of a belt above and encircling the iliac crests to apply traction to the lumbar spine. Its use is uncommon.
— Buck's traction—a form of skin traction exerted by a straight pull on one or both legs. Traction is applied using a prefabricated boot. It is used for hip fracture and dislocation, pelvic injuries, and fractures of the upper or lower leg.
— Russell's traction—a modification of Buck's traction, creating a vertical pull by placing a sling under the leg above the knee. It is used for hip fractures or fractures of the shaft of the femur.

ACUTE AND SUBACUTE CARE

Nursing Management

- Discuss with client the purpose of traction and contraindicated movements or positions.
- Perform baseline neurovascular assessment before insertion of pins or wires.
- Place corks or adhesive tape over protruding ends of pins or wires to prevent injury or damage to clothing.
- Inspect skin around pin sites for odor, redness, or drainage.
- Provide pin site care as ordered (often a daily dressing change with cleansing using antiseptic solution and application of antibiotic ointment).
- Cover the affected limb without interfering with traction.
- Ensure that ropes and pulleys hang free and weights do not reach the floor.
- Ensure that knots in the rope do not catch in the pulleys.
- Add and remove weights per physician order.
- Monitor color, warmth, movement, and sensation of extremity distal to traction every shift.
- Assess distal pulses every shift.
- Monitor degree of pain continually—pain should decrease. If pain increases, notify physician.
- Change linen from top to bottom of bed.
- Provide diversional activities—obtain Occupational Therapy consult.

- Provide normal aids to orientation.
- Use a fracture pan for elimination.
- Provide trapeze for assistance with movement.
- Provide analgesics as ordered (muscle spasms should subside after 48–72 hours).
- Assess skin for breakdown.
- Apply therapeutic mattress to bed.
- Perform range of motion exercises every shift to all joints except those immediately proximal and distal to the fracture.
- Assess lung sounds every shift.
- Instruct client on coughing, deep breathing, and incentive spirometry.
- Monitor for thrombophlebitis.
- Monitor bowel movements and encourage fluids and high-fiber diet.

Following traction removal:
- Assist the client to gradually resume a sitting (and later standing) position (to prevent orthostatic hypotension).
- Prepare client for lack of proprioceptor response (awareness of body position, movement, and posture).
- Discuss that joints may be stiff or unstable and client may feel faint or weak for awhile.

(For more information, see pp. 2137–2146 of Black and Matassarin-Jacobs: *Medical-Surgical Nursing: Clinical Management for Continuity of Care,* 5th ed.)

Transient Ischemic Attacks

OVERVIEW

- Transient ischemic attacks (TIAs) are brief, reversible episodes of neurologic dysfunction caused by temporary, focal cerebral ischemia. By definition, a TIA lasts less than 24 hours. TIAs are also called "mini-strokes" because they often serve as warning signs of an impending stroke.

- During a TIA, a transient decrease occurs in the blood supply to a focal area of the cerebrum or brain stem. Factors that can cause this ischemia include: occlusive disease of the extracranial cerebral vessels; occlusions in the vertebrobasilar system; and emboli. The most frequent site of occlusion is the origin of the internal carotid artery.
- TIAs are often recurrent although some clients have only one or two episodes prior to having a complete stroke. Between episodes, neurologic assessment findings are normal.
- Risk factors and preventive measures are essentially the same as those for cerebrovascular accident (CVA) (see "Cerebrovascular Accident," p. 138).

CLINICAL MANIFESTATIONS

Symptoms are transient, lasting usually from 2–15 minutes to hours. They vary, depending upon which area of the brain is affected.

- decreased vision in one eye
- rapid onset of weakness or numbness in an arm or leg
- alteration in speech pattern
- seizures

ACUTE AND SUBACUTE CARE

Medical Management

(The goal is to prevent the progression of a TIA to a CVA.)

- antihypertensives, antiplatelet drugs, or aspirin
- Warfarin (coumadin) to prevent clot development

Surgical Management

- carotid endarterectomy—opening of the carotid artery to remove obstructing and embolizing plaque. This procedure is performed through an incision on the anterior border of the sternocleidomastoid muscle. A temporary blood supply to the brain may be created by shunting blood through other vessels during the operation.
- extracranial-intracranial bypass—anastomosis of a superficial scalp artery to the middle cerebral

artery, thereby increasing blood flow to the brain. Performed for vascular insufficiency in the distribution of the middle cerebral artery.

Nursing Management

Medical

- Administer antihypertensives, antiplatelet drugs or aspirin as ordered.
- Administer Coumadin as prescribed; monitor prothrombin time (PT) and for any signs/symptoms of bleeding.
- Monitor blood pressure.
- Monitor neurologic status.
- Maintain safety precautions.

Surgical—Postoperative Care

In addition to routine postoperative care:

Extracranial-Intracranial Bypass

Nursing care is the same as for clients undergoing other types of cranial surgery. (See "Intracranial Tumors," p. 431.)

- Monitor vital signs and neurologic status closely, reporting any changes immediately to physician.
- Palpate (or assess by Doppler) pulse created by surgical anastomosis (located just below the curve of the incision) and notify surgeon immediately of any changes in character.
- Monitor BP—hypertension or hypotension may lead to hemorrhage or occlusion of the anastomosis.

Carotid Endarterectomy

- Keep the head in a straight position.
- Elevate the head of the bed when vital signs are stable.
- Maintain systolic blood pressure within 20 mmHg of preoperative values to ensure cerebral perfusion (blood pressure may be labile due to manipulation of the baroreceptors during surgery).
- Monitor for hematoma formation or excessive neck swelling (can cause airway obstruction).

- Apply cold to the operative site as ordered.
- Administer anticoagulant or antiplatelet medications as ordered.
- Assess neurologic status frequently, including pupillary reaction, level of consciousness, motor function and sensory function. Report any changes immediately.
- Assess functioning of the following cranial nerves: facial (VII), vagus (X), spinal accessory (XI), and hypoglossal (XII) because of close proximity to operative site. Cranial nerve damage usually is temporary but may last for months.
- Maintain tracheostomy tray at bedside.

COMMUNITY AND SELF-CARE

Medical Management

Instruct client/significant other regarding:

- Coumadin therapy
  — signs/symptoms of bleeding
  — safety measures
  — importance of follow-up laboratory tests
- antihypertensive or antiplatelet therapy
- signs/symptoms of increasing neurologic deficits to report to physician
- safety measures

Surgical Management

Instruct client/significant other regarding:

- wound care; signs/symptoms of infection
- no constrictive clothing or jewelry around the neck
- driving and lifting restrictions
- need to report persistent or severe headaches, or any manifestations of a TIA
- above information under "Medical Management"

(For more information, see pp. 808–812 of Black and Matassarin-Jacobs: *Medical-Surgical Nursing: Clinical Management for Continuity of Care,* 5th ed.)

Trichomoniasis

OVERVIEW

- Trichomoniasis is a protozoal infection causing vulvovaginitis.
- Trichomoniasis is caused by the parasite protozoan, *Trichomonas vaginalis*.
- The organism likes an alkaline environment, and changes in the vaginal flora make a woman susceptible.
- The organism is almost always transmitted sexually, and recurrence is common.

CLINICAL MANIFESTATIONS

- Female
  - — copious, malodorous, yellow-green vaginal discharge
  - — itching, burning, excoriation, and maceration of the vulvar tissue
  - — cervix may be covered with punctate hemorrhages, "strawberry cervix"
  - — vaginal mucosa is reddened and slightly edematous
  - — pain with intercourse
  - — frequency and burning with urination
- Male
  - — frequency and burning with urination

ACUTE AND SUBACUTE CARE

Medical Management

- single dose of Flagyl (metronidazole) orally for the client and all sexual contacts. A 7-day regime of Flagyl is used for recurrent infection.
- for the pregnant client—Flagyl should not be taken during the first trimester because it may adversely affect fetal development.

Single-dose therapy is usually curative but recurrence is common.

Nursing Management

- Administer Flagyl as ordered.

- Administer PRN medications for pain and itching.
- Instruct regarding perineal care.

COMMUNITY AND SELF-CARE

Instruct the client regarding:

- importance of completing medication regime
- information regarding disease, transmission, treatment, and follow-up
- need to treat all sexual partners
- medication administration
  - — no alcoholic intake during Flagyl administration to prevent the side effects of nausea, vomiting, and headaches
- need for the client to refrain from sexual intercourse or to use a condom while infection is active
- perineal hygiene

(For more information, see pp. 2473–2474 of Black and Matassarin-Jacobs: *Medical-Surgical Nursing: Clinical Management for Continuity of Care,* 5th ed.)

Trigeminal Neuralgia

OVERVIEW

- Trigeminal neuralgia is chronic irritation of the fifth cranial nerve, the trigeminal nerve. The trigeminal nerve has three branches: the ophthalmic, maxillary, and mandibular. Trigeminal neuralgia may occur in any one or more of these branches.
- The causative mechanisms can be divided into intrinsic (abnormalities of the axon or myelin) or extrinsic (mechanical compression from a tumor or from vascular anomalies).
- It is most common between the ages of 50 and 70 years. Approximately 60 per cent of clients are women.

CLINICAL MANIFESTATIONS

- intermittent episodes of intense pain with sudden onset
- pain not relieved by analgesics

- attacks are triggered by tactile stimulation (touch, facial hygiene) and talking
- the right side of face is more commonly affected

ACUTE AND SUBACUTE CARE

Medical Management

- anticonvulsant therapy—carbamazepine (Tegretol), phenytoin (Dilantin)—decrease the reactivity of neurons in the trigeminal nerve
- antispasmodic therapy—baclofen (Liorsal)

Surgical Management

- nerve blocks
- microvascular decompression—craniotomy is performed and the vessel removed from the posterior trigeminal root
- peripheral neurectomy
- rhizotomy—resection of the root of the nerve (requires a craniotomy)
- percutaneous radiofrequency—wave forms create lesions that alter pain transmission

Nursing Management

Medical

- Administer medications as ordered and assess effectiveness.

Surgical

- See care of client following craniotomy, Nursing Management, "Increased Intracranial Pressure," p. 419.

COMMUNITY AND SELF-CARE

Instruct the client regarding:

Medical

- ways to prevent triggering events
- medication regime

- if facial anesthesia is present following surgery, instruct to:
  - test the temperature of food before putting into mouth
  - chew on the unaffected side
  - inspect mucous membranes for irritation
  - use of a water jet device instead of toothbrush for dental hygiene and frequent dental check-ups
- if corneal reflex is impaired, instruct regarding eye care

See care of the client following craniotomy, Nursing Management, "Increased Intracranial Pressure," p. 419.

Tuberculosis, Pulmonary

OVERVIEW

- Tuberculosis (TB) is a chronic infectious disease that is characterized by the formation of tubercles or granulomas in the lungs. It is caused when droplet nuclei of mycobacterium tuberculosis are aerosolized through coughing, laughing, sneezing, or singing and a susceptible client inhales the droplet nuclei. If it penetrates lung tissue, the infection occurs.
- Tuberculosis is a worldwide health problem. After 1940 the incidence of TB declined. From 1985-1993 the number of cases increased due to HIV, immigrants from third world countries, deterioration of the healthcare infrastructure, and the development of multi-drug resistant TB.
- Tuberculosis is a reportable communicable disease. Brief exposure usually does not cause infection. Those having repeated close contact are more prone to infection.

- High risk groups include: immigrants from Asia, Africa, Latin America, and Oceania; the elderly; clients with reduced immunity; clients who are malnourished; Native Americans; Eskimos; and Blacks; economically disadvantaged or homeless; infants and children under the age of five; personnel and residents of long-term care facilities; healthcare workers; clients dependent upon alcohol.
- TB infection may be primary or secondary
  — Primary infection refers to the first time a client is infected with tuberculosis. The primary tubercles heal over a period of months through the formation of fibrous scars and, ultimately, calcified lesions. These lesions may contain certain living bacilli that later can reactivate and cause secondary infection.
  — Secondary infection (or reinfection) occurs when primary sites of infection containing TB bacilli, which may have been latent for years, reactivate when the client's resistance is lowered.

CLINICAL MANIFESTATIONS

- fatigue, anorexia, weight loss
- persistent, long-term, low-grade fever
- chills and sweats (often at night)
- dyspnea, hemoptysis
- chest pain (pleuritic or dull) or chest tightness
- persistent, progressive, and often productive cough

ACUTE AND SUBACUTE CARE

Medical Management

- isoniazid 300 mg daily for 9–12 months for prevention of active TB
- use of three or more medications initially for active TB to destroy resistant organisms; then maintenance therapy with two medications to eliminate most remaining bacilli. Medications used include: isoniazid, ethambutol, rifampin, streptomycin, and pyrazinamide.

- the length of each phase of therapy depends upon the client's compliance and the success of treatment. The course of each treatment phase may be anywhere from 6–24 months.
- TB protocols for noncompliant patients may include medications two to three times weekly.

Nursing Management

- Discuss need for respiratory isolation, if hospitalized.
- Instruct client that public health officials will talk with the client to develop a contact list (persons with whom client has had contact).
- Discuss mode of transmission and methods of preventing spread of disease.
- Monitor for side effects of medications and drug toxicity.
- Collect sputum specimens for acid-fast bacillus smear and culture.
- Discuss mode of transmission of TB and that it is not a shameful disease.

COMMUNITY AND SELF-CARE

Instruct client regarding:

- importance of follow-up visits to ensure that dormant lesions have not reactivated
- signs/symptoms of reinfection (secondary disease)
- importance of compliance with medication regimen
- side effects to report to physician
- need for isolation until 2–4 weeks into treatment
- transmission of TB:
  - — cover mouth and nose when coughing, laughing, or sneezing
  - — TB is not carried on eating utensils or articles
  - — client must wash hands after handling body substances, masks, or soiled tissues
  - — sputum is highly contaminated
  - — need to wear mask and change frequently

(For more information, see pp. 1139–1144 of Black and Matassarin-Jacobs: *Medical-Surgical Nursing: Clinical Management for Continuity of Care,* 5th ed.)

Tympanic Membrane Perforation (Ruptured Eardrum)

- The tympanic membrane is a semitransparent membrane that may become perforated through sports injuries, cleaning the ear with a sharp instrument, falling in water, a hand slap, or middle ear infection.
- A perforation may be acute, as seen with trauma or acute infection, or chronic, as seen in repeated infections.
- Acute perforations usually heal spontaneously. There may be hearing loss associated with the perforation, depending upon the size and location.
- Medical management includes use of systemic and local antibiotics (eardrops).
- Surgical management involves a myringoplasty (closure of the perforation). A tympanoplasty may be performed if the middle ear is also involved.

(For more information, see p. 1007 of Black and Matassarin-Jacobs: *Medical-Surgical Nursing: Clinical Management for Continuity of Care,* 5th ed.)

U

Ulcerative Colitis

OVERVIEW

- Ulcerative colitis is a type of inflammatory bowel disease. It is characterized by periods of exacerbation and remission. This disease spans the entire length of the colon and involves the mucosa and submucosa. It starts in the rectum and distal colon and spreads upward to the sigmoid and descending colon.
- Ulcerative colitis causes inflammation, thickening, congestion, edema, and minute lacerations that ooze blood and eventually develop into abscesses.
- When the inflammatory lesions heal, scarring and fibrosis with narrowing, thickening, and shortening of the colon may occur. Loss of haustral folds also may occur.
- Theories of causation include allergic reaction, altered immunity, bacterial origin, destructive enzymes, and a lack of protective substances in the bowel wall.
- Young adults, women, and Jewish people have a higher incidence of the disease, and it does have a familial tendency.
- Cancer of the colon is more common in clients with ulcerative colitis.
- There are no preventable risk factors, but controlling stress can help keep the disease in remission.

CLINICAL MANIFESTATIONS

- rectal bleeding, anemia may develop
- diarrhea of up to 20 or more stools/day
- liquid stools with tenesmus, blood, mucous, and pus
- urgency, cramping, abdominal pain in lower left quadrant

- nausea, vomiting, dehydration, anorexia, fever, weight loss, and decreased serum potassium
- decreased plasma proteins and prothrombin

ACUTE AND SUBACUTE CARE

Medical Management

- anti-inflammatory therapy, including steroids
- fluid, electrolyte, and blood replacement
- antidiarrheals
- hydrophilic mucilloids
- antispasmodics
- antibiotics and sulfonamides (such as sulfasalazine)
- bowel rest
- total parenteral nutrition
- antacids, histamine receptor antagonists
- anticholinergics
- high protein and calorie diet
- correction of nutritional deficiencies
- decrease physical acitivity

Surgical Management

- total proctocolectomy with a permanent ileostomy
  - — removal of the colon and rectum and closure of the anus
  - — the terminal ileum is brought through the abdominal wall and a permanent ileostomy formed
- ileorectal anastomosis
  - — old procedure performed infrequently
  - — resection of the colon, leaving a rectal stump; the terminal ileum is anastomosed to this stump
- Ileal pouch—anal anastomosis (J Pouch)
  - — excision of the rectal mucosa and colon removal
  - — an ileoanal reservoir is created in the anal canal and a temporary loop ileostomy is formed
  - — after healing takes place, the ileostomy is reversed, and stool drains into the reservoir
  - — prevents the need for an ostomy and preserves the rectal sphincter muscle
- Kock pouch (continent ileostomy)
  - — a reservoir is constructed from a loop of ileum

— stool is retained in the intra-abdominal pouch until the client drains it with a catheter through a special nipple valve
— the stoma is flat and flush with the skin on the right side of the abdomen
— there is no external pouch worn—the internal pouch is drained several times a day

Nursing Management

Medical

- Monitor the number, color, and consistency of stools.
- Hemoccult all stools.
- Administer antidiarrheals as ordered.
- Monitor intake and output; daily weights.
- Provide good perianal skin care—cleanse skin with warm water after each bowel movement and apply protective moisture barrier product.
- Monitor intake of foods and fluids—encourage small servings of bland and easily digested foods.
- Offer nutritional supplements.
- Assess quality, location, severity, and duration of pain—changes in pain may indicate development of complications.
- Administer pain medications as ordered and assess effectiveness.
- Discuss stress management and relaxation techniques (stress may exacerbate).

Surgical

Preoperative Care —if ostomy will be performed

In addition to routine preoperative care:
- Discuss role of enterostomal therapist.
- Arrange for preoperative visit from member of an ostomy association.
- Allow client to wear pouch over selected ostomy site 1–2 days before surgery to ensure comfort with site selected.
- Encourage discussion regarding feelings about change in body image and feelings about loss of a major body part.

Postoperative Care

In addition to routine postoperative care:

- Assess stomal color and contact physician immediately if pale, dusky, or cyanotic.
- Maintain patent nasogastric, gastrostomy, or jejunostomy tube to prevent distention. Measure amount of drainage.
- Clamp tube and start ice chips as ordered when bowel sounds return. After 24 hours start clear liquids.
- Assess for signs/symptoms of intestinal obstruction after ileostomy: anorexia, abdominal cramps, absence of visible peristalsis, absence of ileostomy drainage or a foul, brown, watery discharge in the pouch.
- Monitor for fluid and electrolyte imbalance.
- Monitor for hemorrhage.
- After Kock pouch, assess for suture line leakage and local or generalized peritonitis.
- After continent ileostomy or Kock pouch, assess for start of ileal drainage (3–4 days postoperatively).
- Assist the client to look at and touch the stoma as soon as possible.
- Encourage the client to verbalize feelings about the stoma and its appearance.

COMMUNITY AND SELF-CARE

Medical and Surgical

- Instruct client regarding:
  - — factors that exacerbate: emotional stress, overfatigue, dietary indiscretions, laxatives, antibiotics, physical exertion, respiratory infections
  - — signs/symptoms of fluid and electrolyte imbalance
  - — keeping a record of number of stools, consistency, color, and presence of blood
  - — need for follow-up colonoscopies and barium enemas if have had disease 5 or more years (higher incidence of cancer)
  - — need to report significant weight loss to physician

— side effects of steroids

- Refer to Crohn's and Colitis Foundations of America.
- Refer to American Cancer Society.

SURGICAL

Ileostomy

- Instruct client regarding:
  - — normal appearance of stoma—instruct that stoma will shrink to permanent size within 3–4 months
  - — assessing stoma for signs of irritation or cyanosis
  - — care of the stoma and surrounding skin
  - — signs of fungal skin infection
  - — applying, changing, and emptying pouch
  - — where to purchase ileostomy equipment and supplies
  - — use of deodorizing solutions and tablets
  - — foods that create odor: eggs, fish, onion, cabbage, or greens
  - — foods that reduce odor: spinach, parsley, yogurt, or buttermilk
  - — drinking at least 1500 ml per day
  - — low-residue diet, high in protein, carbohydrates, and calories
  - — foods that may cause problems: berries, whole grains, raw fruits, and vegetables
  - — foods to avoid: rice, bran, coconuts, popcorn, peanuts, skinned vegetables, tough fibrous meats, high-fiber and high-cellulose foods
  - — sexual activity, concerns, and pregnancy—encourage discussion with partner. Discuss emptying pouch before intercourse or wearing soft flannel pouch over it.
  - — need for follow-up with enterostomal therapist
  - — clothing options
  - — medications—enteric coated tablets may not be absorbed in the small intestine
- Encourage to join the Ileostomy Association (associated with American Cancer Society).
- Refer to United Ostomy Association.
- Refer to home health care agency for follow-up ostomy teaching.

Ileorectal Anastomosis

- Instruct client regarding:
  - — importance of defecating before rectum is overly distended
  - — stool will be pasty in consistency
  - — remaining bowel may become diseased
  - — increased risk of rectal cancer
  - — need for regular proctoscopic examinations
  - — need for adequate fluids

Ileal Pouch—Anal Anastomosis

- Instruct client regarding:
  - — need to respond to sensation to defecate so spillage does not occur
  - — need for adequate fluids
  - — stool output—eventually there will be 5–6 stools/day

Continent Ileostomy or Kock Pouch

- Instruct client regarding:
  - — need to empty reservoir every 2 hours for first 2 weeks
  - — evacuation catheter will be removed about 2 weeks after surgery
  - — how to empty the reservoir
  - — need for oral intake of at least eight 8 oz. glasses of water daily
  - — need for Medic-Alert identification and to carry drainage instructions in case of emergency
  - — need to avoid foods such as mushrooms and nuts that could block valve

(For more information, see pp. 1795–1808 of Black and Matassarin-Jacobs: *Medical-Surgical Nursing: Clinical Management for Continuity of Care*, 5th ed.)

Urethritis

OVERVIEW

- Urethritis is an inflammation of the urethra that is commonly associated with sexually transmitted diseases (STDs) and is also seen with cystitis.

- The most common causes are gonorrhea and chlamydial infections in men. In women it is caused by feminine hygiene sprays, perfumed toilet paper, sanitary napkins, spermicidal jellies, urinary tract infections, and changes in the vaginal mucosal lining.

CLINICAL MANIFESTATIONS

- inflamed and painful urethra, swollen meatus
- pyuria—pus in the urine
- with cystitis—dysuria, frequency, urgency, nocturia, low abdominal or perineal pain, and urethral discharge in men

ACUTE AND SUBACUTE CARE

Medical Management

- prevention
- removing the cause
- systemic and topical antibiotics

Surgical Management

- If strictures are severe, surgery is indicated with possible meatotomy for scarring at the meatus.

Nursing Management

- Monitor for signs and symptoms.
- Provide sitz baths with baking soda.
- Encourage an increased fluid intake.

COMMUNITY AND SELF-CARE

Instruct the client regarding:

- signs and symptoms of reoccurrence
- prevention and to avoid irritants
- safe sex practices
- avoid coitus until after the treatment of the STD is completed
- the use of lubrication during intercourse to decrease irritation

(For more information, see p. 1581 of Black and Matassarin-Jacobs: *Medical-Surgical Nursing: Clinical Management for Continuity of Care*, 5th ed.)

Urinary Bladder Calculi (Urolithiasis)

OVERVIEW

- Urinary calculi (urolithiasis) are stones within the urinary system.
- Stones rarely originate in the bladder; most are formed in the kidneys.
- Causative factors include urinary stasis, retention, and supersaturation of urine with poorly soluble crystalloids (such as calcium crystals).
- Risk factors include immobility, dehydration, increase in urine calcium, and prolonged indwelling catheterization.

CLINICAL MANIFESTATIONS

- if the stone remains in the bladder, the client will probably be asymptomatic
- burning, frequency, urgency
- very large stones—heavy feeling in the suprapubic region, decreased bladder capacity or an intermittent urinary stream
- ureteral stones cause severe flank and abdominal pain

ACUTE AND SUBACUTE CARE

Medical Management

- allopurinol for uric acid stones
- straining urine for stones
- forcing fluids up to 3000–4000 ml/day
- extracorporeal lithotripsy (electrically generated shock waves applied externally) to break up the stones

Surgical Management

- removal of small stones transurethrally or with a cystoscope
- litholapaxy (breaking up stones with an instrument) with irrigation for large stones
- laser lithotripsy

Nursing Management

Medical

- Force fluids to 4000 ml/day.
- Strain all urine.
- Administer narcotics and antispasmodics for pain as ordered.
- Lithotripsy—same interventions as "Litholapaxy" below.

Surgical

Litholapaxy

- Monitor for hemorrhage, urinary retention, infection, and stone recurrence.
- Force fluids.
- Perform intermittent irrigations as ordered.
- Strain all urine.

COMMUNITY AND SELF-CARE

Instruct client regarding:
- increasing fluid intake
- voiding every 2 hours
- low-calcium, low-phosphate diet for calcium stones
- low-purine diet for uric acid stones
- maintaining acidic urine pH (except for uric acid stones)
- use of medications for uric acid stones
- signs/symptoms of recurrence

(For more information, see pp. 1595–1598 of Black and Matassarin-Jacobs: *Medical-Surgical Nursing: Clinical Management for Continuity of Care*, 5th ed.)

Urinary Reflux

OVERVIEW

- Urinary reflux is the backward flow of urine within the urinary tract that begins at the vesicoureteral junction, causing backflow into the ureter and frequently into the renal pelvis.

- It frequently occurs in men with benign prostatic hyperplasia (BPH) and congenital vesicoureteral junction abnormalities in younger children or young adults.
- Risk factors include: ectopic ureter, chronic bladder infection secondary to dysfunctional bladder, or outlet obstruction.

CLINICAL MANIFESTATIONS

- pyelonephritis
- distended bladder if the obstruction is in the bladder neck
- renal failure if the obstruction is bilateral and higher than the vesicoureteral junction

ACUTE AND SUBACUTE CARE

Medical Management

- none

Surgical Management

- reimplantation of the ureter
- placement of a uretheral or suprapubic catheter
- uretheral catheter is inserted into the ureter as a splint, which facilitates healing, prevents obstruction from edema, and drains the urine
- prostatectomy as treatment for BPH

Nursing Management

- Routine preoperative and postoperative care.
- Assess for obstruction.
- Assess color and frequency of urine.
- The client will have bright red urine, which will clear over a few days.

COMMUNITY AND SELF-CARE

Instruct the client regarding:
- catheter care at home
- the importance of renal function monitoring

(For more information, see pp. 1599–1600 of Black and Matassarin-Jacobs: *Medical-Surgical Nursing: Clinical Management for Continuity of Care*, 5th ed.)

Urinary Retention

OVERVIEW

- Urinary retention is urine retained in the bladder.
- Benign prostatic hyperplasia, anesthesia, neurologic injury, medications, obstructive strictures, and scarring from chronic urinary tract infections are common causes.

CLINICAL MANIFESTATIONS

- distended bladder with inability to void

ACUTE AND SUBACUTE CARE

Medical Management

- catheterization with a straight catheter or retention catheter
- urethral dilation with progressively larger catheters used each day

Surgical Management

- suprapubic catheter placement
- specific procedures done to relieve obstruction below the bladder

Nursing Management

- Differentiate retention from oliguria and anuria.
- Perform noninvasive methods to stimulate voiding:
  - — place client in a normal sitting or standing position
  - — run water or flush the toilet within earshot of client
  - — pour warm water over perineum or provide warm bath
  - — immerse client's hand in water or have client blow bubbles with a straw in a glass of water
  - — apply ice to or stroke inner thigh to stimulate trigger points.
- Straight catheterize or place retention catheter as ordered.

- Maintain patent drainage system if catheter in place.
- Maintain strict aseptic technique when handling catheter or drainage system.
- Monitor intake and output.

COMMUNITY AND SELF-CARE

Instruct client regarding:
- suprapubic catheter care after discharge (if present):
  - — care of catheter
  - — changing leg bag to conventional drainage bag at night
  - — cleaning of bags and odor control
- self catheterization as appropriate
- signs/symptoms of urinary tract infection and when to call physician
- prevention of infection and need to force fluids

(For more information, see pp. 1600–1604 of Black and Matassarin-Jacobs: *Medical-Surgical Nursing: Clinical Management for Continuity of Care*, 5th ed.)

Urinary Tract Infection

OVERVIEW

- Urinary tract infection refers to an infection within the lower urinary tract, usually affecting the bladder, although the urethra and ureters may be involved.
- Cystitis is an inflammation of the bladder wall, usually caused by ascending bacteria.
- The most common organisms causing urinary tract infections are: *Escherichia coli*, *Enterobacter*, *Pseudomonas*, and *Serratia*.
- Risk factors include: indwelling catheters, pregnancy, aging with associated hormonal changes, and females who are sexually active or who wear synthetic underwear or panty hose.

CLINICAL MANIFESTATIONS

- frequency, urgency, burning on urination, hematuria
- inability to void or voiding in small amounts
- incomplete emptying of the bladder
- low back, suprapubic, abdominal, or flank pain
- positive urine cultures
- chills, fever, malaise, nausea, vomiting
- the elderly may present with mental status changes

ACUTE AND SUBACUTE CARE

Medical Management

- 10–14 day course of antibiotic therapy
- use of medications containing azo dyes to anesthetize the urinary tract mucosa
- chronic urinary tract infection—acidifying the urine through an acid-ash diet to decrease the rate of bacterial multiplication—this may or may not be ordered depending on the specific antiseptic or antibiotic used. (An acid-ash diet is considered more effective in acidifying the urine than use of cranberry juice or ascorbic acid.)

Surgical Management

- Rare, but surgery may include correction of bladder neck strictures or ureteral pelvic junction abnormalities.

Nursing Management

Medical

- Monitor the client's voiding—note frequency, urgency, retention, or dysuria.
- Monitor intake and output.
- Provide warm sitz baths—baking soda may be added for a greater soothing effect.
- Encourage fluids.
- Apply a heating pad to the suprapubic area as ordered to reduce bladder spasms.
- Administer anti-infective agents as ordered—assess for a decrease in the severity of symptoms within 24 hours after the start of medications.
- Monitor culture and sensitivity reports.

- Obtain residuals as ordered.
- Monitor vital signs, consider blood cultures for temperature of 101° F.
- Assess for sepsis (UTIs are the most common cause of gram-negative sepsis).

COMMUNITY AND SELF-CARE

Instruct the client regarding:

- Drinking at least eight 8-ounce glasses of water per day.
- Avoidance of caffeine and alcohol (they irritate the bladder).
- Voiding at the first urge and at least every 2–3 hours during the day.
- Voiding 1–2 times per night.
- Women:
  - — avoidance of synthetic underwear, panty hose, tight jeans
  - — shower instead of tub bath
  - — wearing cotton panties
  - — avoidance of bubble baths, perfumed toilet paper, or sanitary napkins
  - — wiping front to back
  - — if sexually active:
    - wash well before sexual intercourse
    - void immediately after sexual intercourse
    - drink two glasses of water after intercourse.
- Taking the full course of medication, even if symptoms disappear.
- Compliance with the schedule of follow-up urine cultures.
- Following the acid-ash diet as ordered.
- Contacting the physician for signs of persistent infection.

(For more information, see pp. 1571–1579 of Black and Matassarin-Jacobs: *Medical-Surgical Nursing: Clinical Management for Continuity of Care*, 5th ed.)

Urosepsis

OVERVIEW

- Urosepsis is gram-negative (usually *E. Coli*) bacteremia originating in the genitourinary tract.
- The risk factors include: indwelling foley catheter, untreated urinary tract infection, and nursing home clients.
- Urosepsis can lead to septic shock if not treated aggressively.

CLINICAL MANIFESTATIONS

- fever

ACUTE AND SUBACUTE CARE

Medical Management

- culture and sensitivity of the urine
- intravenous (IV) aminoglycosides, B-lactam antibiotics, or third-generation cephalosporins

Nursing Management

- Continue antibiotics until the client has been afebrile for 3-5 days.
- Continue oral antibiotics after IV therapy is finished.
- Nurses need to be aware of the possibility of sepsis with clients who have urinary catheters.

COMMUNITY AND SELF-CARE

- Supply education for nursing home staff regarding symptoms of urosepsis.
- If sepsis is suspected a urine culture should be obtained.
- The elderly may exhibit other more subtle signs of urosepsis such as confusion.

(For more information, see p. 1581 of Black and Matassarin-Jacobs: *Medical-Surgical Nursing: Clinical Management for Continuity of Care*, 5th ed.)

Uterine Prolapse

OVERVIEW

- Uterine prolapse occurs in three stages:
  (1) First degree—the uterus descends into the vaginal canal and the cervix reaches, but does not go through the entrance to the vagina (introitus).
  (2) Second degree—the body of the uterus is within the vagina but the cervix protrudes through the introitus.
  (3) Third degree—the entire uterus and cervix protrude through the introitus and the vaginal canal is inverted (turned inside out).
- Prolapse commonly follows multiple childbirths, childbirth trauma, aging, and failure to maintain the perineal musculature.
- During the stages of prolapse of the uterus, other structures may be pulled down or out of position:
  — cystocele—protrusion of part of the urinary bladder through the vaginal wall due to weakened pelvic muscles
  — rectocele—protrusion of a portion of the rectum through a weak place in the vaginal wall musculature
  — urethrocele—protrusion of a portion of the urethra through the vaginal wall
  — enterocele— herniation of small bowel and/or omentum into the vaginal canal
- When complete prolapse has occurred and involves a cystocele, rectocele, and enterocele, the woman is said to have pelvic relaxation.
- With pelvic relaxation, the cervix protrudes through the vaginal orifice and is constantly irritated, causing inflammation and possible malignant degeneration. The vaginal tissue also is irritated and dry once it is exposed.

CLINICAL MANIFESTATIONS

- feeling that "something is descending internally"
- dyspareunia (pain with intercourse)
- feelings of pressure, dragging, and heaviness

- backaches, bowel and bladder symptoms

Cystocele

- urinary frequency, urgency, urinary tract infections, difficulty emptying the bladder, stress incontinence

Rectocele

- constipation, heaviness, hemorrhoids

ACUTE AND SUBACUTE CARE

Medical Management

- Kegel exercises (see Nursing Management)
- use of a pessary

Surgical Management

Cystocele

- anterior repair or anterior colporrhaphy—tightening the pelvic muscles to provide better bladder support

Rectocele

- posterior repair or posterior colporrhaphy—surgical tightening of the weakened muscles (this also may be performed in conjunction with an anterior repair and then is called an anteroposterior colporrhaphy or anterior-posterior repair)

Enterocele or Urethrocele

- same treatment as for cystocele and rectocele

Complete Uterine Prolapse

- vaginal hysterectomy—removal of the uterus through the vagina

Nursing Management

Medical

- Instruct client on Kegel exercises (alternately tightening and relaxing rectal and vaginal muscles).

These are tightened as if trying to hold back a bowel movement or stop the urinary stream. They should be performed frequently throughout the day or 50–100 times once or twice daily.

Surgical

Postoperative Care

In addition to routine postoperative care:

- Keep urinary catheter patent to keep bladder decompressed and pressure off the anterior vaginal muscles until healing has occurred.
- Instruct client to void every 2 hours after catheter is removed to keep bladder decompressed.
- Monitor for excessive vaginal bleeding, rigid and distended abdomen, or referred shoulder pain. Notify physician if any of these occur.
- Maintain vaginal packing or drain (usually removed after 24–48 hours).
- Provide sitz baths for comfort.

COMMUNITY AND SELF-CARE

Instruct client regarding:

- catheter care (if applicable)
- signs/symptoms to report to physician:
  - — excess bleeding
  - — distended abdomen
  - — inability to void
  - — signs of urinary tract infection
  - — signs of infection
- activity/lifting restrictions
- use of sitz baths for comfort
- use of analgesics
- bleeding may occur on the 4th, 9th, 14th, and 21st days following surgery, as the sutures dissolve
- low-residue diet and stool softeners until healing occurs
- avoidance of constipation, which can cause recurrence

(For more information, see pp. 2409–2411 of Black and Matassarin-Jacobs: *Medical-Surgical Nursing: Clinical Management for Continuity of Care*, 5th ed.)

Uterine Tumors, Benign (Leiomyomas)

OVERVIEW

- Leiomyomas are benign tumors of the uterine muscles. They are the most common tumors of the female genital tract and also are called myomas or fibroids of the uterus.
- They occur in more than 20–30 per cent of all women during their menstrual years. The incidence in black women is two to three times greater than in white women.
- The cause of leiomyomas is unknown, but seems to be related to estrogen stimulation.

CLINICAL MANIFESTATIONS

- frequently asymptomatic
- abnormal uterine bleeding (excessive in amount or duration) with associated anemia, tiredness, weakness, and lethargy
- dysmenorrhea
- urinary frequency
- urinary retention
- constipation
- hydroureter, hydronephrosis, abdominal pain, and dyspareunia are less common symptoms

ACUTE AND SUBACUTE CARE

Medical Management

Treatment depends upon symptoms, age, location, and size of the tumors, onset of complications, and the woman's desire to become pregnant.

Surgical Management

- myomectomy (removal of tumor without removal of the uterus) for small tumors
- total hysterectomy—removal of the uterus and cervix (performed vaginally or abdominally)
- total abdominal hysterectomy with bilateral salpingo-oophorectomy (TAH-BSO)—removal of the uterus, cervix, fallopian tubes, and ovaries

Nursing Management

Medical

- Discuss ways to reduce pain—sitz baths, application of heat to lower abdomen.
- Discuss ways to reduce pain during intercourse—alternate positions, use of water soluble lubricants.

Surgical—Hysterectomy

Preoperative Care

In addition to routine preoperative care:
- Discuss fact that reproductive function will be lost if hysterectomy is performed.
- Instruct that sexual intercourse should be pain-free once healing has occurred, and orgasms are still possible.
- If TAH-BSO will be performed, discuss that surgical menopause will occur.

Postoperative Care

In addition to routine postoperative care:
- Monitor amount of bleeding, number of pads used, and drainage on dressings. Also note color and odor.
- If total abdominal hysterectomy (TAH) was performed, monitor abdominal incision site for redness, drainage, or swelling.
- Encourage turning, coughing, and deep breathing and increase activity as ordered.
- Maintain thigh-high antiembolism stockings.
- Encourage ankle and leg exercises.
- Monitor Homan's sign.
- Maintain urinary catheter to dependent drainage and monitor intake and output.
- Encourage 2–4 liters of fluid daily when tolerating fluids well.
- Monitor for pain on voiding, voiding frequently in small amounts, inability to void, or hematuria when the catheter is removed and report to physician.
- Assess color, odor, and clarity of urine—report any changes.
- Provide analgesics and assess effectiveness.

- Provide good perineal care and catheter care (if present) every shift.
- If abdominal hysterectomy was performed, monitor for return of bowel sounds. Encourage ambulation to stimulate peristalsis.
- Provide open environment for patient to discuss feelings regarding loss of uterus.
- Encourage client to share thoughts/concerns with partner.

COMMUNITY AND SELF-CARE

Instruct client regarding:

Hysterectomy

- performing prescribed abdominal strengthening exercises
- avoidance of heavy lifting for 2 months
- avoidance of activities that increase pelvic congestion (such as dancing, horseback riding, and prolonged standing)
- avoidance of vaginal or rectal sexual activities and douching until permitted by surgeon
- avoidance of constrictive clothing for several months
- symptoms to report to physician—abnormal vaginal discharge, bleeding, signs/symptoms of infection, incision not healing
- possible effects of surgical menopause, and interventions to minimize (if ovaries were removed):
  - vasomotor instability (including hot flashes, night sweats, occasional palpitations, and dizziness)
    - dress in layers so that clothing can be removed during hot flashes
    - avoid hot environments and keep the thermostat around 65° F. or lower
    - avoid highly seasoned, spicy foods, coffee, tea, and alcohol if they trigger hot flashes
    - keep a record of hot flashes to help determine "triggers"
  - vaginal dryness
    - use water soluble jelly for lubrication; estrogen cream if needed
  - osteoporosis
    - take part in weight-bearing exercise
    - increase calcium intake

    - stop smoking
    - decrease caffeine and alcohol intake
  - urinary tract infection
    - drink plenty of fluids
    - void frequently
    - perform good perineal hygiene
- hormone replacement therapy, side effects and precautions (if prescribed)

Myomectomy

- need for routine gynecologic examinations

If surgery was not performed:

- interventions to minimize pain during intercourse (e.g., different positions)
- need for routine gynecologic examinations to monitor the leiomyomas

(For more information, see pp. 2400–2404 of Black and Matassarin-Jacobs: *Medical-Surgical Nursing: Clinical Management for Continuity of Care*, 5th ed.)

Uveitis

OVERVIEW

- Uveitis is an inflammation of the uveal tract that can affect one or more parts of the eye (iris, ciliary body, and choroid).
- Uveitis commonly occurs from a hypersensitivity reaction in its acute form or following microbial infection in its chronic form.

CLINICAL MANIFESTATIONS

- pain (ciliary body muscle spasm)
- blurred vision
- photophobia
- redness of the eye
- constricted pupil

ACUTE AND SUBACUTE CARE

Medical Management

- topical atropine (cycloplegic)—relieves spasm
- topical steroid—to reduce inflammation

- analgesics

Nursing Management

- Administer eye drops.
- Administer PRN analgesics.
- Keep room lights dimmed.
- Implement safety measures.

COMMUNITY AND SELF-CARE

Instruct client regarding:

- technique for instilling eye drops
- measures to relieve photophobia—sunglasses, dimmed lights
- signs/symptoms of increased intraocular pressure (pain, nausea, decreased vision)
- measures for a safe home environment

(For more information, see p. 970 of Black and Matassarin-Jacobs: *Medical-Surgical Nursing: Clinical Management for Continuity of Care*, 5th ed.)

V

Vaginal Cancer

OVERVIEW

- Vaginal cancer is rare, occurring in women over age 50, but is seen in women whose mothers ingested diethylstilbestrol during pregnancy. It typically occurs between menarche and age 30 years.
- Women exposed to diethylstilbestrol in utero should receive twice yearly careful gynecologic examinations beginning at menarche or age 14 years, whichever comes first.
- The prognosis for vaginal cancer is generally poor due to: (1) the rarity of the cancer (making it difficult to identify the best treatment), (2) the typically advanced stage of the cancer when diagnosed, and (3) the difficulty in treating this cancer because of the proximity of important adjacent structures.
- Risk factors also include repeated pregnancies, syphilis, uterine prolapse, pessary use, leukoplakia, and leukorrhea.

CLINICAL MANIFESTATIONS

- foul vaginal discharge
- painless vaginal bleeding
- pruritus
- pain

ACUTE AND SUBACUTE CARE

Medical Management

- external or intravaginal radiation therapy

Surgical Management

- radical hysterectomy, lymphadenectomy, and vaginectomy for early stages (removal of the uterus, cervix, fallopian tubes, ovaries, lymph nodes, upper third of the vagina, and parametrium)

- pelvic exenteration (removal of pelvic organs and formation of an ileostomy and an ileal conduit) for more advanced cancer

Nursing Management

- Discuss the potential impact of the disease process and treatment on sexuality (potential problems include fatigue, pain, dyspareunia, decreased libido, and altered body image).
- Discuss use of alternate positioning and need for adequate lubricant if a partial vaginectomy was performed.
- Discuss use of vaginal dilator to prevent vaginal fibrosis and scarring.

Irradiation

- Discuss need for vaginal penetration to minimize vaginal adhesions and stenosis (may be accomplished by client's own fingers, a vaginal dilator or sexual partner's fingers or penis).
- Discuss need for water soluble lubricant for vaginal dryness.

See "Uterine Tumors, Benign," p. 743, for posthysterectomy care.
See "Radiation Therapy," p. 605.

COMMUNITY AND SELF-CARE

- See nursing management.

(For more information, see pp. 2416–2418 of Black and Matassarin-Jacobs: *Medical-Surgical Nursing: Clinical Management for Continuity of Care,* 5th ed.)

Vaginal Fistulas

OVERVIEW

- Fistulas are abnormal tubelike passages from the vagina to the bladder (vesicovaginal), rectum (rectovaginal), or urethra (urethrovaginal).
- Fistulas may occur: (1) when an abnormal opening is present between two adjacent organs; (2) as a

result of spread of a malignant lesion; (3) following irradiation for cancer; (4) from venereal and other inflammatory diseases; or (5) after a prolonged, difficult labor and delivery.

CLINICAL MANIFESTATIONS

- leakage of urine or feces into the vagina
- excoriation and irritation of the vaginal and vulvar tissues
- infection
- feeling of wetness
- sensation of feeling dirty
- offensive odor (with rectovaginal fistulas)

ACUTE AND SUBACUTE CARE

Surgical Management

Treatment depends upon the location, extent, and cause of the fistula.

- vesicovaginal, urethrovaginal, or rectovaginal fistulectomy—repair of the fistula, which may be performed following a 6-month waiting period during which edema and inflammation subside
- temporary colostomy—may be needed with a rectovaginal fistula

Nursing Management

Preoperative Care

In addition to routine preoperative care:

- Encourage fluid intake if the client has a urinary fistula (restriction of fluids may increase the size of the fistula or the incidence of infection).
- Instruct the client on perineal hygiene measures
  - — cleaning the perineum every 4 hours
  - — sitz baths
  - — douches
  - — changing perineal pads frequently.
- Instruct the client on deodorizing and comfort measures
  - — vitamin A and D ointment
  - — deodorant powders
  - — pouring weak acid or weak base solutions over the perineum, as ordered
  - — deodorizing douches as ordered.

- Instruct client to avoid using excessive pressure when douching.
- Discuss use of ordered enemas for rectovaginal fistulas.

Postoperative Care

In addition to routine postoperative care:

Vesicovaginal or Urethrovaginal Fistulectomy

- Maintain patency of urinary catheter to prevent strain on sutures.
- Encourage fluid intake.
- Do not let urinary catheter become occluded as the pressure could reopen the fistula.

Rectovaginal Fistulectomy

- Instruct not to strain with stools (this may reopen the fistula).
- Discuss use of stool softeners and laxatives.

COMMUNITY AND SELF-CARE

- See nursing management.

(For more information, see pp. 2414–2416 of Black and Matassarin-Jacobs: *Medical-Surgical Nursing: Clinical Management for Continuity of Care,* 5th ed.)

Vaginosis, Bacterial

OVERVIEW

- Bacterial vaginosis is caused by the organism, *Gardnerella vaginalis.*

CLINICAL MANIFESTATIONS

- mild to moderate amount of malodorous ("fishy"), gray, homogenous, thin vaginal discharge
- vaginal irritation and burning

ACUTE AND SUBACUTE CARE

Medical Management

- Flagyl (metronidazole) by mouth for 7 days (unless pregnant, due to adverse effect Flagyl may have on fetal development).

Nursing Management

- Administer Flagyl as ordered.
- Instruct regarding perineal care.
- Instruct regarding palliative measures—PRN medication for pain and itching, sitz baths, etc.

COMMUNITY AND SELF-CARE

Instruct client regarding:

- importance of completing medication regime
- information regarding disease, transmission, treatment, and follow-up
- medication administration:
  - — no alcohol intake during Flagyl administration to prevent side effects of nausea, vomiting, and headaches
- need to treat male partners only if recurrent or resistant infection
- need to avoid sexual intercourse during the treatment and condom use to prevent recurrence
- perineal hygiene

(For more information, see pp. 2474–2475 of Black and Matassarin-Jacobs: *Medical-Surgical Nursing: Clinical Management for Continuity of Care,* 5th ed.)

Valvular Heart Disease

OVERVIEW

- The four heart valves maintain the one-way flow of blood through the heart and lungs. Dysfunction occurs when the heart valves are unable to fully open or close. A stenosed valve may impede the flow of one chamber to the next. An insufficient valve may allow blood to regurgitate back into the chamber from which the blood is being pumped.

- Valvular heart disease remains fairly common in the United States even though the incidence is steadily decreasing as the incidence of rheumatic fever decreases. Aortic valve disease is far less common than mitral valve disease, however, it often occurs in conjunction with mitral valve disease. Pure lesions of the tricuspid valve are uncommon. Tricuspid stenosis or regurgitation usually develops in combination with other structural disorders. Abnormalities of the pulmonic valve are usually congenital defects with few developing after birth. Only mitral and aortic disease will be covered here because of their higher incidence.
- *Mitral stenosis* is a block in blood flow into the left ventricle resulting from an abnormality of the leaflets, which prevents opening of the valve during diastole.
- *Mitral regurgitation* occurs when blood from the left ventricle is ejected back into the left atrium during systole because of an incompetent mitral valve.
- *Mitral valve prolapse* occurs when one or both of the valve leaflets bulge into the left atrium during ventricular systole.
- *Aortic stenosis* is an obstruction to flow across the aortic valve during systole, creating resistance to ejection and increased pressure in the left ventricle.
- *Aortic regurgitation* —blood ejected into the aorta during systole re-enters the left ventricle due to an incompetent aortic valve.
- Risk factors include:
  — acute rheumatic fever
  — coronary artery disease
  — age—calcification of the valve
  — connective tissue disorders
  — infective endocarditis
- Acquired valvular dysfunction is usually caused by inflammation of the endocardium due to acute rheumatic fever or infectious endocarditis. The inflammation causes the valve leaflets and chordae tendineae to become fibrous. The chordae tendineae shorten. In valvular stenosis, the valve

orifice narrows and the valve leaflets may become fused or thickened in such a way that the valve cannot open freely. With valvular insufficiency, scarring and retraction of the valve leaflets results in incomplete closure. Either problem increases the heart's workload. The heart may compensate with dilation and hypertrophy, however, if the damage worsens, without intervention the heart will fail.

CLINICAL MANIFESTATIONS

- Mitral stenosis
  — low-pitched murmur (diastolic)
  — loud S_1
  — dyspnea, orthopnea, paroxysmal nocturnal dyspnea (PND)
  — fatigue
  — palpitations
  — pulmonary crackles
  — hemoptysis, cough
  — narrowed pulse pressure
  — atrial fibrillation
  — peripheral edema
- Mitral regurgitation
  — high-pitched murmur (systolic)
  — weakness, fatigue
  — left ventricular failure; dyspnea, orthopnea, PND, crackles, S_3, and S_4
  — right ventricular failure; neck vein distention, peripheral edema, hepatomegaly
  — atrial fibrillation
- Mitral valve prolapse
  — not uncommon to be asymptomatic with only a regurgitant murmur on physical examination
  — tachycardia, lightheadedness, syncope
  — fatigue, weakness
  — dyspnea, chest discomfort
- Aortic stenosis:
  Clinical manifestations occur gradually and late in the disease. There is a long latent period in which the client is asymptomatic.
  — systolic, harsh murmur
  — dyspnea, orthopnea, PND
  — S_3 and S_4
  — fatigue

- — vertigo, syncope
  - — chest pain
  - — bradycardia
- Aortic regurgitation
  - — diastolic, blowing murmur
  - — dyspnea, orthopnea, PND
  - — fatigue, weakness
  - — syncope
  - — palpitations
  - — pulmonary congestion
  - — wide pulse pressure
  - — sinus tachycardia, PVCs
  - — S_3 and S_4
  - — neck vein distention, peripheral edema, hepatomegaly

ACUTE AND SUBACUTE CARE

Medical Management

- Mitral stenosis
  - — oral diuretics
  - — sodium-restricted diet
  - — digitalis preparations and beta-blockers to slow heart rate and improve activity tolerance
- Mitral regurgitation
  - — restriction of physical activities that produce fatigue and dyspnea
  - — sodium-restricted diet
  - — diuretics and nitrates
- Mitral valve prolapse
  - — beta-blockers to relieve syncope, palpitations, and chest pain
- Aortic stenosis
  - — activity restrictions
  - — pharmacologic management of dysrhythmias
- Aortic regurgitation
  - — same as aortic stenosis

Surgical Management

- Mitral stenosis
  - — valve replacement
  - — valve reconstruction (commissurotomy)
- Mitral regurgitation
  - — valve replacement

— valve reconstruction

- Mitral valve prolapse
  — surgical intervention usually is not needed
- Aortic stenosis
  — valve replacement
  — balloon valvuloplasty to dilate valve orifice
- Aortic regurgitation
  — valve replacement

Nursing Management

Medical

- Auscultate heart and lung sounds.
- Monitor intake and output.
- Monitor for decreased cardiac output—rise in heart rate, drop in BP, or decrease in urinary output.
- Daily weights.
- Monitor activity tolerance.
- Assess for peripheral edema, neck vein distention, and hepatomegaly.

Surgical

- See "Cardiac Surgery," p. 122.

COMMUNITY AND SELF-CARE

Instruct client regarding:

- activity restrictions
- dietary restrictions
- importance of adequate rest
- prophylactic antibiotics before and after dental or surgical procedures
- need for follow-up appointments.

(For more information, see pp. 1342–1350 of Black and Matassarin-Jacobs: *Medical-Surgical Nursing: Clinical Management for Continuity of Care,* 5th ed.)

Varicose Veins

OVERVIEW

- Varicose veins are caused by the loss of valvular competence and the constant elevation of venous pressure, which results in distention and tortuosity of the superficial veins.

- The greater and lesser saphenous veins and perforator veins in the ankle are common sites of varicosities.
- Varicose veins may be either primary or secondary. Primary varicose veins result from a congenital or familial predisposition that leads to loss of elasticity of the vein wall. Secondary varicosities occur when trauma, obstruction, deep vein thrombosis, or inflammation damages valves.
- The prevalence increases with age and peaks between the fifth and sixth decades of life. Varicose veins are more common in women.

CLINICAL MANIFESTATIONS

- complaint of aching, heaviness, itching
- moderate swelling of the extremity
- dilated tortuous skin veins

ACUTE AND SUBACUTE CARE

Surgical Management

- ligation (tying off) of the greater saphenous vein at the saphenofemoral junction, combined with saphenous vein stripping and ligation of incompetent perforator veins. Removal of the vein is performed through multiple, short incisions. An incision is made at the ankle over the saphenous vein and a nylon wire is threaded up the vein to the groin. The wire is brought out through the groin, capped, and then the wire and vein are pulled out through the ankle incision.
- sclerotherapy—injection of a sclerosing agent into varicosed veins that damages the vein and endothelium, causing aseptic thrombosis that closes the veins. This treatment is palliative and is performed for cosmetic reasons to close small, residual varicosities after surgery.

Nursing Management

Postoperative Care

In addition to routine postoperative care:

- Maintain firm elastic pressure over the whole limb.

- Elevate foot of bed 6–9 inches.
- Ambulate as ordered (usually 24–48 hours after surgery).
- Instruct client to walk rather than to stand or sit.
- Assess for possible complications:
  — hemorrhage
  — infection
  — nerve damage
  — deep vein thrombosis

COMMUNITY AND SELF-CARE

Instruct client regarding:
- signs/symptoms to report to physician
- measures to prevent venous stasis:
  — no crossing legs
  — no constrictive clothing
  — avoid standing or sitting for prolonged periods of time
  — elevate legs when sitting or lying down
  — elastic stockings

(For more information, see pp. 1438–1439 of Black and Matassarin-Jacobs: *Medical-Surgical Nursing: Clinical Management for Continuity of Care,* 5th ed.)

Venous Stasis Ulcers

- Venous stasis ulcers represent the end stage of chronic venous insufficiency. Over a period of years, the excess venous pressure causes small skin veins and venules to rupture, with creation of stasis ulcers. Stasis ulcers are characteristically located in the malleolar area.
- Once the skin is broken, infection occurs, usually due to staphylococcus or streptococcus.
- Interventions include:
  — antibiotic therapy
  — bedrest with leg elevated
  — Unna boot—bandage impregnated with calamine, zinc oxide, and glycerin
  — hydrocolloid dressing used to promote epithelization
  — ulcer debridement

— skin grafting
- Instruct the client regarding:
  — wound care
  — elevation of legs above level of heart whenever possible when sitting or lying down
  — not crossing legs
  — use of elastic stockings after wound is healed
  — avoidance of constrictive clothing
  — avoidance of standing or sitting for prolonged periods of time
  — importance of daily skin inspection

(For more information, see pp. 1436–1438 of Black and Matassarin-Jacobs: *Medical-Surgical Nursing: Clinical Management for Continuity of Care,* 5th ed.)

Vincent's Angina (Trench Mouth, Necrotizing Ulcerative Gingivitis)

OVERVIEW

- Vincent's angina is an acute bacterial infection of the gingiva in adults.
- It is caused by resident flora in the mouth, fusiform bacteria, and spirochetes.
- Major risk factors are poor oral hygiene, nutritional deficiencies, lack of rest and sleep, local tissue damage, and debilitative diseases. It is not contagious.

CLINICAL MANIFESTATIONS

- oral ulcers covered with a pseudomembrane
- elevated white blood count
- oral pain, foul taste, pain, choking sensation
- thick secretions, anorexia, lymphadenopathy

ACUTE AND SUBACUTE CARE

Medical Management

- removal of devitalized tissue
- correction of underlying cause
- pain medications
- peroxide mouthwashes

(For more information, see pp. 1724–1725 of Black and Matassarin-Jacobs: *Medical-Surgical Nursing: Clinical Management for Continuity of Care,* 5th ed.)

Vulvar Cancer

OVERVIEW

- Cancer of the vulva accounts for 5 per cent of female genital carcinoma and is found mainly in women over 50 years of age.
- Vulvar cancer has a slow growth rate and remains localized for a long time.
- The prognosis is poor for vulvar invasive lesions.
- Risk factors include: vulvar leukoplakia, sexually transmitted disease, kraurosis (vulvar and mucous membrane skin atrophy and dryness), diabetic vulvitis, and other primary malignancies (such as cervical cancer).

CLINICAL MANIFESTATIONS

- pruritus
- vulvar soreness
- tissue irritation, bleeding
- vulvar edema
- pelvic lymphadenopathy

ACUTE AND SUBACUTE CARE

Medical Management

- chemotherapy is used less often than surgical intervention
- irradiation generally is not used, as the tissue tolerates it poorly

Surgical Management

- simple vulvectomy—removal of the labia majora and minora and possibly the glans clitoris
  — the perineal area also may be removed
- radical vulvectomy—excision of tissue from the anus to a few centimeters from the symphysis pubis (skin, labia majora and minora, and clitoris)

— may also involve bilateral dissection of groin lymph nodes

Nursing Management

Surgical

Preoperative Care

In addition to routine preoperative care:

- Discuss fears and concerns of client, such as fear of disfigurement, grief over the loss of a body part, fear of death, and concerns regarding sex.
- Discuss preoperative procedures, which will include an enema, douche, and insertion of a Foley catheter.

Postoperative Care

In addition to routine postoperative care:

- Maintain patency of drains and monitor color and quantity of output.
- Provide wound care as ordered.
- Provide frequent dressing changes.
- Provide meticulous perineal care.
- Maintain patency of urinary catheter (usually left in place 7–14 days or until adequate healing has occurred).
- Provide sitz baths as ordered.
- Monitor urinary patterns and bowel movements.
- Use bed cradle to keep bed linens away from the incision.
- Provide antiembolism or sequential compression stockings to prevent leg edema and thrombophlebitis.
- Encourage client to perform leg exercises and elevate legs when possible to prevent edema.
- Provide opportunities for client to discuss: fears and concerns regarding change in body image, possibility of recurrence or metastasis, concern over change in sexual function, and fear of her partner's rejection.
- Discuss physical changes that may affect sexuality
  - — removal of clitoris may result in loss of ability to achieve orgasm
  - — may be a loss of sensation in vagina
  - — introital stenosis may occur making intercourse painful or difficult (dilators or plastic surgery may be used to treat)

COMMUNITY AND SELF-CARE

- Instruct client regarding:
  - — lower extremity lymph edema and ways to prevent
  - — use of antiembolism stockings
  - — avoidance of sitting or standing for long periods or crossing the legs
  - — avoidance of constrictive clothing
  - — elevating the legs as much as possible
  - — urinating into a funnel to avoid wetting clothes if direction of urine stream is unpredictable
  - — avoidance of strenuous exercises involving the legs and pelvis
  - — gradually resuming normal physical activities
  - — resuming sexual activity, when restrictions are discontinued
    - need for water soluble lubricant
    - top or side positions for intercourse
    - use of dilators as ordered by physician
  - — use of showers rather than tub baths
  - — avoidance of douching until permitted
  - — perineal and wound care
  - — notification of the physician if the following occur:
    - perineal pain unrelieved by prescribed analgesics
    - foul-smelling perineal discharge
    - heavy bleeding or clots
    - foul odor from the incision
    - change in color of incision (especially signs of decreased circulation)
    - swelling of groin or genital area
    - frequent urination, urinating in small amounts, and discomfort or burning on urination
    - temperature of 100° F. or higher
    - pain, tenderness, or redness in the calves
- Refer for sexual counseling if desired by the client.

(For more information, see pp. 2418–2422 of Black and Matassarin-Jacobs: *Medical-Surgical Nursing: Clinical Management for Continuity of Care,* 5th ed.)

APPENDICES

APPENDIX A. COMPARISON OF FIVE TYPES OF VIRAL HEPATITIS

Factor	**Hepatitis A**	**Hepatitis B**	**Hepatitis C**	**Hepatitis D** (Delta Agent)	Hepatitis E
Incidence	Endemic in areas of poor sanitation. Common in fall and early winter	Worldwide, especially in drug addicts, homosexuals, people exposed to blood and blood products. Occurs all year	Posttransfusion, those working around blood and blood products. Occurs all year	Causes hepatitis only in association with hepatitis B and only in presence of HB_sAg. Endemic in Mediterranean	Parts of Asia, Africa, and Mexico where there is poor sanitation
Incubation period	2–6 wk	6 wk–6 mo (12–14 wk avg.)	6–7 wk	Same as hepatitis B	2–9 wk
Risk factors	Close personal contact or by handling feces-contaminated wastes	Healthcare workers in contact with body secretions, blood, and blood products. Hemodialysis and posttransfusion clients. Homosexually active males and drug abusers	Similar to hepatitis B	Same as hepatitis B	Traveling or living in areas where incidence is high
Transmission	Infected feces, fecal-oral route. May be airborne if copious secretions. Shellfish from contaminated water. Also rarely parenteral				

Table continues on following page

Factor	Hepatitis A	Hepatitis B	Hepatitis C	Hepatitis D (Delta Agent)	Hepatitis E
Severity	Mortality low. Rarely causes fulminating hepatic failure	More serious, may be fatal. Mortality rate up to 60%	Can lead to chronic hepatitis	Similar to hepatitis B. More severe if occurs with chronic active hepatitis B	Illness self-limiting. Mortality rate in pregnant women 10%–20%.
Diagnostic tests	Anti-HAV, IgM positive in acute hepatitis; IgG positive after infection	HB_sAg or anti-HB_c-IgM.	Anti-HCV or anti-HDV. Recombinant immunoblot assay	HDAg-positive	Anti-HEV.
Prophylaxis and active or passive immunity	Hygiene. Immune globulin (passive). Vaccine under development (active)	Hygiene, avoidance of risk factors. Immune globulin (passive). Hepatitis B vaccine (active)	Hygiene. Immune globulin (passive)	Hygiene. Hepatits B vaccine (active)	Hygiene, sanitation. No immunity

anti-HAV, antibody to hepatitis A virus; anti-HB_c-IgM, antibody to hepatitis B—IgM; anti-HCV, antibody to hepatitis C virus; anti-HEV, antibody to hepatitis E virus; HBs-Ag, hepatitis B surface antigen.

APPENDIX B. RISK PREDICTORS FOR SKIN BREAKDOWN

Patient's Name	Evaluator's Name				Date of Assessment			
SENSORY PERCEPTION ability to respond to discomfort	**1. Completely limited:** Unresponsive to painful stimuli, either because of state of unconsciousness or severe sensory impairment, which limits ability to feel pain over most of body surface	**2. Very limited:** Responds only to painful stimuli (but not verbal commands) by opening eyes or flexing extremities. Cannot communicate discomfort verbally, OR has a sensory impairment which limits the ability to feel pain or discomfort over one half of body surface	**3. Slightly limited:** Responds to verbal commands by opening eyes and obeying some commands, but cannot always communicate discomfort or need to be turned, OR has some sensory impairment which limits ability to feel pain or discomfort in one or two extremities.	**4. No impairment:** Responds to verbal commands by obeying. Can communicate needs accurately. Has no sensory deficit which would limit ability to feel pain or discomfort				
MOISTURE degree to which skin is exposed to moisture	**1. Very Moist:** Skin is kept moist almost constantly by perspiration and urine. Dampness is detected every time patient is moved or turned. Linen must be changed more than one time each shift	**2. Occasionally Moist:** Skin is frequently, but not always kept moist, linen must be changed two to three times every 24 hours	**3. Rarely Moist:** Skin is rarely moist more than three to four times a week, but linen does require changing at that time	**4. Never Moist:** Perspiration and incontinence is never a problem, linen changed at routine intervals only				

Table continues on following page

ACTIVITY degree of physical activity	**1. Bedfast:** Confined to bed	**2. Chairfast:** Ability to walk severely impaired or nonexistant and must be assisted into chair or wheelchair when not in bed	**3. Walks occasionally:** Walks occasionally during day, but for very short distances, with or without assistance. Spends majority of each shift in bed or chair	**4. Walks frequently:** Walks a moderate distance at least once every 1 to 2 hours during waking hours			
MOBILITY ability to change and control body position	**1. Completely immobile:** Unable to make even slight changes in position without assistance	**2. Very limited:** Makes occasional slight changes in position without help but unable to make frequent or significant changes in position independently	**3. Slightly limited:** Makes frequent though slight changes in position without assistance but unable to make or maintain major changes in position independently	**4. No limitations:** Makes major and frequent changes in position without assistance			
NUTRITION usual food intake pattern	**1. Very poor:** Never eats a complete meal. Rarely eats more than 1/3 of any food offered. Takes even fluids poorly. Does not take a liquid dietary supplement, OR is NPO and/or maintained on clear liquids or IV for more than 5 days	**2. Probably inadequate:** Rarely eats a complete meal and generally eats only about one half of any food offered. Protein intake is poor. Occasionally will take a liquid dietary supplement, OR receiving less than optimum amount of liquid diet or tube feeding	**3. Adequate:** Eats over half of most meals. Eats moderate amount of protein source one to two times daily. Occasionally will refuse a meal. Will usually take a dietary supplement if offered, OR is on a tube feeding or TPN regimen which probably meets most of nutritional needs	**4. Excellent:** Eats most of every meal. Never refuses a meal. Frequently eats between meals. Does not require a dietary supplementation			

FRICTION AND SHEAR	**1. Problems:** Requires moderate to maximum assistance in moving. Complete lifting without sliding against sheets is impossible. frequently slides down in bed or chair, requiring frequent repositioning with maximum assistance. Either spasticity, contractures or agitation leads to almost constant friction	**2. Potential Problem:** Moves feebly independently or requires minimum assistance. Skin probably slides against bedsheets or chair to some extent when movement occurs. Maintains relatively good position in chair or bed most of time but occasionally slides down	**3. No Apparent Problem:** Moves in bed and in chair independently and has sufficient muscle strength to lift up completely during move. Maintains good position in bed or chair at all times.			

Key: 16, minimum risk; 13–14, moderate risk; 12 or less, high risk; NPO, nothing by mouth; IV, intravenously, TPN, total parenteral nutrition.
The Braden Scale. (Courtesy of Barbara Braden and Nancy Bergstrom. Copyright 1988.)

APPENDIX C. CRITICAL MONITORING

Acid-Base Imbalances

Respiratory Acidosis	Metabolic Acidosis
Defining Signs	**Defining Signs**
Hypoventilation	Hyperventilation (Kussmaul's respiration [air hunger])
Increasing $Paco_2$	Decreasing HCO_3^-
Decreasing pH	Decreasing pH
Commonly Seen	**Commonly Seen**
Hypoxemia	Stress response followed by lethargy
Hyperkalemia	Increasing serum Cl^- and anion gap
Increased cardiac output	Hyperkalemia
Hypertension	
Verbalized sensation of dyspnea	
Stress response, followed by decreasing level of consciousness	
Seen with Severe Imbalance	**Seen with Severe Imbalance**
Papilledema	Bradycardia or other dysrhythmias
Seizures	Gastrointestinal distention
Dysrhythmias	Abdominal pain
Muscle tremors	Nausea and vomiting
Cor pulmonale (with chronic respiratory acidosis)	Decreased cardiac output
	Hypotension

Respiratory Alkalosis	Metabolic Alkalosis
Defining Signs	**Defining Signs**
Hyperventilation Decreasing $Paco_2$ Increasing pH	Increasing HCO_3^- Increasing pH Hypoventilation
Commonly Seen	**Commonly Seen**
Lightheadedness Confusion	Confusion Decreasing level of consciousness Numbness and tingling of extremities Hypochloremia Hypovolemia Hypokalemia
Seen with Severe Imbalance	**Seen with Severe Imbalance**
Numbness and tingling of extremities and around the mouth Muscle weakness Tachycardia	Muscle tremors Muscle cramping or tetany Seizures Dysrhythmias Decreased cardiac output Hypotension

APPENDIX D. ANALYSIS OF ARTERIAL BLOOD GASES (ABGS)

Step 1: Classify the pH

Normal: 7.35–7.45
Acidemia: <7.35
Alkalemia: >7.45

Step 2: Assess $Paco_2$

Normal: 35–45 mm Hg
Respiratory acidosis: >45 mm Hg
Respiratory alkalosis: <35 mm Hg

Step 3: Assess HCO_3^-*

Normal: 22–26 mEq/L
Metabolic acidosis: <22 mEq/L
Metabolic alkalosis: >26 mEq/L

Step 4: Determine Presence of Compensation

Compensation present: $Paco_2$ and HCO_3^- are abnormal (or nearly so) in *opposite* directions, e.g., one is acidotic and the other alkalotic.†
Compensation absent: One component ($Paco_2$ or HCO_3^-) is abnormal, the other normal.

Step 5: Identify Primary Disorder, if Possible

If pH is clearly abnormal: The acid-base component most consistent with pH is the primary disorder.
If pH is normal or near-normal: The more deviant component is probably primary.†† To verify, note whether pH is on acidotic or alkalotic side of 7.4. The more deviant value should be consistent with this pH.

Step 6: Classify Degree of Compensation, if Present
Limits of complete compensation:

Metabolic acidosis: The decrease in $Paco_2$ is approximately equal to the last two digits of the pH.
Metabolic alkalosis: The $Paco_2$ is approximately equal to 0.6 times the increase in HCO_3^-.
Respiratory acidosis: For every 10-mm Hg increase in $Paco_2$, the HCO_3^- is increased by 1 mEq/L (in acute acidosis) or 4 mEq/L (in chronic acidosis).
Respiratory alkalosis: For every 10-mm Hg decrease in $Paco_2$, the HCO_3^- is decreased by 2 mEq/L (in acute alkalosis) or 5 mEq/L (in chronic alkalosis).
"Compensation" beyond these limits suggests the presence of a complex disorder.

---

* Base excess (BE) is also reported with ABGs and is a second index of metabolic status. Normal BE is –2 to +2. Because fluctuation in BE exactly parallels that of bicarbonate, it is not necessary to classify both.

† It is possible, but less likely, that two opposing primary imbalances (e.g., a complex disorder) are present, which results in the appearance of compensation. The detection of complex disorders is facilitated by the use of acid-base maps or nomograms and by the formulas in Step 6, but a complex disorder cannot always be differentiated from compensation.

†† It is unlikely that the more deviant value represents compensation, because the body does not overcompensate for imbalance. When pH approaches the normal range, compensatory mechanisms are no longer triggered.

APPENDIX E. FUNCTIONS AND TYPES OF CRANIAL NERVES

	Name	Function	Type
I	Olfactory	Olfaction (smell)	Sensory
II	Optic	Vision	Sensory
III	Oculomotor	Extraocular eye movement	Motor
		Elevation of eyelid	
		Pupil constriction	Parasympathetic
IV	Trochlear	Extraocular eye movement	Motor
V	Trigeminal		
	Ophthalmic division	Somatic sensations of cornea, nasal mucous membranes, face	Sensory
	Maxillary division	Somatic sensations of face, oral cavity, anterior two thirds of tongue, teeth	Sensory
	Mandibular division	Somatic sensation of lower face	Sensory
		Mastication (chewing)	Motor
VI	Abducens	Lateral eye movement	Motor
VII	Facial	Facial expression	Motor
		Taste, anterior two thirds of tongue	Sensory
		Salivation	Parasympathetic

Table continues on following page

	Name	Function	Type
VIII	Vestibulocochlear		
	Vestibular	Equilibrium	Sensory
	Cochlear	Hearing	Sensory
IX	Glossopharyngeal	Taste, posterior third of tongue	Sensory
		Swallowing	Motor
X	Vagus	Sensation in pharynx, larynx, external ear	Sensory
		Swallowing	Motor
		Thoracic and abdominal visceral parasympathetic nervous system activities	Parasympathetic
XI	Spinal accessory	Neck and shoulder movement	Motor
XII	Hypoglossal	Tongue movement	Motor

APPENDIX F. CHAMPION TRAUMA SCORE

Glasgow Coma Scale (GCS)

Eye-opening response	Spontaneous	4
	To voice	3
	To pain	2
	None	1
Best verbal response	Oriented	5
	Confused	4
	Inappropriate words	3
	Incomprehensible sounds	2
	None	1
Best motor response	Obeys command	6
	Localizes pain	5
	Withdraws (pain)	4
	Flexion (pain)	3
	Extension (pain)	2
	None	1
Total	Apply this score to GCS portion of Trauma Score	3–15

Trauma Score

GCS (total points from above)	14–15	5
	11–13	4
	8–10	3
	5–7	2
	3–4	1
Respiratory rate	10–24/min	4
	25–35/min	3
	36/min or greater	2
	1–9/min	1
	None	0
Respiratory expansion	Normal	1
	Retractive/none	0
Systolic blood pressure	90 mm Hg or greater	4
	70–89 mm Hg	3
	50–69 mm Hg	2
	0–49 mm Hg	1
	No pulse	0
Capillary refill	Normal	2
	Delayed	1
	None	0
Total trauma score		1–16

Trauma score	16	15	14	13	12	11	10	9	8	7	6	5	4	3	2	1
Percentage survival	99	98	96	93	87	76	60	42	26	15	8	4	2	1	0	0

From Moore, E.F., et al. (1990). *Early care of the injured patient.* Philadelphia: B.C. Decker.

APPENDIX G. REFERENCE VALUES IN HEMATOLOGY (For some procedures the reference values may vary, depending on the method used)

Test		Conventional Units	SI Units
Acid hemolysis test (Ham)		No hemolysis	No hemolysis
Alkaline phosphatase, leukocyte		Total score 14 to 100	Total score 14 to 100
Cell counts			
Erythrocytes			
Males		4.6 to 6.2 million/mm^3	4.6 to 6.2 × 10^{12}/L
Females		4.2 to 5.4 million/mm^3	4.2 to 5.2 × 10^{12}/L
Children		4.5 to 5.1 million/mm^3	4.5 to 5.1 × 10^{12}/L
Leukocytes, total		4500 to 11,000/mm^3	4.5 to 11.0 × 10^9/L
Leukocytes, differential	***Percentage***	***Absolute***	***Absolute***
Myelocytes	0	0/mm^3	O/L
Band neutrophils	3 to 5	150 to 400/mm^3	150 to 400 × 10^6/L
Segmented neutrophils	54 to 62	3000 to 5800/mm^3	3000 to 5800 × 10^6/L
Lymphocytes	25 to 33	1500 to 3000/mm^3	1500 to 3000 × 10^6/L
Monocytes	3 to 7	300 to 500/mm^3	300 to 500 × 10^6/L
Eosinophils	1 to 3	50 to 250/mm^3	50 to 250 × 10^6/L
Basophils	0 to 0.75	15 to 50/mm^3	15 to 50 × 10^6/L
Platelets		150,000 to 350,000/mm^3	150 to 350 × 10^9/L
Reticulocytes		25,000 to 75,000/mm^3	25 to 75 × 10^9/L
		0.5% to 1.5% of erythrocytes	
Coagulation tests			
Bleeding time (template)		2.75 to 8.0 min	2.75 to 8.0 min

Coagulation time (glass tubes)	5 to 15 min	5 to 15 min
Factor VIII and other coagulation factors	50% to 150% of normal	0.5 to 1.5 of normal
Fibrin split products (Thrombo-Welco test)	<10 µg/ml	<10 mg/L
Fibrinogen	200 to 400 mg/dl	2.0 to 4.0 g/L
Partial thromboplastic time (PTT)	20 to 35 sec	20 to 35 sec
Prothrombin time (PT)	12.0 to 14.0 sec	12.0 to 14.0 sec
Coombs' test		
Direct	Negative	Negative
Indirect	Negative	Negative
Corpuscular values of erthrocytes		
Mean corpuscular hemoglobin (MCH)	26 to 34 pg	0.40 to 0.53 fmol
Mean corpuscular volume (MCV)	80 to 96 μm^3	80 to 96 fL
Mean corpuscular hemoglobin concentration (MCHC)	32% to 36%	0.32% to 0.36%
Haptoglobin	26 to 185 mg/dl	260 to 1850 mg/L
Hematocrit		
Males	40 to 54 ml/dl	0.40 to 0.54 volume fraction
Females	37 to 47 ml/dl	0.37 to 0.47 volume fraction
Newborns	49 to 54 ml/dl	0.49 to 0.54 volume fraction
Children (varies with age)	35 to 49 ml/dl	0.35 to 0.49 volume fraction
Hemoglobin		
Males	14.0 to 18.0 g/dl	2.17 to 2.79 mmol/L
Females	12.0 to 16.0 g/dl	1.86 to 2.48 mmol/L
Newborns	16.5 to 19.5 g/dl	2.56 to 3.02 mmol/L
Children (varies with age)	11.2 to 16.5 g/dl	1.74 to 2.56 mmol/L

Table continues on following page

Test	Conventional Units	SI Units
Hemoglobin		
Males	14.0 to 18.0 g/dl	2.17 to 2.79 mmol/L
Females	12.0 to 16.0 g/dl	1.86 to 2.48 mmol/L
Newborns	16.5 to 19.5 g/dl	2.56 to 3.02 mmol/L
Children (varies with age)	11.2 to 16.5 g/dl	1.74 to 2.56 mmol/L
Hemoglobin, fetal	<1.0% of total	<0.01% of total
Hemoglobin A_{1C}	3% to 5% of total	0.03% to 0.05% of total
Hemoglobin A_2	1.5% to 3.0% of total	0.015% to 0.03% of total
Hemoglobin, plasma	0 to 5.0 mg/dl	0 to 0.8 µmol/L
Methemoglobin	30 to 130 mg/dl	4.7 to 20 µmol/L
Sedimentation rate (ESR)		
Wintrobe		
Males	0 to 5 mm/hr	0 to 5 mm/hr
Females	0 to 15 mm/hr	0 to 15 mm/hr
Westergren		
Males	0 to 15 mm/hr	0 to 15 mm/hr
Females	0 to 20 mm/hr	0 to 20 mm/hr

APPENDIX H. REFERENCE VALUES FOR BLOOD, PLASMA, AND SERUM (For some procedures the reference values may vary, depending on the method used)

Test	Conventional Units	SI Units
Acetoacetate plus acetone		
Qualitative	Negative	Negative
Quantitative	0.3 to 2.0 mg/dl	3 to 20 mg/L
Acid phosphatase, serum (thymolphthalein monophosphate substrate)	0.11 to 0.60 U/L	0.11 to 0.60 U/L
Adrenocorticotropin, plasma (ACTH)		
6:00 AM	10 to 80 pg/ml	10 to 80 ng/L
6:00 PM	<50 pg/ml	<50 ng/L
Alanine aminotransferase, serum (ALT, SGPT)	7 to 35 U/L	7 to 35 U/L
Albumin, serum	3.5 to 5.5 g/dl	35 to 55 g/L
Aldolase, serum	1.5 to 12.0 U/L	1.5 to 12.0 U/L
Aldosterone, plasma		
Supine	3 to 10 ng/dl	0.08 to 0.30 nmol/L
Standing		
Males	6 to 22 ng/dl	0.17 to 0.61 nmol/L
Females	5 to 30 ng/dl	0.14 to 0.83 nmol/L
Alkaline phosphatase, serum (ALP)	20 to 90 U/L (30° C)	20 to 90 U/L (30° C)
Ammonia nitrogen, plasma	15 to 49 μg/dl	11 to 35 μmol/L
Amylase, serum	25 to 125 U/L	25 to 125 U/L
Anion gap	8 to 16 mEq/L	8 to 16 mmol/L
Ascorbic acid, blood	0.4 to 1.5 mg/dl	23 to 85 μml/L

Table continues on following page

Test	Conventional Units	SI Units
Aspartate aminotransferase, serum (AST, SGOT)	7 to 40 U/L	7 to 40 U/L
Base excess, blood	0 ± 2 mEq/L	0 ± 2 mmol/L
Bicarbonate		
Venous plasma	23 to 29 mEq/L	23 to 29 mmol/L
Arterial blood	18 to 23 mEq/L	18 to 23 mmol/L
Bile acids, serum	0.3 to 3.0 mg/dl	3 to 30 mg/L
Bilirubin, serum		
Conjugated	0.1 to 0.4 mg/dl	1.7 to 6.8 μmol/L
Unconjugated	0.2 to 0.7 mg/dl	3.4 to 12 μmol/L
Total	0.3 to 1.1 mg/dl	5.1 to 19 μmol/L
Calcium, serum	9.0 to 11.0 mg/dl	2.25 to 2.75 mmol/L
Calcium, ionized, serum	4.25 to 5.25 mg/dl	1.05 to 1.30 mmol/L
Carbon dioxide, total, serum or plasma	24 to 30 mEq/L	24 to 30 mmol/L
Carbon dioxide tension, blood P_{CO_2}	35 to 45 mm Hg	35 to 45 mm Hg
β-Carotene serum	40 to 200 μg/dl	0.74 to 3.72 μmol/L
Catecholamines, plasma		
Epinephrine	15 to 55 pg/ml	82 to 300 pmol/L
Norpinephrine	65 to 400 pg/ml	384 to 2364 pmol/L
Ceruloplasmin, serum	23 to 44 mg/dl	230 to 440 mg/L
Chloride, serum or plasma	96 to 106 mEq/L	96 to 106 mmol/L
Cholesterol, serum or EDTA plasma		
Desirable range	<200 mg/dl	<5.18 mmol/L
LDL Cholesterol	60 to 180 mgdl	600 to 1800 mg/L
HDL Cholesterol	30 to 80 mg/dl	300 to 800 mg/L

Copper		
Males	70 to 140 μg/dl	11 to 22 μmol/L
Females	85 to 155 μg/dl	13 to 24 μmol/L
Cortisol, plasma		
8:00 AM	6 to 23 μg/dl	170 to 635 nmol/L
4:00 PM	3 to 15 μg/dl	82 to 413 nmol/L
10:00 PM	<50% of 8 AM value	<0.5% of 8 AM value
Creatine, serum	0.2 to 0.8 mg/dl	15 to 61 μmol/L
Creatine kinase, serum (CK, CPK)		
Males	55 to 170 U/L	55 to 170 U/L
Females	30 to 135 U/L	30 to 135 U/L
Creatine kinase MB isozyme, serum	0.0 to 4.7 ng/ml	0.0 to 4.7 μg/L
Creatinine, serum	0.6 to 1.2 mg/dl	53 to 108 μmol/L
Ferritin, serum	20 to 200 ng/ml	20 to 200 μg/L
Fibrinogen, plasma	200 to 400 mg/dl	2.0 to 4.0 g/L
Folate		
Serum	1.8 to 9.0 ng/ml	4.1 to 20.4 nmol/L
Erythrocytes	150 to 450 ng/ml	340 to 1020 nmol/L
Follicle-stimulating hormine, plasma (FSH)		
Males	4 to 25 mU/ml	4 to 25 U/L
Females	4 to 30 mU/ml	4 to 30 U/L
Postmenopausal	40 to 250 mU/ml	40 to 250 U/L

Table continues on following page

Test	Conventional Units	SI Units
γ-Glutamyltransferase, serum		
Males	5 to 38 U/L	5 to 38 U/L
Females	5 to 29 U/L	5 to 29 U/L
Gastrin, serum	0 to 200 pg/ml	0 to 200 ng/L
Glucose (fasting), plasma or serum	70 to 115 mg/dl	3.89 to 6.38 mmol/L
Growth hormone, plasma (HGH)	0 to 10 ng/ml	0 to 10 μg/L
Haptoglobin, serum	26 to 185 mg/dl	260 to 1850 mg/L
Immunoglobulins, serum		
IgG	550 to 1900 mg/dl	5.5 to 19.0 g/L
IgA	60 to 333 mg/dl	0.60 to 3.3 g/L
IgM	45 to 145 mg/dl	0.45 to 1.5 g/L
IgD	0.5 to 3.0 mg/dl	5 to 30 mg/L
IgE	<500 ng/ml	<500 μg/L
Insulin (fasting), plasma	5 to 25 μU/ml	36 to 179 pmol/L
Iron, serum	75 to 175 ng/dl	13 to 31 μmol/L
Iron-binding capacity, serum		
Total	250 to 410 μg/dl	45 to 73 μmol/L
Saturation	20% to 55%	0.20 to 0.55
Lactate		
Venous blood	4.5 to 19.8 mg/dl	0.50 to 2.2 mmol/L
Arterial blood	4.5 to 14.4 mg/dl	0.50 to 1.6 mmol/L
Lactate dehydrogenase, serum (LD, LDH)	100 to 190 U/L	100 to 190 U/L
Lipase, serum	10 to 140 U/L	10 to 140 U/L

Lipids, total, serum	450 to 850 mg/dl	4.5 to 8.5 g/L
Luteinizing hormone, serum (LH)		
Males	6 to 18 mU/ml	6 to 18 U/L
Females		
Premenopausal	5 to 22 mU/ml	5 to 22 U/L
Midcycle	3 × baseline	3 × baseline
Postmenopausal	>30 mU/ml	>30 U/L
Magnesium, serum	1.8 to 3.0 mg/dl	0.75 to 1.25 mmol/L
Osmolality	286 to 295 mOsm/kg H_2O	2.85 to 295 mOsm/kg H_2O
Oxygen, blood		
Capacity (varies with hemoglobin)	16 to 24 vol%	7.14 to 10.7 mmol/L
Content, arterial	15 to 23 vol%	6.69 to 10.3 mmol/L
Saturation, arterial	94% to 100%	0.94 to 1.00
Tension, Po2	75 to 100 mm Hg	75 to 100 mm Hg
P_50	26 to 27 mm Hg	26 to 27 mm Hg
pH, arterial blood	7.35 to 7.45	7.35 to 7.45
Phenylalanine, serum	<3 mg/dl	<0.18 mmol/L
Phosphate, inorganic, serum	3.0 to 4.5 mg/dl	1.0 to 1.5 mmol/L
Potassium, serum or plasma	3.5 to 5.0 mEq/L	3.5 to 5.0 mmol/L
Prolactin, serum		
Males	1 to 20 ng/ml	1 to 20 µg/L
Females	1 to 25 ng/ml	1 to 25 µg/L
Protein, serum		
Total	6.0 to 8.0 g/dl	60 to 80 g/L
Albumin	3.5 to 5.5 g/dl	35 to 55 g/L
α_1-Globulin	0.2 to 0.4 g/dl	2 to 4 g/L

Table continues on following page

Test	Conventional Units	SI Units
α_2-Globulin	0.5 to 0.9 g/dl	5 to 9 g/L
β-Globulin	0.6 to 1.1 g/dl	6 to 11 g/L
γ-Globulin	0.7 to 1.7 g/dl	7 to 17 g/L
Pyruvate, blood	0.3 to 0.9 mg/dl	0.03 to 0.10 mmol/L
Sodium, serum or plasma	136 to 145 mEq/L	136 to 145 mmol/L
Testosterone, plasma		
Males	275 to 875 ng/dl	9.0 to 10.0 nmol/L
Females	23 to 75 ng/dl	0.8 to 2.6 nmol/L
Pregnant	38 to 190 ng/dl	1.3 to 6.6 nmol/L
Thyroid-stimulating hormone, serum (TSH)	0 to 7 μU/ml	0 to 7 mU/L
Thyroxine, free, serum (FT_4)	1.0 to 2.1 ng/dl	13 to 27 pmol/L
Thyroxine, serum (T_4)	4.4 to 9.9 μg/dl	57 to 128 nmol/L
Triglycerides, serum	40 to 150 mg/dl	0.4 to 1.5 g/L
Triiodothyronine, serum (T_3)	150 to 250 ng/dl	2.3 to 3.9 nmol/L
Triiodothyronine uptake, resin (T_3RU)	25% to 38% uptake	0.25 to 0.38 uptake
Urate		
Males	2.5 to 8.0 mg/dl	0.15 to 0.48 mmol/L
Females	1.5 to 7.0 mg/dl	0.09 to 0.42 mmol/L
Urea, serum or plasma	24 to 49 mg/dl	4.0 to 8.2 mmol/L
Urea nitrogen, serum or plasma	11 to 23 mg/dl	3.9 to 8.2 mmol/L
Viscosity, serum	1.4 to 1.8 × water	1.4 to 1.8 × water
Vitamin A, serum	20 to 80 μg/dl	0.70 to 2.80 μmol/L
Vitamin B_{12}, serum	180 to 900 pg/ml	133 to 664 pmol/L

APPENDIX I. REFERENCE VALUES FOR URINE (For some procedures the reference values may vary, depending on the method used)

Test	Conventional Units	SI Units
Acetone and acetoacetate, qualitative	Negative	Negative
Albumin		
Qualitative	Negative	Negative
Quantitative	10 to 100 mg/24 hr	10 to 100 mg/24 hr
Aldosterone	3 to 20 µg/24 hr	8.3 to 55 nmol/24 hr
δ-Aminolevulinic acid	1.3 to 7.0 mg/24 hr	10 to 53 µmol/24 hr
Amylase	3 to 20 U/hr	3 to 20 U/hr
Amylase/creatinine clearance ratio	1% to 4%	0.01% to 0.04%
Bilirubin, qualitative	Negative	Negative
Calcium (usual diet)	<250 mg/24 hr	<6.3 mmol/24 hr
Catecholamines		
Epinephrine	<10 µg/24 hr	<55 nmol/24 hr
Norepinephrine	<100 µg/24 hr	<590 nmol/24 hr
Total free catecholamines	4 to 126 µg/24 hr	24 to 745 nmol/24 hr
Total metanephrines	0.1 to 1.6 mg/24 hr	0.5 to 8.1 µmol/24 hr
Chloride (varies with intake)	110 to 250 mEq/24 hr	110 to 250 nmol/24 hr
Copper	0 to 50 µg/24 hr	0 to 0.80 µmol/24 hr
Cortisol, free	10 to 100 µg/24 hr	27.6 to 276 nmol/24 hr
Creatinine	15 to 25 mg/kg body weight/24 hr	0.13 to 0.22 mmol/kg body weight/24 hr

Table continues on following page

Test	Conventional Units	SI Units
Creatinine clearance (corrected to 1.73 m2 body surface area)		
Males	110 to 150 ml/min	110 to 150 ml/min
Females	105 to 132 ml/min	105 to 132 ml/min
Dehydroepiandrosterone		
Males	0.2 to 2.0 mg/24 hr	0.7 to 6.9 µmol/24 hr
Females	0.2 to 1.8 mg/24 hr	0.7 to 6.2 µmol/24 hr
Estrogens, total		
Males	4 to 25 µg/24 hr	14 to 90 nmol/24 hr
Females	5 to 100 µg/24 hr	18 to 360 nmol/24 hr
Glucose (as reducing substance)	<250 mg/24 hr	<250 mg/24 hr
Hemoglobin and myoglobin, qualitative	Negative	Negative
17-Hydroxycorticosteroids		
Males	3 to 9 mg/24 hr	8.3 to 25 µmol/24 hr
Females	2 to 8 mg/24 hr	5.5 to 22 µmol/24 hr
5-Hydroxyindoleacetic acid		
Qualitative	Negative	Negative
Quantitative	<9 mg/24 hr	<47 µmol/24 hr
17-Ketosteroids		
Males	6 to 18 mg/24 hr	21 to 62 µmol/24 hr
Females	4 to 13 mg/24 hr	14 to 45 µmol/24 hr
Magnesium	6.0 to 8.5 mEq/24 hr	3.0 to 4.2 mmol/24 hr
Metanephrines (see Catecholamines)		
Osmolality	38 to 1,400 mOsm/kg H_2O	38 to 1,400 mOsm/kg H_2O

pH	4.6 to 8.0	4.6 to 8.0
Phenylpyruvic acid, qualitative	Negative	Negative
Phosphate	0.9 to 1.3 g/24 hr	29 to 42 mmol/24 hr
Porphobilinogen		
Qualitative	Negative	Negative
Quantitative	<2.0 mg/24 hr	<9 µmol/24 hr
Porphyrins		
Coproporphyrin	50 to 250 µg/24 hr	77 to 380 nmol/24 hr
Uroporphyrin	10 to 30 µg/24 hr	12 to 36 nmol/24 hr
Potassium	25 to 100 mEq/24 hr	25 to 100 mmol/24 hr
Pregnanediol		
Males	0.4 to 1.4 mg/24 hr	1.2 to 4.4 µmol/24 hr
Females		
Proliferative phase	0.5 to 1.5 mg/24 hr	1.6 to 4.7 µmol/24 hr
Luteal phase	2.0 to 7.0 mg/24 hr	6.2 to 22 µmol/24 hr
Postmenopausal	0.2 to 1.0 mg/24 hr	0.6 to 3.1 µmol/24 hr
Pregnanetriol	<2.5 mg/24 hr	<7.4 µmol/24 hr
Protein		
Qualitative	Negative	Negative
Quantitative	10 to 150 mg/24 hr	10 to 150 mg/24 hr
Sodium	130 to 260 mEq/24 hr	130 to 260 mmol/24 hr
Specific gravity	1.003 to 1.030	1.003 to 1.030
Urate	200 to 500 mg/24 hr	1.2 to 3.0 mmol/24 hr
Urobilinogen	<4.0 mg/24 hr	<6.8 µmol/24 hr
Vanillylmandelic acid (VMA) (4-hydroxy-3-methoxymandelic acid)	1 to 8 mg/24 hr	5 to 40 µmol/24 hr

APPENDIX J. BLOOD COMPONENTS

Whole Blood	Red Blood Cells	Platelet Concentrates	Fresh Frozen Plasma	Cryoprecipitate	Granulocyte Concentrates	Plasma Derivatives	Coagulation Factor Concentrates
Composition							
RBC, plasma, plasma proteins (globulins, antibodies), 63 ml of anticoagulant-preservative	RBC with CPDA-1 solution (anticoagulant-preservative only), final hematocrit no higher than 80% (80% RBC, 20% plasma) RBC with 100 ml additive solution, final hematocrit about 55%–60%	Single-unit platelets contain a minimum of 5.5 $\times 10^{10}$ (1 unit) platelets in 50–70 ml of plasma obtained by separating platelet-rich plasma from 1 unit of fresh whole blood; 6–10 units may be pooled for 1 transfusion Single-donor platelets contain a minimum of 3.0 $\times 10^{11}$ platelets (6 units) obtained from single donor by use of automated cell separator during apher-	91% water, 7% protein (globulin, antibodies, clotting factors), and 2% carbohydrates Freezing within 8 hr of collection preserves all clotting factors	Each unit contains about 80–120 units of factor VIII (antihemophilic factor) that represents 50% of antihemophilic factor originally present in unit, vWF, 250 mg of fibrinogen, and 20%–30% of factor XIII present in a unit of whole blood, suspended in 10–20 ml of plasma	Unit obtained by granulocytaphresis contains a minimum of 1.0 $\times$ 10^{10} granulocytes, variable amounts of lymphocytes (usually <10%), 30–50 ml of RBC and 100–400 ml of plasma, and 6–10 units of platelets; the platelets can be separated from the unit if the granulocyte recipient is not thrombocytopenic	*Albumin:* 96% albumin, 4% globulin and other proteins extracted from plasma; available as a 5% solution, oncotically equivalent to plasma, and also a concentrated 25% solution *Plasma protein fraction:* 83% albumin and 17% globulins extracted from plasma; less pure than albumin and has higher degree of contamination with other plasma proteins; in 5% solution only	*Factor VIII:* Lyophilized concentrate containing large quantities of factor VIII; prepared from large pools of donor plasma, but heat treatment during fractionation process significantly reduces risk of transmitting viral disease *Factor IX:* Lyophilized concentrate containing large quantities of factor IX; also contains factors II, VII, and X; product prepared from

		esis; recipient exposed to fewer donors, which decreases complications					large pools of donor plasma, but heat treatment during fractionation process significantly reduces risk of transmitting viral disease
Volume							
500 ml/unit	250–350 ml/uinit 350–400 ml/unit	50–70 ml/unit 200–400 ml/unit	200–250 ml	5–10 ml/unit	200–400 ml with platelets 100–200 ml without platelets	Albumin: 250 and 500 ml (5%); 50 and 100 ml (25%)	Multiple-dose vial
Equipment							
19- to 20-gauge needle, standard straight or Y-type blood administration set with minimum 170-μm filter, 0.9% saline	19- to 20-gauge needle, standard straight or Y-type blood administration set with minimum 170-μm filter, 0.9% saline	19- to 21-gauge needle, component administration set with standard 170-μm filter, 0.9% saline	19- to 23-gauge needle, component administration set with standard 170-μm filter, 0.9% saline	19- to 21-gauge needle, component administration set with standard 170-μm filter, 0.9% saline	19- to 21-gauge needle, component administration set with standard 170-μm filter, 0.9% saline *Never* use a leukocyte-depleting filter to infuse granulocytes	19- to 21-gauge needle and standard IV infusion set A filter may be required by some manufacturers; check product insert for specific instructions Administration set with filter may be supplied with the albumin	IV push through filtered needle or IV drip using component recipient set

Table continues on following page

Whole Blood	Red Blood Cells	Platelet Concentrates	Fresh Frozen Plasma	Cryoprecipitate	Granulocyte Concentrates	Plasma Derivatives	Coagulation Factor Concentrates
ABO/Rh Compatibility							
The ABO type of the donor should be identical with the recipient's Rh– blood can be given to an Rh– or Rh+ recipient	A can match with A or O; B can match with B or O; O can match only with O; AB can match with A, B, or O Rh– blood can be given to either Rh+ or Rh– recipient	Whereas platelets have no ABO or Rh antigens, they are suspended in 200–400 ml of plasma containing donor antibodies and a small number of RBC There is evidence that platelet survival decreases if donor plasma is incompatible, and large volumes of incompatible plasma may cause a positive direct Coombs' test It is also possible for even a small number of Rh+ RBC to stimulate anti-D in an Rh– recipient; therefore, plasma ABO and Rh compatibility is recommended	A can match with A or AB; B can match with B or AB; AB can match only with AB; O can match with A, B, AB, or O Rh– and Rh+ blood can be given to either Rh+ or Rh– recipient	Cryoprecipitate contains no RBC and a small volume of plasma ABO crossmatching not needed, and plasma compatibility preferred but not required	Granulocytes contain a significant number of RBC and plasma; therefore, ABO of donor should be identical with recipient's RH– components may be transfused to an Rh+ recipient	Antibodies destroyed during processing; therefore, compatibility not a factor	Antibodies destroyed during processing, so compatibility not a factor

Special Considerations							
Whole blood transfusion is rarely indicated Treatment with specific blood components is usually recommended	RBC may be viscous, so 0.9% saline may be added to achieve optimal flow rates For some clients, a leukocyte depletion filter may be used to prevent complications	Because platelet concentrates contain few RBC, crossmatch testing is not required Plasma ABO and Rh compatibility is recommended, especially when the total volume of the transfusion exceeds 150–200 ml Only filters specially designed for platelet transfusion should be used	Plasma carries same risk of disease transmission as does whole blood If only volume expansion is required, products of choice are crystalloid or colloid solutions, such as saline or albumin Plasma contains no RBC, and Rh compatibility and crossmatching are not required ABO compatibility must be confirmed before administration	Single units of cryoprecipitate may be pooled into 1 container by the blood collection center If individual bags are issued, 0.9% saline may need to be added to rinse residual cryoprecipitate from bags and tubing	Granulocytes have short survival (<24 hr); infuse as soon as possible Granulocyte concentrates contain a significant number of RBC; pretransfusion testing ordinarily the same as for RBC transfusion Increased incidence of febrile, nonhemolytic reactions with granulocyte transfusions; infuse slowly, observe client closely; premedication with an antihistamine, acetaminophen, steroids, or meperidine may be indicated to prevent repeat reactions	PPF and albumin cannot transmit hepatitis or HIV infection; the pasteurization process used to prepare the products destroys such viruses Hypotension has been associated with rapid infusion of PPF; 25% albumin can cause a significantly increased blood pressure because of its ability to draw fluid into the intravascular space	Factor VIII and factor IX assays should be performed at appropriate intervals to assess response Factor VIII concentration lacks vWF and should not be used in treatment of von Willebrand's disease

Table continues on following page

Whole Blood	Red Blood Cells	Platelet Concentrates	Fresh Frozen Plasma	Cryoprecipitate	Granulocyte Concentrates	Plasma Derivatives	Coagulation Factor Concentrates
Expected Outcomes							
Prevention or resolution of hypovolemic shock and anemia In a nonbleeding adult, 1 unit of whole blood should increase hematocrit by 3% and hemoglobin by 1 g/dl	Resolution of symptoms of anemia In a nonbleeding adult, 1 unit of RBC should increase hematocrit by 3% and hemoglobin by 1 g/dl	Prevention or resolution of bleeding due to thrombocytopenia or platelet dysfunction 1 unit should raise peripheral platelet count 5000–10,000/mm^3 if underlying cause is resolved or controlled Efficacy of platelet transfusion can be determined by obtaining platelet counts at 1 hr and 18–24 after infusion	Treatment effectiveness is assessed by monitoring coagulation function, specifically, PT and PTT, or by specific factor assays	Correction of factor VIII, vWF, factor XIII, and fibrinogen deficiency; cessation of bleeding in uremic clients Laboratory values required to assess effectiveness of treatment	Do not administer amphotericin B within 4 hr of granulocyte transfusion (pulmonary insufficiency seen with concurrent administration) Improvement in or resolution of infection No increase in peripheral WBC count usually seen after granulocyte transfusion in adults, although increase may be seen in children	The client will acquire and maintain adequate blood pressure and volume support	The client will develop hemostasis because of increased levels of factor VIII and factor IX activity

An improvement in clinical condition because of resolving infection is the only measure of treatment effectiveness

CPDA-1, citrate-phosphate-dextrose-adenine; FFP, fresh-frozen plasma; HIV, human immunodeficiency virus; IV, intravenous; PPF, plasma protein fraction; PT, prothrombin time; PTT, partial thromboplastin time; RBC, red blood cells; vWF, von Willebrand's factor; WBC, white blood cells.

INDEX

C